Respiratory Medicine and Surgery

Editors

SARAH M. REUSS
A. BERKLEY CHESEN

VETERINARY CLINICS OF NORTH AMERICA: EQUINE PRACTICE

www.vetequine.theclinics.com

Consulting Editor
THOMAS J. DIVERS

April 2015 • Volume 31 • Number 1

ELSEVIER

1600 John F. Kennedy Boulevard ● Suite 1800 ● Philadelphia, Pennsylvania, 19103-2899

http://www.vetequine.theclinics.com

VETERINARY CLINICS OF NORTH AMERICA: EQUINE PRACTICE Volume 31, Number 1
April 2015 ISSN 0749-0739, ISBN-13: 978-0-323-35988-7

Editor: Patrick Manley
Developmental Editor: Donald Mumford

Veterinary Clinics of North America: Equine Practice (ISSN 0749-0739) is published in April, August, and December by Elsevier Inc., 360 Park Avenue South, New York, NY 10010-1710. Business and Editorial Offices: 1600 John F. Kennedy Blvd., Suite 1800, Philadelphia, PA 19103-2899. Subscription prices are $270.00 per year (domestic individuals), $431.00 per year (domestic institutions), $130.00 per year (domestic students/residents), $315.00 per year (Canadian individuals), $543.00 per year (Canadian institutions), $365.00 per year (international individuals), $543.00 per year (international institutions), and $180.00 per year (international and Canadian students/residents). To receive student/resident rate, orders must be accompanied by name of affiliated institution, date of term, and the signature of program/residency coordinator on institution letterhead. Orders will be billed at individual rate until proof of status is received. Foreign air speed delivery is included in all *Clinics* subscription prices. All prices are subject to change without notice. **POSTMASTER:** Send address changes to *Veterinary Clinics of North America: Equine Practice*, 3251 Riverport Lane, Maryland Heights, MO 63043. Customer Service (orders, claims, online, change of address): Elsevier Health Sciences Division, Subscription Customer Service, 3251 Riverport Lane, Maryland Heights, MO 63043. Tel: 1-800-654-2452 (U.S. and Canada); 314-447-8871 (outside U.S. and Canada). Fax: 314-447-8029. E-mail: journalscustomerservice-usa@elsevier.com (for print support); E-mail: journalsonlinesupport-usa@elsevier.com (for online support).

Reprints. For copies of 100 or more of articles in this publication, please contact the Commercial Reprints Department, Elsevier Inc., 360 Park Avenue South, New York, NY 10010-1710. Tel.: 212-633-3874; Fax: 212-633-3820; E-mail: reprints@elsevier.com.

Veterinary Clinics of North America: Equine Practice is covered in *MEDLINE/PubMed (Index Medicus), Excerpta Medica, Current Contents/Agriculture, Biology and Environmental Sciences, and ISI.*

Contributors

CONSULTING EDITOR

THOMAS J. DIVERS, DVM
Diplomate, American College of Veterinary Internal Medicine; Diplomate, American
College of Veterinary Emergency and Critical Care; Steffen Professor of Veterinary
Medicine, Section Chief, Section of Large Animal Medicine, College of Veterinary
Medicine, Cornell University, Ithaca, New York

EDITORS

SARAH M. REUSS, VMD
Diplomate, American College of Veterinary Internal Medicine; Service Chief of Large
Animal Internal Medicine; Clinical Assistant Professor, Department of Large Animal
Clinical Sciences, University of Florida College of Veterinary Medicine, Gainesville,
Florida

A. BERKLEY CHESEN, DVM
Diplomate, American College of Veterinary Surgery - Large Animal; Equine Comprehensive
Wellness, Santa Fe, New Mexico

AUTHORS

KIRSTEN E. BAILEY, BVSc (Hons)
Member of the Australian and New Zealand College of Veterinary Scientists; Centre for
Equine Infectious Disease, The University of Melbourne, Australia

ELIZABETH J. BARRETT, DVM, MS
Diplomate, American College of Veterinary Surgery - Large Animal; Hagyard Equine
Medical Institute, Lexington, Kentucky

A. BERKLEY CHESEN, DVM
Diplomate, American College of Veterinary Surgery - Large Animal; Equine Comprehensive
Wellness, Santa Fe, New Mexico

NOAH D. COHEN, VMD, MPH, PhD
Diplomate, American College of Veterinary Internal Medicine; Professor, Department of
Large Animal Clinical Sciences, Texas A&M University College of Veterinary Medicine,
Texas

ROSEMARY S. CUMING, BVSc
Member Australian and New Zealand College of Veterinary Scientists (Equine Medicine);
Resident Large Animal Internal Medicine, J.T. Vaughan Large Animal Teaching Hospital,
Department of Clinical Sciences, Auburn University College of Veterinary Medicine,
Auburn, Alabama

ANDRÉS DIAZ-MÉNDEZ, MedVet, MSc, PhD
Centre for Equine Infectious Disease, The University of Melbourne, Australia

DAVID E. FREEMAN, MVB, PhD
Diplomate, American College of Veterinary Surgeons; Large Animal Clinical Sciences, College of Veterinary Medicine, University of Florida, Gainesville, Florida

STEEVE GIGUÈRE, DVM, PhD
Diplomate, American College of Veterinary Internal Medicine; Professor and Marguerite Thomas Hodgson Chair in Equine Studies, Department of Large Animal Medicine, University of Georgia College of Veterinary Medicine, Athens, Georgia

JAMES R. GILKERSON, BVSc, BSc (Vet), PhD
Centre for Equine Infectious Disease, The University of Melbourne, Australia

CAROL A. HARTLEY, BSc (Hons), PhD
Centre for Equine Infectious Disease, The University of Melbourne, Australia

KENNETH HINCHCLIFF, BVSc, MS, PhD
Diplomate, American College of Veterinary Internal Medicine; Professor and Dean, Equine Centre, Faculty of Veterinary and Agricultural Sciences, The University of Melbourne, Werribee, Victoria, Australia

KARA M. LASCOLA, DVM, MS
Diplomate, American College of Veterinary Internal Medicine (Large Animal Internal Medicine); Assistant Professor of Equine Medicine, Department of Veterinary Clinical Medicine, University of Illinois College of Veterinary Medicine, Urbana, Illinois

MARTHA MALLICOTE, DVM
Diplomate, American College of Veterinary Internal Medicine (Large Animal); Clinical Assistant Professor, Large Animal Clinical Science, College of Veterinary Medicine, University of Florida, Gainesville, Florida

MELISSA R. MAZAN, DVM
Diplomate, American College of Veterinary Internal Medicine; Associate Professor and Section Head, Large Animal Department of Clinical Sciences, Cummings School of Veterinary Medicine at Tufts University, North Grafton, Massachusetts

TARALYN M. McCARREL, DVM
Diplomate, American College of Veterinary Surgeons; Assistant Professor, Large Animal Clinical Sciences, University of Florida College of Veterinary Medicine, Mount Hope, Ontario, Canada

SARAH M. REUSS, VMD
Diplomate, American College of Veterinary Internal Medicine; Service Chief of Large Animal Internal Medicine; Clinical Assistant Professor, Department of Large Animal Clinical Sciences, University of Florida College of Veterinary Medicine, Gainesville, Florida

KIM A. SPRAYBERRY, DVM
Diplomate, American College of Veterinary Internal Medicine; Associate Professor, Animal Science Department, Cal Poly University San Luis Obispo, San Luis Obispo, California

ALLISON J. STEWART, BVSc, MS
Diplomate, American College of Veterinary Internal Medicine; Diplomate, American College of Veterinary Emergency and Critical Care; Professor Equine Medicine, J.T. Vaughan Large Animal Teaching Hospital, Department of Clinical Sciences, Auburn University College of Veterinary Medicine, Auburn, Alabama

STACEY SULLIVAN, BVSc, MVS
Member of the Australian and New Zealand College of Veterinary Scientists; Equine Centre, Faculty of Veterinary and Agricultural Sciences, The University of Melbourne, Werribee, Victoria, Australia

CANAAN WHITFIELD-CARGILE, DVM
Diplomate, American College of Veterinary Surgery - Large Animal; Diplomate, American College Veterinary Sports Medicine; Graduate Research Assistant, Department of Large Animal Clinical Sciences, College of Veterinary Medicine and Biomedical Sciences, Texas A&M University, College Station, Texas

PAMELA A. WILKINS, DVM, MS, PhD
Diplomate, American College of Veterinary Internal Medicine (Large Animal Internal Medicine); Diplomate, American College of Veterinary and Emergency Critical Care; Professor of Equine Medicine, Department of Veterinary Clinical Medicine, University of Illinois College of Veterinary Medicine, Urbana, Illinois

J. BRETT WOODIE, DVM, MS
Diplomate, American College of Veterinary Medicine; Rood and Riddle Equine Hospital, Lexington, Kentucky

Contents

This article reviews dorsal displacement of the soft palate (DDSP) and nasopharyngeal cicatrix. Palatial instability results in exercise intolerance and upper respiratory noise in performance horses. Palatial instability can progress to DDSP either permanently or only during exercise. There have been advancements related to the etiopathogensis, diagnosis, and treatment of DDSP. The laryngeal tie-forward has gained popularity and is the most widely accepted treatment option for this condition, either alone or in combination with other procedures. Nasopharyngeal cicatrix affects a small geographic region. Diagnosis is definitively made via endoscopy. The most effective treatment of this condition is a permanent tracheostomy.

Laryngeal disorders are relatively common in the horse, and thorough diagnostic evaluation is essential to make an accurate definitive diagnosis and selection of appropriate treatment. The value of exercising endoscopy must not be overlooked, and the recent development of dynamic (overground) endoscopy is providing new insights into dynamic laryngeal lesions. The focus of this article will be on recently described disorders and treatments or modifications to existing treatments. It summarizes the numerous investigations attempting to perfect the laryngoplasty procedure for treatment of laryngeal hemiplegia. The newly described conditions, bilateral dynamic laryngeal collapse, and dynamically flaccid epiglottis will also be discussed.

There are few diseases that ignite as much fervor among horse owners as strangles. *Streptococcus equi* subsp *equi* (strangles) infections frequently require the treating veterinarian to manage not only the clinical cases but also the biosecurity and provision of information to all involved parties. Although the disease is typically characterized by low mortality and high morbidity, restrictions of horse movement that result from appropriate quarantine procedures often frustrate the involved parties. The aims of this article are to provide clinically relevant information for diagnosis, treatment, and biosecurity management of strangles infection.

antimicrobial selection results in a good prognosis for both survival and return to athletic function in most horses.

Sarah M. Reuss and Noah D. Cohen

Bacterial pneumonia is a common cause of disease in both neonatal and weanling foals. The causal organism or organisms differ with the age of the foal, should be identified via microbiologic culture, and will ultimately dictate appropriate treatment. Initial treatment in neonates should be broad spectrum and bactericidal, whereas weanling age foals may receive more targeted treatment. The combination of a macrolide antibiotic and rifampin remains the gold standard for treatment of *Rhodococcus equi* pneumonia; however, resistance to these antimicrobials is a concern.

Pamela A. Wilkins and Kara M. Lascola

Interstitial pneumonias encompass a wide variety of acute and chronic respiratory diseases and include the specific diseases equine multinodular pulmonary fibrosis and acute lung injury and acute respiratory distress. These diseases have been diagnosed in all age groups of horses, and numerous agents have been identified as potential causes of interstitial pneumonia. Despite the varied causes, interstitial pneumonia is uniformly recognized by the severity of respiratory disease and often poor clinical outcome. This article reviews the causal agents that have been associated with the development of interstitial pneumonia in horses. Pathophysiology, clinical diagnosis, and treatment options are discussed.

Melissa R. Mazan

Inflammatory airway disease and recurrent airway obstruction are 2 non-septic diseases of the equine respiratory system with a shared cause of exposure to particulate matter. They appear to occupy 2 ends of a spectrum of disease, but are differentiated by history, clinical signs, and response to treatment. Diagnosis can be made by sampling of respiratory fluids and lung function testing. Treatment consists of environmental modification and pharmacologic treatment with systemic or inhaled corticosteroids and bronchodilators.

Stacey Sullivan and Kenneth Hinchcliff

Exercise-induced pulmonary hemorrhage (EIPH) is an important disease of horses that perform high-intensity athletic activity. EIPH is an ongoing concern for the racing industry because of its high prevalence; potential impact on performance; welfare concerns; and use of prophylactic medications, such as furosemide, on race day. During the last 10 years, significant progress has been made in understanding the pathogenesis and risk factors for EIPH and the impact of the disease on performance and career. This article summarizes the most recent advances in EIPH.

VETERINARY CLINICS OF NORTH AMERICA: EQUINE PRACTICE

VETERINARY CLINICS OF
NORTH AMERICA, EQUINE PRACTICE

FORTHCOMING ISSUES

August 2015
Equine Pathology and Laboratory
Diagnostics
Colleen Duncan and
Bruce Wobeser, Editors

December 2015
Rehabilitation of the Equine Athlete
Melissa King and Narelle Stubbs, Editors

RECENT ISSUES

December 2014
New Perspectives in Infectious Diseases
Robert H. Mealey, Editor

August 2014
Emergency and Critical Care
Vanessa L. Cook and Diana Hassel, Editors

RELATED ISSUE

Veterinary Clinics of North America: Exotic Animal Practice
September 2013 (Vol. 16, No. 3)
New and Emerging Diseases
Sue Chen and Nicole R. Wyre, Editors

Foreword

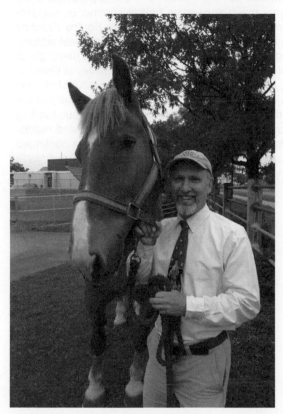

Thomas J. Divers, DVM
Consulting Editor

Dr Simon Turner has, as consulting editor, successfully guided *Veterinary Clinics of North America: Equine Practice* for the past 26 years. Dr Turner has recently retired from the position as consulting editor and, on behalf of hundreds of equine practitioners who were consistent readers of the journal, I thank him for his enormous efforts in developing the popularity and value of this scientific journal.

I am very much looking forward to trying to fill Dr Turner's shoes as I assume the duties of consulting editor of *Veterinary Clinics of North America: Equine Practice*, a journal that aims to provide state-of-the-art, topic-based discussions, with important and practical information directly applicable to equine practice. As we move forward, I believe the future issues should continue to focus on topics of the greatest interest to the largest number of practicing equine veterinarians and should contain new and clinically applicable information in all aspects of equine practice. My background, primary professional interests, and experiences are in equine internal medicine, emergency

Vet Clin Equine 31 (2015) xiii–xiv
http://dx.doi.org/10.1016/j.cveq.2015.01.002
0749-0739/15/$ – see front matter © 2015 Published by Elsevier Inc.

vetequine.theclinics.com

medicine, ambulatory medicine, and critical care, but I will be consulting with my colleagues in all areas of equine practice to help select the most appropriate issue topics. Most importantly, I would very much appreciate having comments, suggestions, and feedback from all *Veterinary Clinics of North America: Equine Practice* readers: suggestions you may have for topics to be covered, authors or guest editors, and any changes of format. Through the past efforts of Dr Turner, the many guest editors, article contributors, and editors, John Vassallo and Patrick Manley at Elsevier, *Veterinary Clinics of North America: Equine Practice* has been listed on PubMed. This highlights both the scientific quality of the publication and the technical quality of the digital files. This accomplishment makes it somewhat easier to recruit outstanding article editors, knowing that an abstract of the material will be widely and readily available on PubMed. With your help and suggestions along with Elsevier's continued support, I hope that we together can continue to make *Veterinary Clinics of North America: Equine Practice* a highly valued and treasured journal for as many equine practitioners as possible.

Thomas J. Divers, DVM
Section of Large Animal Medicine
Cornell University
College of Veterinary Medicine
Ithaca, NY 14853, USA

E-mail address:
tjd8@cornell.edu

Preface

Updates on Respiratory Medicine and Surgery

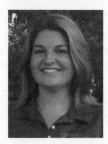 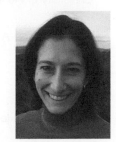

Sarah M. Reuss, VMD, DACVIM   A. Berkley Chesen, DVM, DACVS-LA
Editors

It has been our privilege to serve as Guest Editors for this issue of *Veterinary Clinics of North America: Equine Practice*. The last issue that focused specifically on the respiratory system was the April 2003 issue edited by Eric Parente. While various conditions and treatments have been covered individually in issues since then, we hope this issue presents a comprehensive update on the medical and surgical conditions of the equine respiratory tract.

In the past decade, there have been significant strides in the diagnosis, treatment, and prevention of many conditions affecting the upper and lower airways of the horse. Vast advances in technology have allowed for improved diagnostic imaging with the routine use of digital radiography and ultrasound as well as increased availability of dynamic endoscopy, computed tomography, and MRI. Researchers have furthered our knowledge of the etiologic organisms causing many of the infectious diseases of the respiratory tract, thus allowing for improved preventative strategies. They have also further elucidated the pathophysiology of frustrating diseases such as recurrent airway obstruction, inflammatory airway disease, and exercise-induced pulmonary hemorrhage. New antimicrobials have been discovered and validated for use in equines, and novel surgical procedures have been devised to offer hope to the owner of the equine athlete. Despite these many advances, however, the respiratory system continues to be a challenge for veterinarians and horse owners.

We would like to offer a sincere thank-you to all of the many contributors to this issue. It was an honor to work with such a diverse group of experts who were willing to share their time and knowledge with others. Thanks also to Drs A. Simon Turner

Vet Clin Equine 31 (2015) xv–xvi
http://dx.doi.org/10.1016/j.cveq.2015.01.001
0749-0739/15/$ – see front matter © 2015 Published by Elsevier Inc.

vetequine.theclinics.com

and Jeremiah Easley at Colorado State University and the editorial staff at Elsevier (especially Patrick Manley, Don Mumford, and Nicole Congleton) for their help and support.

Sarah M. Reuss, VMD, DACVIM
Department of Large Animal Clinical Sciences
University of Florida's College of Veterinary Medicine
Gainesville, FL 32610, USA

A. Berkley Chesen, DVM, DACVS-LA
Equine Comprehensive Wellness
Santa Fe, NM 87508, USA

E-mail addresses:
sreuss@ufl.edu (S.M. Reuss)
berkleychesen@gmail.com (A.B. Chesen)

Update on Diseases and Treatment of the Pharynx

A. Berkley Chesen, DVM[a],*, Canaan Whitfield-Cargile, DVM[b]

KEYWORDS

- Pharynx • Palatial Instability • Dorsal displacement of the soft palate
- Exercise intolerance • Laryngeal tie-forward • Nasopharyngeal cicatrix
- Permanent tracheostomy

KEY POINTS

- Palatial instability can progress to dorsal displacement of the soft palate (DDSP).
- Laryngohyoid apparatus position seems to be a factor associated with DDSP.
- The laryngeal tie-forward is the most widely accepted treatment option for this condition, either alone or in combination with other procedures.
- Nasopharyngeal cicatrix most commonly affects older horses living primarily on pasture in the areas around the Gulf in the Southern United States.
- Standing permanent tracheostomy is the best long-term treatment of affected horses.

UPDATE ON DORSAL DISPLACEMENT OF THE SOFT PALATE IN HORSES
Background

Palatial instability (PI) is the most common dynamic obstruction of the upper respiratory tract (URT) of horses.[1] PI is typically defined as instability of the caudal portion of the soft palate resulting in its billowing into the nasopharynx and obstruction of the normal flow of air.[2] This can further progress to dorsal displacement of the soft palate (DDSP) as occurs when the caudal margin of the soft palate displaces dorsally, over the epiglottis, resulting in more severe URT obstruction (**Fig. 1**).[3] DDSP is reported to occur in 1.3% of horses in general but is estimated to occur in a much higher prevalence in race horses.[4,5] This condition is typically described as intermittent, occurring only during exercise, or persistent, where the condition is present at rest.[6] The exact cause of DDSP is unclear and the subject of much debate and recent publications.[7] Factors implicated in the etiopathogenesis of DDSP include neuromuscular dysfunction, URT inflammation or infection, anatomic abnormalities and variations, and complications

The authors have nothing to disclose.
[a] Equine Comprehensive Wellness, 118 Camino Los Abuelos, Santa Fe, NM 87508, USA;
[b] Department of Large Animal Clinical Sciences, College of Veterinary Medicine and Biomedical Sciences, Texas A&M University, 4475 TAMU, College Station, TX 77843, USA
* Corresponding author.
E-mail address: berkleychesen@gmail.com

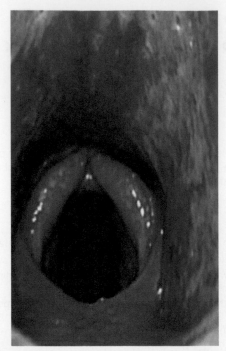

Fig. 1. Characteristic image of the nasopharynx of a horse with DDSP at rest.

of URT surgery for other conditions.[8–13] The unclear etiopathogenesis of this common condition has resulted in a large number of treatment options directed at each of the proposed causes. Recent improvements and changes in technology have resulted in new information related to the etiopathogenesis of DDSP and more diagnostic options.

Updates on Etiopathogenesis

Epiglottis

The epiglottis has long been discussed as a factor involved in the etiopathogenesis of DDSP. This has been demonstrated in several publications where either intermittent DDSP or poor performance was associated with an abnormal appearance of the epiglottis.[14–16] However, other authors suggest that the abnormal-appearing epiglottis is a result and not a cause of DDSP.[5] This is further highlighted by the fact that horses with experimentally induced epiglottic retroversion fail to develop DDSP.[17] Therefore epiglottic augmentation is no longer recommended as a routine treatment option for DDSP.

Tongue position

Similarly, tongue position has been discussed as a potential cause of DDSP and is the basis for use of the tongue-tie to prevent DDSP. Tongue retraction is thought to simultaneously result in caudal retraction of the larynx and dorsal pressure on the soft palate "pushing" it dorsal to the epiglottis. Although an occasional horse can benefit from the use of a tongue-tie in regards to DDSP, this is not the expected response and there remains no sound scientific evidence to its use.[18,19]

Neuromuscular dysfunction

Neuromuscular dysfunction as a cause for DDSP is supported by recreation of the disorder with specific nerve blocks (pharyngeal branch of the vagus nerve or the hypoglossal nerve) or muscle belly transection (thyrohyoideus).[8,9,20] A potential cause of neuromuscular dysfunction resulting in DDSP is inflammation caused by URT infection. This is supported by reports of increased prevalence of DDSP following URT infections.[13,14]

Laryngeal/hyoid position

The relative positions of the larynx and hyoid apparatus is another speculated cause of DDSP supported by reports demonstrating a more ventrally located basihyoid bone in horses with DDSP as determined ultrasonographically, and horses with persistent DDSP have a more caudally located larynx than those with less severe, intermittent DDSP.[6,21] Furthermore, increased head and neck flexion increases the incidence of DDSP by a combination of increased negative pressures in the airway and caudal retraction of the larynx.[22,23] Improving the position of the larynx and hyoid apparatus is the basis of the laryngeal tie forward procedure, which aims to move the larynx dorsal and rostral and the basihyoid dorsal and caudal. The goal of this repositioning is to stabilize the soft palate.[24]

Postoperative implications

PI leading to DDSP has been reported following laryngoplasty to treat recurrent laryngeal neuropathy and surgery to correct epiglottic entrapment.[12] The cause of this is unknown; it is possible that DDSP was present, but not diagnosed, preoperatively or that these disorders represent progression of a common neuromuscular dysfunction syndrome affecting the URT of horses. It is also possible that DDSP postoperatively is a complication of the surgery either caused by iatrogenic nerve damage during surgery or a result of chronic URT inflammation postoperatively.[12]

Summary of etiopathogenesis

Clearly the root cause of DDSP is complex and incompletely understood. Although there are isolated cases where the cause of DDSP is obvious, such as persistent epiglottic frenulum, epiglottic entrapment, and subepiglottic cysts, this is the exception rather than the rule. The more common phenotype of this disease begins with PI of undetermined cause. As the disease progresses PI becomes more severe until clinical DDSP occurs resulting in poor performance.[16]

Updates on Diagnosis of Dorsal Displacement of the Soft Palate

DDSP is most commonly diagnosed via endoscopy of the URT where the soft palate obscures visualization of the epiglottic cartilage. The affected horse usually swallows frequently, which temporarily replaces the epiglottis dorsal to the soft palate.[25] Endoscopy is performed either at rest or while exercising. In general, observation of DDSP at rest is a fairly reliable positive predictive test but a very poor negative predictive test for DDSP.[14,26] In all cases the gold standard diagnostic modality is videoendoscopy while exercising, which can be performed using a high-speed treadmill or dynamic over-the-ground endoscopy. It has been shown that DDSP occurs most commonly during, or at the end of, strenuous exercise. Although both modalities are widely accepted, a higher diagnostic rate of DDSP has been reported with high-speed treadmill endoscopy presumably because of failure of over-the-ground endoscopy to create the exertion of high-speed treadmill.[27] In contrast, there is strong evidence that head and neck position influences DDSP and therefore over-the-ground endoscopy, although being ridden under normal conditions including head and neck positioning, is more likely to result in an accurate diagnosis.[22] Therefore, the recommendation to achieve the most accurate diagnosis is to make every effort to recreate race or performance conditions including speed, duration, tack, and head and neck positions.

Recently ultrasonographic and radiographic evaluation of the equine upper airway has gained popularity.[28] Position of the larynx and basihyoid bone has been associated with DDSP. Ultrasonographic determination of a more ventrally located basihyoid bone, measured at the lingual process, has been reported as a predictor of DDSP; with every centimeter of increasing depth, the odds of DDSP decrease by 17-fold.[21] Similarly, radiographs of the laryngeal region can provide some information regarding the position of the larynx and basihyoid bone and DDSP.[6,24] When performing radiographs of the laryngeal region of the horse to assess positioning of the larynx and hyoid apparatus it is important to use a standardized head position with extension being most useful for this purpose.[29]

Updates on Treatment of Dorsal Displacement of the Soft Palate

Management of DDSP remains controversial because of the lack of a clear cause of this disorder, resulting in several treatment strategies each directed toward one of the proposed causes. As with any disease, it is imperative that any underlying cause is first addressed including antimicrobials in the case of concurrent URT infection, and appropriate treatment of and concurrent structural abnormalities. Typically, medical management consisting of rest, anti-inflammatory drugs, and time is recommended for any young horse (<2–3 years old) and certainly for any animal with ongoing upper respiratory inflammation for any cause.[30] If there are no concurrent structural or anatomic abnormalities and medical therapy has failed to result in improvement then specific intervention for DDSP can be initiated. Specific interventions for DDSP are summarized in **Table 1**. Management of DDSP ranges from simple tack changes, attempts to decrease pliability of the soft palate and/or epiglottis, attempts to prevent

Table 1
Summary of treatment options for DDSP

Treatment	Aim of Treatment	Reported Success Rates
Figure-of-eight noseband	Keeps mouth shut preventing positive pressure in the oropharynx	Unreported
W-bit, serena-song bit	Prevent retraction of the tongue	Unreported
Tongue-tie	Prevent retraction of the tongue	53%–61%[31,35]
Laryngohyoid support device	Support larynx in a more dorsal and rostral position	7/7 horses with experimentally induced DDSP[34]
Staphylectomy (not routinely recommended)	Reduce epiglottic length and/or stiffen caudal edge of the soft palate	Not performed alone but in combination with other procedures 60%–63%[36,37]
Palatoplasty	Increase soft palate stiffness	28%–51%[31,32]
Strap muscle myectomy	Reduce caudal retraction of the larynx	58%[38]
Laryngeal tie-forward	Reposition the laryngohyoid apparatus	66%–81% (treated horses were as likely race as normal horses)[24]
Combination surgeries	Combined aims of other treatments	Varied but no dramatic improvement over single therapies

caudal traction of the larynx, and repositioning of the larynx and basihyoid bone with a prosthetic suture. Because of the uncertainty of cause it can be difficult to choose a management strategy but every effort should be made to choose a treatment strategy based on the most likely cause in the patient being examined and scientific, evidence-based information.[7]

Table 1 highlights the modest success rates of most therapies aimed at DDSP. Additionally, there has been new information that continues to build a body of evidence against use of staphylectomy and various forms of palatoplasty for most horses with this condition.[5,31–33] There is increasing support implicating laryngohyoid positioning as a factor associated with DDSP.[5,6,9,20,21,24,34] As such currently the most widely accepted surgical intervention, following failed conservative therapy, is laryngeal tie-forward with or without myectomy of the sternohyoideus and sternothyrohyoideus. Success rates approaching upward of 80% have been reported for this treatment strategy and there seems to be minimal detrimental effects to the horse.[5,6,24]

UPDATE ON NASOPHARYNGEAL CICATRIX IN THE HORSE

Nasopharyngeal cicatrix is scarring of the pharynx, guttural pouch openings, epiglottis, and/or arytenoid cartilages caused by inflammation. In acute cases, the mucosa appears hyperemic on endoscopic examination.[39] Chronic cases show dense weblike strands of tissue attached to the pharynx (**Fig. 2**).

This condition is typically seen in the Gulf States, specifically Eastern and Southern Texas. It was thought that mares had a predilection for the condition; however, according to a recent publication, there is not an association with the sex of the horse.[40] Other risk factors thought to contribute to this disease include age (older horses are more often affected) and those housed on pasture.[40]

The incidence tends to be in horses that are older and kept primarily on pasture. Because of this and being in a specific geographic area, although unproved, the cause is thought to be an allergen.[39]

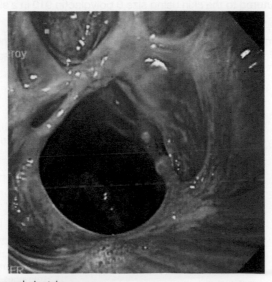

Fig. 2. Nasopharyngeal cicatrix.

Risk Factors for Nasopharyngeal Cicatrix

Aged horses, horses kept on pasture, and geographic location (Gulf States, especially Southern and Eastern Texas) are risk factor for nasopharyngeal cicatrix. Clinical signs typically include upper respiratory noise, exercise intolerance, and much less often, dysphagia.[39,41] With acute inflammation, nasal discharge is often apparent.[41] Acute inflammation is associated with horses who present in respiratory distress and have narrowing of the airway diameter by at least 50%.[41] Compared with control animals, coughing is not associated with nasopharyngeal cicatrix.[41]

Early diagnosis is beneficial, because changing the management of the horse may stop the progression of the condition. Horses should be removed from pasture and placed in a dry lot and or stall. There have been attempts to remove portions of the scarred tissue using a diode laser or other; however, recurrence and progression are common. The most effective treatment is a standing permanent tracheostomy,[42] the procedure for which is as follows:

- Standing sedation with detomidine and butorphanol
- Horse's head is suspended while in stocks to extend and raise the head to gain access to the neck
- Local anesthetic infiltrated in an inverted U surrounding the second to sixth tracheal rings
- 4 × 7 cm elliptical incision through skin and subcutaneous tissue is made, centered on the ventral midline
- Portions of the sternohyoideus, sternothyroideus, and omohyoideus muscles are crushed at the proximal and distal ends of the incision using Ferguson angiotrib forceps
- Electrocoagulation is ideal to resect the muscle at the crushed locations (**Fig. 3**)
- Approximately 20 mL of 2% lidocaine is injected into the tracheal lumen
- Desired tracheal rings are incised on midline (**Fig. 4**)
- The ring is then undermined in both directions to free approximately one-third of the ring (do not penetrate the mucosa during dissection) (**Fig. 5**)
- Mucosa is incised in a double Y (**Fig. 6**)
- Mucosa is sutured to the skin using size 0 polyglactin 910 in a simple interrupted pattern (**Fig. 7**)

Broad-spectrum antibiotics are recommended for 5 to 7 days, and flunixin meglumine (1.1 mg/kg twice a day).[42] The stoma is to be gently cleaned with warm

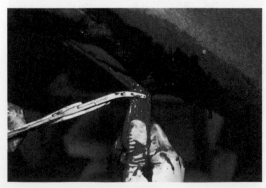

Fig. 3. Using electrocoagulation to remove muscle.

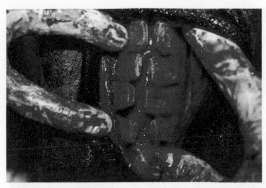

Fig. 4. Tracheal rings incised on midline.

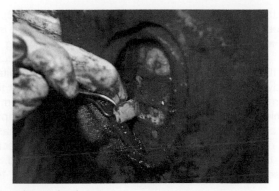

Fig. 5. Undermining the tracheal rings.

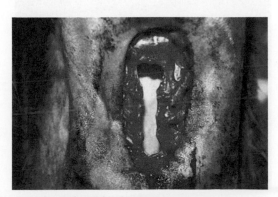

Fig. 6. Double Y incision through tracheal mucosa.

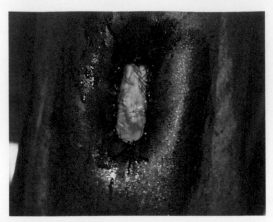

Fig. 7. Sutured skin to tracheal mucosa.

compresses until the site has completely healed (30–60 days) (**Fig. 8**). Removal of the sutures after 2 weeks tends to decrease discharge from the site. It is also important to keep horses away from fences or doorways where rubbing the incision is possible.[42]

It is imperative that horses be kept away from deep water indefinitely. Results of a retrospective study showed that although it was previously thought that potential issues resulting from a permanent tracheostomy could pose a problem with parturition in broodmares, this was not found to be an issue.[42] Tracheal collapse has also not been an issue according to the results in this study; however, it has been seen by the author more often in Miniature Horses after a permanent tracheostomy. This may be caused by other anatomic abnormalities in this breed. The long-term outcome for horses with this condition undergoing a permanent tracheostomy is very good.[42]

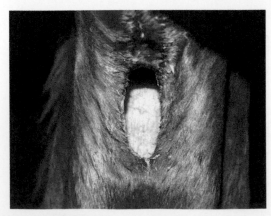

Fig. 8. Healed permanent tracheostomy.

REFERENCES

1. Lane JG, Bladon B, Little DR, et al. Dynamic obstructions of the equine upper respiratory tract. Part 1: observations during high-speed treadmill endoscopy of 600 Thoroughbred racehorses. Equine Vet J 2006;38:393–9.
2. Tan RH, Dowling BA, Dart AJ. High-speed treadmill videoendoscopic examination of the upper respiratory tract in the horse: the results of 291 clinical cases. Vet J 2005;170:243–8.
3. Allen K, Franklin S. The effect of palatal dysfunction on measures of ventilation and gas exchange in Thoroughbred racehorses during high intensity exercise. Equine Vet J 2013;45:350–4.
4. Raphel CF. Endoscopic findings in the upper respiratory tract of 479 horses. J Am Vet Med Assoc 1982;181:470–3.
5. Ducharme NG. Pharynx. In: Auer JA, Stick JA, editors. Equine surgery. 4th edition. St Louis (MO): Elsevier; 2012. p. 569–91.
6. Ortved KF, Cheetham J, Mitchell LM, et al. Successful treatment of persistent dorsal displacement of the soft palate and evaluation of laryngohyoid position in 15 racehorses. Equine Vet J 2010;42:23–9.
7. Allen KJ, Christley RM, Birchall MA, et al. A systematic review of the efficacy of interventions for dynamic intermittent dorsal displacement of the soft palate. Equine Vet J 2012;44:259–66.
8. Holcombe SJ, Derksen FJ, Stick JA, et al. Effect of bilateral blockade of the pharyngeal branch of the vagus nerve on soft palate function in horses. Am J Vet Res 1998;59:504–8.
9. Ducharme NG, Hackett RP, Woodie JB, et al. Investigations into the role of the thyrohyoid muscles in the pathogenesis of dorsal displacement of the soft palate in horses. Equine Vet J 2003;35:258–63.
10. Tulleners E, Stick JA, Leitch M, et al. Epiglottic augmentation for treatment of dorsal displacement of the soft palate in racehorses: 59 cases (1985–1994). J Am Vet Med Assoc 1997;211:1022–8.
11. Yarbrough TB, Voss E, Herrgesell EJ, et al. Persistent frenulum of the epiglottis in four foals. Vet Surg 1999;28:287–91.
12. Barnett TP, O'Leary JM, Dixon PM, et al. Characterisation of palatal dysfunction after laryngoplasty. Equine Vet J 2014;46:60–3.
13. Courouce-Malblanc A, Deniau V, Rossignol F, et al. Physiological measurements and prevalence of lower airway diseases in Trotters with dorsal displacement of the soft palate. Equine Vet J Suppl 2010;(38):246–55.
14. Kelly PG, Reardon RJ, Johnston MS, et al. Comparison of dynamic and resting endoscopy of the upper portion of the respiratory tract in 57 Thoroughbred yearlings. Equine Vet J 2013;45:700–4.
15. Garrett KS, Pierce SW, Embertson RM, et al. Endoscopic evaluation of arytenoid function and epiglottic structure in Thoroughbred yearlings and association with racing performance at two to four years of age: 2,954 cases (1998 2001). J Am Vet Med Assoc 2010;236:669–73.
16. Allen K, Franklin S. Characteristics of palatal instability in Thoroughbred racehorses and their association with the development of dorsal displacement of the soft palate. Equine Vet J 2013;45:454–9.
17. Holcombe SJ, Derksen FJ, Stick JA, et al. Effects of bilateral hypoglossal and glossopharyngeal nerve blocks on epiglottic and soft palate position in exercising horses. Am J Vet Res 1997;58:1022–6.

18. Barakzai SZ, Finnegan C, Boden LA. Effect of "tongue tie" use on racing performance of thoroughbreds in the United Kingdom. Equine Vet J 2009;41:812–6.
19. Beard WL, Holcombe SJ, Hinchcliff KW. Effect of a tongue-tie on upper airway mechanics during exercise following sternothyrohyoid myectomy in clinically normal horses. Am J Vet Res 2001;62:779–82.
20. Cheetham J, Pigott JH, Hermanson JW, et al. Role of the hypoglossal nerve in equine nasopharyngeal stability. J Appl Physiol (1985) 2009;107:471–7.
21. Chalmers HJ, Yeager AE, Ducharme N. Ultrasonographic assessment of laryngohyoid position as a predictor of dorsal displacement of the soft palate in horses. Vet Radiol Ultrasound 2009;50:91–6.
22. Van Erck E. Dynamic respiratory videoendoscopy in ridden sport horses: effect of head flexion, riding and airway inflammation in 129 cases. Equine Vet J Suppl 2011;(40):18–24.
23. Fjordbakk CT, Chalmers HJ, Holcombe SJ, et al. Results of upper airway radiography and ultrasonography predict dynamic laryngeal collapse in affected horses. Equine Vet J 2013;45:705–10.
24. Cheetham J, Pigott JH, Thorson LM, et al. Racing performance following the laryngeal tie-forward procedure: a case-controlled study. Equine Vet J 2008;40:501–7.
25. Pigott JH, Ducharme NG, Mitchell LM, et al. Incidence of swallowing during exercise in horses with dorsal displacement of the soft palate. Equine Vet J 2010;42:732–7.
26. Lane JG, Bladon B, Little DR, et al. Dynamic obstructions of the equine upper respiratory tract. Part 2: comparison of endoscopic findings at rest and during high-speed treadmill exercise of 600 thoroughbred racehorses. Equine Vet J 2006;38:401–7.
27. Allen KJ, Franklin SH. Comparisons of overground endoscopy and treadmill endoscopy in UK thoroughbred racehorses. Equine Vet J 2010;42:186–91.
28. Chalmers HJ. Ultrasonographic examination of the upper airway. In: Auer JA, Stick JA, editors. Equine surgery. 4th edition. St Louis (MO): Elsevier; 2012. p. 546–52.
29. McCluskie LK, Franklin SH, Lane JG, et al. Effect of head position on radiographic assessment of laryngeal tie-forward procedure in horses. Vet Surg 2008;37:608–12.
30. Parente EJ, Martin BB, Tulleners EP, et al. Dorsal displacement of the soft palate in 92 horses during high-speed treadmill examination (1993–1998). Vet Surg 2002;31:507–12.
31. Barakzai SZ, Boden LA, Hillyer MH, et al. Efficacy of thermal cautery for intermittent dorsal displacement of the soft palate as compared to conservatively treated horses: results from 78 treadmill diagnosed horses. Equine Vet J 2009;41:65–9.
32. Reardon RJ, Fraser BS, Heller J, et al. The use of race winnings, ratings and a performance index to assess the effect of thermocautery of the soft palate for treatment of horses with suspected intermittent dorsal displacement. A case-control study in 110 racing Thoroughbreds. Equine Vet J 2008;40:508–13.
33. Alkabes KC, Hawkins JF, Miller MA, et al. Evaluation of the effects of transendoscopic diode laser palatoplasty on clinical, histologic, magnetic resonance imaging, and biomechanical findings in horses. Am J Vet Res 2010;71:575–82.
34. Woodie JB, Ducharme NG, Hackett RP, et al. Can an external device prevent dorsal displacement of the soft palate during strenuous exercise? Equine Vet J 2005;37:425–9.
35. Barakzai SZ, Dixon PM. Conservative treatment for thoroughbred racehorses with intermittent dorsal displacement of the soft palate. Vet Rec 2005;157:337–40.

36. Smith JJ, Embertson RM. Sternothyroideus myotomy, staphylectomy, and oral caudal soft palate photothermoplasty for treatment of dorsal displacement of the soft palate in 102 thoroughbred racehorses. Vet Surg 2005;34:5–10.
37. Barakzai SZ, Johnson VS, Baird DH, et al. Assessment of the efficacy of composite surgery for the treatment of dorsal displacement of the soft palate in a group of 53 racing Thoroughbreds (1990–1996). Equine Vet J 2004;36:175–9.
38. Harrison IW, Raker CW. Sternothyrohyoideus myectomy in horses: 17 cases (1984–1985). J Am Vet Med Assoc 1988;193:1299–302.
39. Auer JA, Stick JA. Equine surgery. 4th edition. St Louis (MO): Elsevier Saunders; 2012.
40. Norman TE, Chaffin MK, Bissett WT, et al. Risk factors associated with nasopharyngeal cicatrix syndrome in horses. J Am Vet Med Assoc 2013;242:1267–70.
41. Norman TE, Chaffin MK, Bisset WT, et al. Association of clinical signs with endoscopic findings in horses with nasopharyngeal cicatrix syndrome: 118 cases (2003–2008). J Am Vet Med Assoc 2012;240:734–9.
42. Chesen AB, Rakestraw PC. Indications for and short- and long-term outcome of permanent tracheostomy performed in standing horses: 82 cases (1995–2005). J Am Vet Med Assoc 2008;232:1352–6.

Update on Laryngeal Disorders and Treatment

Taralyn M. McCarrel, DVM[a], J. Brett Woodie, DVM, MS[b],*

KEYWORDS

- Larynx • Dynamic endoscopy • Laryngeal hemiplegia • Prosthetic laryngoplasty
- Epiglottis

KEY POINTS

- Thorough diagnostic evaluation, including exercising endoscopy when appropriate, is essential for accurate diagnosis and appropriate selection of treatment.
- Exercising endoscopy should recreate conditions under which clinical signs manifest, and resting endoscopy may not be an accurate reflection of dynamic lesions.
- Arytenoid cartilage abduction loss is the most common complication of prosthetic laryngoplasty, but it does not necessarily indicate laryngoplasty failure.
- Surgical procedures of the epiglottis and subepiglottic tissue are preferably performed through transnasal or transoral approaches because of higher complication rates following laryngotomy.

INTRODUCTION

The larynx is positioned between the pharynx and trachea and is comprised of 5 cartilages (epiglottis, thyroid, cricoid, and left and right arytenoids) with a mucous membrane lining the luminal surface. The stability and movement of the cartilages are controlled by the extrinsic and intrinsic laryngeal muscles, allowing the larynx to dilate during exercise, occlude the trachea during swallowing, and function during vocalization. The predominant clinical significance of laryngeal disorders relates to airway obstruction, resulting in poor performance and respiratory noise. However, primary laryngeal disorders and complications of upper airway surgery can present as dysphagia, nasal discharge, and coughing. Given that most laryngeal disorders are caused by disruption of normal anatomy or function, treatment is predominantly surgical. However, medical therapy, in the form anti-inflammatories and broad spectrum antimicrobials, often accompanies surgical treatment when infection and inflammation are part of the disease process.

The authors have nothing to disclose.
[a] Large Animal Clinical Sciences, University of Florida College of Veterinary Medicine, PO Box 100136, Gainesville, Florida 32610, USA; [b] Rood and Riddle Equine Hospital, PO Box 12070, Lexington, KY 40580, USA
* Corresponding author.
E-mail address: bwoodie@roodandriddle.com

The following text is intended to provide the reader with the most current information regarding diagnostic evaluation of the larynx, recently described abnormalities, and new treatments or modifications of existing treatments. The review will not be exhaustive, but rather, will focus on topics that have received significant attention in recent literature.

PATIENT EVALUATION

Diagnostic evaluation of a patient with suspected laryngeal pathology is summarized in **Box 1**. The unsedated horse should be restrained for assessing resting laryngeal function, while the remainder of the examination may be performed sedated. Interestingly, detomidine and acepromazine impair left arytenoid function, but had no effect on right arytenoid function.[1] A recent postmortem survey of 91 Thoroughbred racehorses found laryngopharyngeal pathology in 14.3%, and approximately half (7.7%) involved the subepiglottic tissue, emphasizing the importance of elevating the epiglottis under sedation and topical local anesthesia during resting examination.[2] A definitive diagnosis may be attained following resting endoscopy (**Fig. 1**). However, further diagnostic investigation as outlined in **Box 1** can be of great value.

Exercising Upper Airway Endoscopic Examination—Treadmill and Dynamic

Exercising endoscopic examination is the gold standard for diagnosis of functional upper airway disorders. Approximately 50% of horses presented for evaluation with normal resting endoscopy will have dynamic obstruction diagnosed on exercising examination, and 19% to 56% of horses will have multiple abnormalities.[3–6] Several studies have utilized treadmill endoscopy to describe dynamic abnormalities in Thoroughbred and Standardbred racehorses, and sport horses of various breeds.[3,6–13] However, the recent introduction of the dynamic (overground) respiratory endoscope has paved the way for new insights into disorders of the larynx, and the upper airway in general. A selection of lesions diagnosed on exercising endoscopy is depicted in **Fig. 2**.

Dynamic respiratory endoscopy uses a portable endoscope and video capture system to allow the horse to be ridden or driven in its normal environment, unlike the treadmill, which does not allow simulation of exercising surface or effect of other horses. Additionally, rider or driver intervention is limited, as is the effect of pulling for driven horses. Poll flexion and rider intervention (use of spurs, change of gait, and tight turns) affect upper airway instability and complex upper airway obstruction in ridden sport horses.[4] Poll flexion had a significant effect on vocal cord collapse (VCC) (odds ratio [OR] 10.28), axial deviation of the aryepiglottic folds (ADAF) (OR 8.56), and multiple upper airway obstruction (MAO) (OR 13.31) in 1 study.[4] Furthermore, rider intervention had a significant effect on arytenoid cartilage collapse (OR 3.62), VCC (OR 9.11), ADAF (OR 3.63), and MAO (OR 10.83).[4] Although poll flexion can be reproduced on a treadmill, rider interventions cannot.[10,11,13–15] Further advantages of the dynamic respiratory endoscope include lower equipment cost and potential for wider availability. A major disadvantage of dynamic examination is the lack of standardization of the exercise test. Recreating exercise conditions during which clinical signs manifest is critical to an accurate examination. A dynamic endoscopy study of Thoroughbred racehorses in the United Kingdom found that 82% of horses presented for respiratory noise during training demonstrated clinical signs during the test, while horses presented for noise during racing or poor performance only demonstrated clinical signs during 61% and 7% of examinations respectively.[16] Horses were trained and the examinations performed predominantly in intervals over short straight gallops, which may explain greater success reproducing lesions that occurred during training and not those occurring only during longer race distances.

> **Box 1**
> **Diagnostic evaluation of the larynx**
>
> *History—Key Questions*
> - Presenting complaint, clinical signs
> - Use or intended use
> - When do clinical signs occur?
>   - At rest
>   - During exercise
>   - Effect of tack, poll flexion
> - Prior surgery, disease, or trauma of head or neck
>
> *Physical Examination*
> - Auscultate heart and lungs
> - Palpate jugular furrow and asses jugular fill (evidence surgery, trauma, thrombosis of vein)
> - Palpate larynx (evidence of prior surgery, prominence of muscular process, laryngeal dysplasia)
> - Assess airflow from nostrils
> - Character of nasal discharge if any
>
> *Resting Endoscopy*
> - Arytenoids—function, thickness, mucosal lesions
> - Epiglottis—position, thickness, ulceration, entrapping membrane
>   - Sedation and local block of palate and epiglottis may be required to elevate epiglottis to assess subepiglottic region once entire upper airway has been assessed
> - Remainder of airway (pharynx, guttural pouches, nasal passages, trachea)
>
> *Exercising Endoscopy[a]*
> - Treadmill or overground
> - Recreate conditions under which clinical signs occur
>
> *Oral Examination[a]*
> - Palpation and/or oral endoscopy of epiglottis/subepiglottic tissue
>
> *Imaging Modalities[a]*
> - Ultrasound
> - Radiography
> - Computed tomography
> - Magnetic resonance imaging
>
> [a] Modalities that may be useful depending on findings of history, physical examination, and resting endoscopy.

DISORDERS OF THE ARYTENOIDS
Abnormal Arytenoid Abduction at Rest

When assessing the horse with submaximal arytenoid abduction, recurrent laryngeal neuropathy (RLN) is usually the first diagnosis to come to mind. However, all causes of impaired arytenoid abduction should be considered to guide appropriate diagnostic

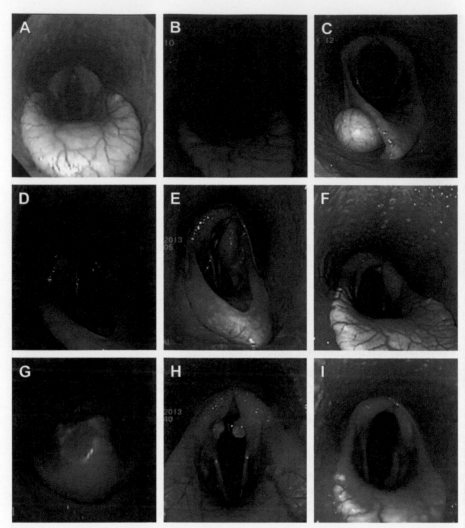

Fig. 1. Abnormalities identified on resting endoscopy. (*A*) Normal larynx at rest. (*B*) Normal larynx after stimulated swallow. (*C*) Subepiglottic cyst. (*D*) Bilateral arytenoid chondritis and thin nonulcerated epiglottic entrapment; this horse was treated with permanent tracheostomy. (*E*) Same horse as in *D* 1 year later; note inflammation has resolved. There is no change in cartilage deformation. (*F*) Grade 4 recurrent laryngeal neuropathy. (*G*) Thick ulcerated epiglottic entrapment. (*H*) Arytenoid granuloma; ultrasound confirmed this horse did not have arytenoid chondropathy. (*I*) After left prosthetic laryngoplasty and ventriculocordectomy with rostral displacement of the palatopharyngeal arch (RDPA), this horse does not have laryngeal dysplasia, and RDPA resolved during exercising examination.

evaluation and treatment (**Box 2**). Laryngeal ultrasound following resting endoscopy is tremendously valuable for making a definitive diagnosis of RLN, arytenoid chondropathy, and laryngeal dysplasia. There have been no major advancements in the diagnosis or management of arytenoid chondropathy or laryngeal dysplasia beyond recent imaging studies. The reader is referred to the article, "Diagnostic Imaging of the Upper Airway," in this edition for further information on these topics.

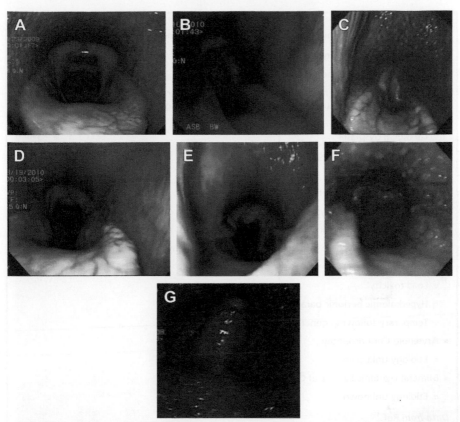

Fig. 2. Abnormalities identified on exercising endoscopy. (*A*) Normal maximal symmetric arytenoid abduction. (*B*) Left arytenoid collapse and axial deviation of the aryepiglottic folds (right > left). (*C*) Bilateral dynamic laryngeal collapse. (*D*) Sagittal folding of the epiglottis. (*E*) Axial overriding of the corniculate processes. (*F*) Ventromedial deviation of the corniculate processes. (*G*) Epiglottic retroversion.

Recurrent laryngeal neuropathy

The most common cause of impaired left arytenoid abduction is RLN. Treatment options for RLN have classically included prosthetic laryngoplasty (tie-back) (PL), partial arytenoidectomy, laryngeal reinnervation, and ventriculectomy or ventriculocordectomy (alone of combined with PL).[17] The value of ventriculocordectomy for reducing respiratory noise is broadly accepted, and the procedure is routinely combined with PL.[18,19] Electrical stimulation of nerve or muscle may become a viable option in the future, although arytenoid abduction was not achieved in horses with grade 4 RLN in 1 study.[20–22]

Prosthetic laryngoplasty, whereby a suture is placed through the cricoid and arytenoid cartilages to achieve arytenoid abduction, remains the hallmark treatment for RLN and will be the focus of the following text. The major goal of PL is to optimize and maintain arytenoid position, maximizing airflow while minimizing aspiration. To this end, numerous studies are performed focusing on suture type, position, number, and force; causes of laryngoplasty failure and abduction loss; and methods to stabilize the cricoarytenoid joint.

Box 2
Disorders resulting in abnormal arytenoid abduction and causes

- Left Laryngeal Hemiplegia
  - Recurrent laryngeal neuropathy (most common)
  - Recurrent laryngeal nerve injury (perivascular jugular vein injection, guttural pouch infection/mycosis, trauma or surgery of the neck, impingement by neoplasms in neck or thorax)
  - Laryngeal dysplasia
- Right Laryngeal Hemiplegia
  - Laryngeal dysplasia
  - Recurrent laryngeal nerve injury
- Bilateral Laryngeal Paralysis
  - Organophosphate toxicity
  - Central nervous system disease (ie, equine protozoal myeloencephalitis)
  - Hepatic disease
  - Lead toxicity
  - Hyperkalemic periodic paralysis
  - Temporary following general anesthesia
- Arytenoid Chondropathy
  - Etiology unknown
- Bilateral Dynamic Laryngeal Collapse
  - Etiology unknown

Data from Ref.[1]

Ideal arytenoid cartilage abduction was determined to be that which achieves 88% of maximal cross-sectional area of the laryngeal lumen in vitro; however, submaximally exercising horses likely do not require this degree of abduction to perform.[23] Clinical recommendations range from 80% to 90% of maximal abduction in racehorses and 60% to 80% of maximal abduction in nonperformance horses.[24] The cricoarytenoideus dorsalis muscle (CAD), the only abductor of the larynx, is comprised of medial and lateral bellies that exert different effects on arytenoid position.[25] Recent studies have concluded that the prosthetic suture should mimic the path of the lateral belly to achieve optimal abduction, although 1 study found no difference between sutures following the path of the medial or lateral belly when only 1 suture was tied.[25–27] Two sutures achieve greater cross-sectional area than a single suture, but addition of a third suture confers no advantage.[27,28] The force required to achieve maximal arytenoid abduction has been reported to be 20 N in cadaveric larynges, and 27.6 N to achieve optimal abduction in vivo.[27,29] Perkins and colleagues[24] evaluated the effect of performing ventriculocordectomy before PL on force to achieve arytenoid abduction. Importantly the adductor muscles were cut, which may have contributed to an overall lower mean force (12 N) to achieve maximal abduction. Although ventriculocordectomy prior to PL resulted in 12% and 45% less force to achieve 0.8 left–right quotient and cross-sectional area respectively, the overall highest force measured during the study to achieve maximal abduction was only 18 N.[24]

The authors recommend ventriculocordectomy prior to PL to minimize suture forces on cartilage, which could result in cartilage failure. However, as an example of perspective, PL sutures undergo forces of 46.6 N during swallowing, which occurs more than 1000 times per day.[29] Therefore, the one-time force at the time of tying appears to pale in comparison to the long-term effect of swallowing.

The most common complication of PL is abduction loss; however, the specific causes are unknown in most cases.[30] Dahlberg and colleagues[31] proposed that variations in cricoid conformation may contribute to abduction loss, particularly if the suture slips down the caudal lateral surface of a cricoid with a large lateral cricoid angle (slope of the caudal lateral cricoid surface). Further investigation is warranted to substantiate this theory. Cartilage failure (fracture or suture cut-through) is thought to occur secondary to high suture forces. Indeed, failure of the muscular process has been reported to result in PL failure.[29,32] The theory that abduction loss was caused by suture forces generated by the adductor muscles led to the recommendation to delay PL until complete paralysis; this theory has been disproven.[33] Swallowing, as already described, thus far has been shown to exert the greatest force on laryngoplasty sutures and may be a major mechanism contributing to abduction loss. One strategy to minimize long-term cyclic forces on laryngoplasty sutures is stabilization of the cricoarytenoid joint (CAJ). Polymethylmethacrylate was injected into the CAJ of cadaveric larynges and resulted in maintenance of tracheal pressure and flow with and without the suture in place, and significantly lesser increase in suture strain with increasing translaryngeal pressures.[34] Parente and colleagues[35] described a modified PL with 2 key differences from traditional PL; first the muscular process was approached caudal to the cricopharyngeus and the insertion of the CAD transected compared with the traditional approach, whereby the crico- and thyropharyngeus muscles are separated to expose the muscular process, and second the CAJ was opened and cartilage debrided. The modified PL had significantly less abduction loss and lower impedance compared with traditional PL after 3 months. Furthermore, there was no difference in impedance with the suture intact or cut in modified PL samples, which demonstrated histologic evidence of joint fusion.[35] Importantly, the study author recommends repeat PL within 2 weeks if postoperative abduction loss does occur because of an inability to alter abduction once joint fusion is complete.[35]

There are 2 important questions to consider when evaluating horses following PL:

- Does arytenoid cartilage abduction loss equate to laryngoplasty failure?
- Are all cases of laryngoplasty failure caused by abduction loss?

Endoscopic grades of surgical laryngeal abduction are described on a scale from 1 to 5, where grade 1 represents excessive abduction (80°–90° to sagittal plane), and grade 5 represents no abduction.[36] Abduction loss progresses for several weeks, with 93% of horses experiencing abduction loss between 6 days and 6 weeks.[37] Arytenoid abduction grade stabilizes 6 weeks postoperatively at a median of grade 3 (moderate abduction, 45° to sagittal plane).[37,38] Postoperative arytenoid abduction grade was not correlated with return to racing, lifetime starts, earnings in 5 postoperative races, or arytenoid cartilage stability during exercise.[37,38] However, these results can only be applied to horses with grade 1 to 3 abduction, because there were insufficient grade 4s and 5s for evaluation. Between 87% and 91% of horses presented for PL failure had multiple abnormalities on exercising endoscopy.[39,40] Therefore, the answer to both questions is no. Although abduction loss should not be ignored, it does not define PL failure, and exercising endoscopy provides the most accurate information regarding arytenoid stability and causative abnormalities manifesting as PL failure.

Reports of outcome following PL are highly variable, with 48% to 94% of horses starting 1 race, while others suggest reasonable estimates for success range from 50% to 70% in racehorses, and 86% to 93% in nonracehorses.[17,41] Interestingly, Barakzai and colleagues[42] and Mason and colleagues[43] reported significantly shorter racing careers following PL, while Aceto and Parente[44] reported no difference in racing longevity between horses undergoing modified PL and cohorts. Following modified laryngoplasty, there was no difference in number of race starts or dollars earned between treated horses and cohorts with the exception of the first quarter after returning to racing.[44] The reason for these differences is unknown but may be related to arytenoid stabilization or differences in approach minimizing postoperative complications. Complications of PL have been thoroughly reviewed and are summarized in **Box 3**.[30,36,45]

Bilateral Dynamic Laryngeal Collapse

Bilateral dynamic laryngeal collapse (DLC) is defined as collapse of both arytenoid cartilages and vocal folds during exercise.[10] Norwegian Coldblooded Trotters (NCTs) are predisposed compared with Standardbreds (45.3% and 2.4% of examined horses, respectively).[10,14,15,46–49] Bilateral dynamic laryngeal collapse has been reported sporadically in other publications, and the authors have also diagnosed DLC in various breeds of gaited horses (unpublished data).[6] Resting endoscopy is normal, and DLC manifests only during exercising endoscopy with forced poll flexion. Laryngeal conformation returns to normal when the head is extended.[14] The etiology is unknown; however, affected horses have a more rostral position of the larynx during poll flexion compared with unaffected horses, which may result in physical compression of the larynx.[48] Affected horses also have more negative tracheal peak inspiratory pressures when exercising with the poll flexed compared with controls.[14]

There are no large studies evaluating treatment of DLC. One investigation compared conservative treatment, which consisted of a variety of unspecified tack or training changes, with bilateral ventriculocordectomy.[49] The authors hypothesized that VCC preceded arytenoid collapse and the arytenoid collapse could thus be prevented by preventing VCC. This hypothesis was disproven, and there was no difference in return to racing or racing performance between treatment groups, with 11 of 26 horses being retired.[49] The development of a modified checkrein to prevent poll flexion appears promising for use in harness horses. Horses with DLC were evaluated with conventional and modified checkrein during treadmill endoscopy. The modified checkrein successfully prevented poll flexion and improved endoscopic scores; additionally, tracheal peak inspiratory pressures were significantly less negative.[46] Larger clinical

---

Box 3
Postoperative complications of laryngoplasty

- Loss of arytenoid abduction
- Dysphagia and coughing
- Upper esophageal incompetence (rare)
- Seroma
- Surgical site inflammation/infection
- Arytenoid inflammation
- Postoperative airway obstruction (rare)

Data from Refs.[30,36,45]

studies are needed to confirm improvement in racing performance. Unfortunately for many breeds of sport horses, poll flexion is essential during competition, which negates the modified checkrein as a treatment option. One author (JBW) has treated these horses with left PL (or right PL if the right arytenoid is more severely affected) and unilateral or often bilateral ventriculocordectomy. However, results have not yet been objectively assessed. In cases that did not respond favorably to surgical intervention and continued to have respiratory obstruction during exercise, the most common causes were continued DLC or collapse of the arytenoid not subjected to PL.

DISORDERS OF THE EPIGLOTTIS
Epiglottic Entrapment

Epiglottic entrapment (EE) occurs when the loose subepiglottic mucosal tissue becomes persistently or intermittently entrapped over the dorsal surface of the epiglottis. Upper airway noise is the most common complaint in racehorses, with a smaller subset of horses demonstrating exercise intolerance.[50–53] EE may also be identified on routine endoscopy with no clinical signs. Mature nonracehorses with epiglottic abnormalities display multiple clinical signs with respiratory noise (9 of 13 horses) and coughing (7 of 13 horses) occurring with similar frequency.[54] The endoscopic appearance of EE in racehorses is highly variable; however, the nature of the entrapment in mature non-racehorses was reported to be chronic, thick, and ulcerated in all cases.[51,52,54]

There have been no clinical studies evaluating medical therapy alone for treatment of EE. One study reported successful treatment of 3 of 4 horses using anti-inflammatory therapy alone; however, conclusions cannot be drawn from this small sample size.[55] Anti-inflammatory therapy in the form of systemic nonsteroidal anti-inflammatories, systemic corticosteroids, and topical anti-inflammatory throat spray used alone or in combination are consistently given for 7 to 14 days postoperatively, or longer if deemed necessary based on clinical signs and repeated endoscopic examination.[51,52,54] Administration of antimicrobials is more variable and dependent on clinician preference.

Surgical treatment options for EE are presented in **Box 4**. When selecting a surgical procedure several factors should be taken into consideration:

- Surgeon experience and available equipment
- Nature of the entrapment (thickness, scaring, curling of the epiglottic cartilage)
- Horse temperament
- Surgeon's hand size relative to the horse (oral, hand-assisted techniques)
- Complications and outcome associated with surgical approach

---

Box 4
Surgical treatment options for epiglottic entrapment

- Transnasal laser axial division
- Transnasal or transoral endoscope guided axial division with a curved hook bistoury
- Transnasal endoscope-guided axial division with a shielded hook bistoury
- Transoral hand-assisted axial division with a hook bistoury
- Transnasal electrosurgical axial division
- Surgical excision through a laryngotomy

Data from Refs.[17,50–57]

Three recent publications have described modifications of established surgical procedures. Perkins and colleagues[56] described an endoscope-guided, transoral axial division of EE using a hook bistoury in standing sedated horses. A hand must be placed in the mouth to displace the soft palate dorsal to the epiglottis. One horse had to be anesthetized, and all horses had resolution of clinical signs with no recurrence for 1 year. The ability and desire of the surgeon to reach his or her hand to the epiglottis in an awake horse, and risk of inadvertent injury caused by movement or swallowing during release of the entrapping tissue need to be carefully considered. An oral, hand-assisted technique using a hook bistoury in anesthetized horses has also been described.[57] Transnasal axial division of entrapping tissue was described in 8 horses using a shielded hook bistoury designed to prevent laceration of unintended structures.[50] All surgeries were successful, and there were no short- or long-term complications. However, larger studies are needed to draw firm conclusions regarding the safety and efficacy of all techniques.

Most horses return to racing at the same or higher level following surgical correction of EE using transnasal or transoral hook or laser techniques.[41] Release of EE through a laryngotomy is associated with a higher complication rate and significantly decreased success (27%–33%).[53,54] Laryngotomy is currently only recommended for cases with severely thick and fibrotic entrapments.[17,53] Re-entrapment ranges from 0% to 10% with axial division using a hook bistoury, and is approximately 5% for axial division using Nd:YAG laser.[51,52,56,57] Recurrence following electrosurgical axial division of tissue reached 40% and is not recommended.[17] The most common complication following EE correction is postoperative dorsal displacement of the soft palate, which has been reported to occur in up to 10% of hook or laser axial division procedures.[51,52] There is a risk of laceration of unintended structures when a hook bistoury is used in a sedated horse, as well as with transnasal use in an anesthetized horse. One report described lacerations of the epiglottis or soft palate in 4 of 33 procedures using a conventional hook transnasally in sedated horses.[50]

Dynamically Flaccid Epiglottis

Two recent publications by Strand and colleagues define and report the frequency of dynamically flaccid epiglottis (DFE) alone or in combination with other dynamic upper airway lesions in NCT and Standardbred racehorses undergoing treadmill endoscopy.[10,15] DFE is defined as a medial collapse of the lateral margins of the epiglottis and may be primary or secondary[15]:

- Primary DFE—the center of tissue collapse is along the margin of the epiglottis
- Secondary DFE—the center of tissue collapse is along the aryepiglottic folds, and the margins of the epiglottis are drawn medially by the aryepiglottic fold

Resting endoscopy is normal; DFE is a dynamic lesion and is induced or exacerbated by poll flexion. A DFE may occur alone or may be associated with ADAF or DLC.[10] NCTs were diagnosed with DFE significantly more often than Standardbreds (45.3% and 17.1%, respectively).[15] The authors of this article have also observed a similar manifestation in gaited horses with folding of the epiglottis in the sagittal plane (McCarrel & Woodie 2014). The etiology of DFE is unknown, and there is no defined treatment.

SUMMARY

Thorough diagnostic evaluation, including exercising endoscopy when appropriate, is essential for accurate diagnosis and appropriate selection of treatment. Exercising endoscopy should recreate conditions under which clinical signs manifest, and it should be noted that resting endoscopy may not be an accurate reflection of dynamic lesions. Arytenoid cartilage abduction loss is the most common complication of PL but does not necessarily indicate laryngoplasty failure. Surgical procedures of the epiglottis and subepiglottic tissue are preferably performed through transnasal or transoral approaches because of higher complication rates following laryngotomy.

REFERENCES

1. Lindegaard C, Husted L, Ullum H, et al. Sedation with detomidine and acepromazine influences the endoscopic evaluation of laryngeal function in horses. Equine Vet J 2007;39(6):553–6.
2. Diab S, Pascoe J, Shahriar M, et al. Study of laryngopharyngeal pathology in Thoroughbred horses in southern california. Equine Vet J 2009;41(9):903–7.
3. Tan RH, Dowling BA, Dart AJ. High-speed treadmill videoendoscopic examination of the upper respiratory tract in the horse: the results of 291 clinical cases. Vet J 2005;170(2):243–8.
4. Van Erck E. Dynamic respiratory videoendoscopy in ridden sport horses: effect of head flexion, riding and airway inflammation in 129 cases. Equine Vet J Suppl 2011;40:18–24.
5. Witte SH, Witte TH, Harriss F, et al. Association of owner-reported noise with findings during dynamic respiratory endoscopy in thoroughbred racehorses. Equine Vet J 2011;43(1):9–17.
6. Davidson EJ, Martin BB, Boston RC, et al. Exercising upper respiratory videoendoscopic evaluation of 100 nonracing performance horses with abnormal respiratory noise and/or poor performance. Equine Vet J 2011;43(1):3–8.
7. Lane JG, Bladon B, Little DR, et al. Dynamic obstructions of the equine upper respiratory tract. Part 1: observations during high-speed treadmill endoscopy of 600 Thoroughbred racehorses. Equine Vet J 2006;38(5):393–9.
8. Martin BB Jr, Reef VB, Parente EJ, et al. Causes of poor performance of horses during training, racing, or showing: 348 cases (1992-1996). J Am Vet Med Assoc 2000;216(4):554–8.
9. Barakzai SZ, Dixon PM. Correlation of resting and exercising endoscopic findings for horses with dynamic laryngeal collapse and palatal dysfunction. Equine Vet J 2011;43(1):18–23.
10. Strand E, Skjerve E. Complex dynamic upper airway collapse: associations between abnormalities in 99 harness racehorses with one or more dynamic disorders. Equine Vet J 2012;44(5):524–8.
11. Franklin SH, Naylor JR, Lane JG. Videoendoscopic evaluation of the upper respiratory tract in 93 sport horses during exercise testing on a high-speed treadmill. Equine Vet J Suppl 2006;36:540–5.
12. Dart AJ, Dowling BA, Hodgson DR, et al. Evaluation of high-speed treadmill videoendoscopy for diagnosis of upper respiratory tract dysfunction in horses. Aust Vet J 2001;79(2):109–12.
13. Kannegieter NJ, Dore ML. Endoscopy of the upper respiratory tract during treadmill exercise: a clinical study of 100 horses. Aust Vet J 1995;72(3):101–7.
14. Strand E, Fjordbakk CT, Holcombe SJ, et al. Effect of poll flexion and dynamic laryngeal collapse on tracheal pressure in Norwegian coldblooded trotter racehorses. Equine Vet J 2009;41(1):59–64.
15. Strand E, Fjordbakk CT, Sundberg K, et al. Relative prevalence of upper respiratory tract obstructive disorders in two breeds of harness racehorses (185 cases: 1998–2006). Equine Vet J 2012;44(5):518–23.

16. Allen KJ, Franklin SH. Assessment of the exercise tests used during overground endoscopy in UK Thoroughbred racehorses and how these may affect the diagnosis of dynamic upper respiratory tract obstructions. Equine Vet J Suppl 2010; 38:587–91.
17. Fulton IC, Anderson BH, Stick JA, et al. Larynx. In: Auer JA, Stick JA, editors. Equine surgery. 4th edition. St Louis (MO): Elsevier; 2012. p. 592–623.
18. Brown JA, Derksen FJ, Stick JA, et al. Ventriculocordectomy reduces respiratory noise in horses with laryngeal hemiplegia. Equine Vet J 2003;35(6):570–4.
19. Cramp P, Derksen FJ, Stick JA, et al. Effect of ventriculectomy versus ventriculocordectomy on upper airway noise in draught horses with recurrent laryngeal neuropathy. Equine Vet J 2009;41(8):729–34.
20. Ducharme NG, Cheetham J, Sanders I, et al. Considerations for pacing of the cricoarytenoid dorsalis muscle by neuroprosthesis in horses. Equine Vet J 2010; 42(6):534–40.
21. Cheetham J, Regner A, Jarvis JC, et al. Functional electrical stimulation of intrinsic laryngeal muscles under varying loads in exercising horses. PLoS One 2011;6(8):e24258.
22. Vanschandevijl K, Nollet H, Vonck K, et al. Functional electrical stimulation of the left recurrent laryngeal nerve using a vagus nerve stimulator in a normal horse. Vet J 2011;189(3):346–8.
23. Rakesh V, Ducharme NG, Cheetham J, et al. Implications of different degrees of arytenoid cartilage abduction on equine upper airway characteristics. Equine Vet J 2008;40(7):629–35.
24. Perkins JD, Meighan H, Windley Z, et al. In vitro effect of ventriculocordectomy before laryngoplasty on abduction of the equine arytenoid cartilage. Vet Surg 2011;40(3):305–10.
25. Cheetham J, Radcliffe CR, Ducharme NG, et al. Neuroanatomy of the equine dorsal cricoarytenoid muscle: surgical implications. Equine Vet J 2008;40(1):70–5.
26. Perkins JD, Raffetto J, Thompson C, et al. Three-dimensional biomechanics of simulated laryngeal abduction in horses. Am J Vet Res 2010;71(9):1003–10.
27. Bischofberger AS, Hadidane I, Wereszka MM, et al. Effect of age and prostheses location on rima glottidis area in equine cadaveric larynges. Vet Surg 2013;42(3): 286–90.
28. Dart A, Tee E, Brennan M, et al. Effect of prosthesis number and position on rima glottidis area in equine laryngeal specimens. Vet Surg 2009;38(4):452–6.
29. Witte TH, Cheetham J, Soderholm LV, et al. Equine laryngoplasty sutures undergo increased loading during coughing and swallowing. Vet Surg 2010; 39(8):949–56.
30. Ahern BJ, Parente EJ. Surgical complications of the equine upper respiratory tract. Vet Clin North Am Equine Pract 2008;24(3):465–84.
31. Dahlberg JA, Valdes-Martinez A, Boston RC, et al. Analysis of conformational variations of the cricoid cartilages in thoroughbred horses using computed tomography. Equine Vet J 2011;43(2):229–34.
32. Hardcastle MR, Pauwels FE, Collett MG. Clinicopathologic observations on laryngoplasty failure in a horse. Vet Surg 2012;41(5):649–53.
33. Witte TH, Mohammed HO, Radcliffe CH, et al. Racing performance after combined prosthetic laryngoplasty and ipsilateral ventriculocordectomy or partial arytenoidectomy: 135 Thoroughbred racehorses competing at less than 2400 m (1997–2007). Equine Vet J 2009;41(1):70–5.
34. Cheetham J, Witte TH, Rawlinson JJ, et al. Intra-articular stabilisation of the equine cricoarytenoid joint. Equine Vet J 2008;40(6):584–8.

35. Parente EJ, Birks EK, Habecker P. A modified laryngoplasty approach promoting ankylosis of the cricoarytenoid joint. Vet Surg 2011;40(2):204–10.
36. Dixon RM, McGorum BC, Railton DI, et al. Long-term survey of laryngoplasty and ventriculocordectomy in an older, mixed-breed population of 200 horses. Part 1: maintenance of surgical arytenoid abduction and complications of surgery. Equine Vet J 2003;35(4):389–96.
37. Barakzai SZ, Boden LA, Dixon PM. Postoperative race performance is not correlated with degree of surgical abduction after laryngoplasty in national hunt Thoroughbred racehorses. Vet Surg 2009;38(8):934–40.
38. Barnett TP, O'Leary JM, Parkin TD, et al. Long-term maintenance of arytenoid cartilage abduction and stability during exercise after laryngoplasty in 33 horses. Vet Surg 2013;42(3):291–5.
39. Davidson EJ, Martin BB, Rieger RH, et al. Exercising videoendoscopic evaluation of 45 horses with respiratory noise and/or poor performance after laryngoplasty. Vet Surg 2010;39(8):942–8.
40. Compostella F, Tremaine WH, Franklin SH. Retrospective study investigating causes of abnormal respiratory noise in horses following prosthetic laryngoplasty. Equine Vet J Suppl 2012;43:27–30.
41. Beard WL, Waxman S. Evidence-based equine upper respiratory surgery. Vet Clin North Am Equine Pract 2007;23(2):229–42.
42. Barakzai SZ, Boden LA, Dixon PM. Race performance after laryngoplasty and ventriculocordectomy in national hunt racehorses. Vet Surg 2009;38(8): 941–5.
43. Mason BJ, Riggs CM, Cogger N. Cohort study examining long-term respiratory health, career duration and racing performance in racehorses that undergo left-sided prosthetic laryngoplasty and ventriculocordectomy surgery for treatment of left-sided laryngeal hemiplegia. Equine Vet J 2013;45(2): 229–34.
44. Aceto H, Parente EJ. Using quarterly earnings to assess racing performance in 70 thoroughbreds after modified laryngoplasty for treatment of recurrent laryngeal neuropathy. Vet Surg 2012;41(6):689–95.
45. Froydenlund TJ, Dixon PM. A review of equine laryngoplasty complications. Equine Vet Educ 2014;26(2):98–106.
46. Fjordbakk CT, Holcombe S, Fintl C, et al. A novel treatment for dynamic laryngeal collapse associated with poll flexion: the modified checkrein. Equine Vet J 2012; 44(2):207–13.
47. Strand E, Hanche-olsen S, Grønvold AM, et al. Dynamic bilateral arytenoid and vocal fold collapse associated with head flexion in 5 Norwegian coldblooded trotter racehorses. Equine Vet Educ 2004;16(5):242–50.
48. Fjordbakk CT, Chalmers HJ, Holcombe SJ, et al. Results of upper airway radiography and ultrasonography predict dynamic laryngeal collapse in affected horses. Equine Vet J 2013;45(6):705–10.
49. Fjordbakk CT, Strand E, Hanche-Olsen S. Surgical and conservative management of bilateral dynamic laryngeal collapse associated with poll flexion in harness race horses. Vet Surg 2008;37(6):501–7.
50. Lacourt M, Marcoux M. Treatment of epiglottic entrapment by transnasal axial division in standing sedated horses using a shielded hook bistoury. Vet Surg 2011;40(3):299–304.
51. Ross MW, Gentile DG, Evans LE. Transoral axial division, under endoscopic guidance, for correction of epiglottic entrapment in horses. J Am Vet Med Assoc 1993; 203(3):416–20.

52. Tulleners EP. Transendoscopic contact neodymium: yttrium aluminum garnet laser correction of epiglottic entrapment in standing horses. J Am Vet Med Assoc 1990;196(12):1971–80.
53. Lumsden JM, Stick JA, Caron JP, et al. Surgical treatment for epiglottic entrapment in horses: 51 cases (1981–1992). J Am Vet Med Assoc 1994;205(5):729–35.
54. Aitken MR, Parente EJ. Epiglottic abnormalities in mature nonracehorses: 23 cases (1990-2009). J Am Vet Med Assoc 2011;238(12):1634–8.
55. Greet TR. Experiences in treatment of epiglottal entrapment using a hook knife per nasum. Equine Vet J 1995;27(2):122–6.
56. Perkins JD, Hughes TK, Brain B. Endoscope-guided, transoral axial division of an entrapping epiglottic fold in fifteen standing horses. Vet Surg 2007;36(8):800–3.
57. Russell T, Wainscott M. Treatment in the field of 27 horses with epiglottic entrapment. Vet Rec 2007;161(6):187–9.

Update on *Streptococcus equi* subsp *equi* Infections

Martha Mallicote, DVM

KEYWORDS

- Lymphadenopathy • Guttural pouch • Empyema • Strangles
- *Streptococcus equi* subsp *equi*

KEY POINTS

- The classic form of strangles includes fever and lymphadenopathy that develop within 3 to 14 days of initial exposure. Less common complications include metastatic abscesses, purpura hemorrhagica (PH), myositis, and other immune-mediated conditions.
- Samples (purulent debris or nasopharyngeal wash samples) should be submitted for both routine culture and polymerase chain reaction (PCR) testing to provide the highest diagnostic sensitivity.
- Chronically infected horses, with no outward clinical signs, are a likely source of new strangles outbreaks. Identification of these horses requires screening with upper airway endoscopy.
- Application of good biosecurity measures is integral to the successful resolution of a strangles outbreak.

PATHOGENESIS AND EPIDEMIOLOGY

The clinical syndrome referred to as strangles is caused by infection with *Streptococcus equi* subsp *equi*, a β-hemolytic, Lancefield group C *Streptococcus*. Unlike other *Streptococcus* sp (and particularly *S equi* subsp *zooepidemicus*), this grampositive agent is not considered a normal commensal in the equine respiratory tract and is generally associated with disease.

Several microbiologic traits of *S equi* subsp *equi* contribute to its pathogenicity. Unlike many other β-hemolytic *Streptococcus* sp, *S equi* subsp *equi* is able to evade phagocytosis. This avoidance is specifically associated with a hyaluronic acid capsule and SeM surface protein.[1,2] Several cell surface antigens are also thought to contribute to virulence and can assist with serologic diagnosis. Significant experimental efforts have been directed toward leveraging these various cell surface antigens for better diagnostic testing.

The author has nothing to disclose.
Large Animal Clinical Science, College of Veterinary Medicine, University of Florida, PO Box 100136, Gainesville, FL 32610, USA
E-mail address: mallicotem@ufl.edu

Vet Clin Equine 31 (2015) 27–41
http://dx.doi.org/10.1016/j.cveq.2014.11.003
0749-0739/15/$ – see front matter © 2015 Elsevier Inc. All rights reserved.

Successful infection begins with bacterial entry to the oral or nasal passage of the horse. Bacteria access pharyngeal tonsillar tissue and directly colonize deeper tissue via this location. Bacterial cell surface antigens mediate the entry of bacteria into tonsillar epithelial cells. Within a few hours of initial colonization, S equi subsp equi is no longer evident on the epithelial tissue but can be found within subepithelial cells and the lymph nodes responsible for draining the pharyngeal region.[3]

Bacterial arrival into the local lymph nodes stimulates an influx of neutrophils, but because of evasion of phagocytosis these cells are generally unable to prevent bacterial multiplication and colonization of the node. These accumulated neutrophils eventually contribute to the typical lymph node abscesses seen with the disease. Streptolysin S and streptokinase also seem to contribute to cell membrane damage and the ultimate formation of abscesses.[4] Although uncommon, distant or metastatic infection and abscessation can occur after lymphatic or hematogenous spread.

The time delay between exposure and initial colonization of local lymph nodes is short. Fever develops within 3 to 14 days of exposure. Bacteremia has been demonstrated for 6 to 12 days after experimental infection with a virulent strain.[5] After the onset of fever, nasal shedding can be expected within 2 to 3 days and typically persists for 2 to 3 weeks. Shedding can continue beyond this point, particularly in animals that develop an infection of the guttural pouch (GP).

Although relatively few organisms are present at the time of initial colonization, there is evidence of substantial bacterial propagation by the time of onset of fever. Abscessation and subsequent rupture of the abscesses allows for easy contamination of the environment and infection of other horses.

CLINICAL SYNDROME

The classic signs of strangles include fever and lymphadenopathy, which develop within 3 to 14 days of initial exposure to disease. Submandibular and retropharyngeal lymph nodes are most frequently affected, but any node in the head and neck is theoretically susceptible. Periorbital swellings are reported, and involvement of the lymph nodes at the thoracic inlet may result in substantial and dangerous restriction of tracheal airflow. Lymphadenopathy progresses to abscesses that, if allowed to mature, generally rupture and drain a tenacious purulent material. Depending on the direction of rupture (retropharyngeal lymph nodes can drain into the GP or pharynx) purulent material may drain via the nasal passages or directly externally. Retropharyngeal lymph nodes that drain into the GP may also establish a chronic empyema. Ocular discharge may also be present. The occasional horse develops such significant lymphadenopathy that pharyngeal or tracheal airflow is restricted.

Fever typically occurs before maturation and rupture of abscesses and resolves after the establishment of drainage. Some horses become depressed and inappetant at the initial stage of infection; this is most likely because of fever, but dysphagia can also occur. Cough is occasionally present and may be worsened by secondary pharyngitis or laryngitis.

Routine blood testing is not required for straightforward cases of strangles. Complete blood cell count typically reveals a hyperfibrinogenemia and mature neutrophilia.[6] Blood chemistry is generally unremarkable.

Complications

Most strangles cases progress as described above and resolve within several weeks after rupture of the abscessed lymph nodes. However, various sequelae can occur including establishment of chronic carriers, metastatic abscessation, and immuno-logic complications.

A subset of horses with simple strangles infections are chronically infected and may become intermittent shedders of S equi subsp equi. These shedders most likely serve as the source of infection in outbreaks that occur in a closed herd. During the first 4 to 6 weeks after acute infection, some horses continue to shed organisms simply because of delayed clearance. A smaller subset becomes true chronic, long-term shedders (as many of 10% of affected horses in an outbreak). By far, the most common location for this chronic infection is within the GP. Retropharyngeal lymph nodes often drain into the GP, and this material may form a GP empyema. If the purulent debris is allowed to remain in the pouch, it forms inspissated purulent material termed chondroids. Both empyema and chondroids act as chronic sources of S equi subsp equi that can be shed into the environment. Unfortunately, many horses with chronic infection localized within the GP are outwardly normal, with no evidence of nasal drainage or fever. Identification and treatment of horses with insidious GP infection is important to successful control of outbreaks.[7–9]

Metastatic Infections

Commonly referred to as bastard strangles, these infections occur in sites remote to the usual head and neck involvement of S equi subsp equi infection. Spread is most likely via hematogenous or lymphatic routes, although local invasion is also possible. Infection of the lymph nodes within the cranial mediastinum or thoracic inlet can result in serious complications related to tracheal impingement and respiratory distress. Intrathoracic abscesses can be seen as the sole infection or in conjunction with pneumonia. Bronchopneumonia is also a possible form of metastatic disease.[10] Metastatic abscesses can form within the abdominal cavity resulting in a presenting complaint of colic or weight loss, with or without a recent history of respiratory infection. In a report of 5 horses treated surgically for abdominal abscesses greater than 15 cm in diameter, 4 cases had a history of strangles outbreak involvement within the past 3 months, while the fifth horse had no such history for at least the prior year.[11] Intra-abdominal abscesses can be found associated with abdominal lymph nodes or organs, including the liver, kidneys, and spleen.[12,13]

Theoretically, abscesses can form at any lymph node site, and individual reports can be found of unique metastatic locations that are attributed to invasion of a regional lymph node.[14] Other rarely reported infections include meningitis, myocarditis, endocarditis, panophthalmitis, keratitis, funiculitis, and septic arthritis.[15–19]

There is anecdotal suggestion that the use of antimicrobial therapy early in the course of an uncomplicated strangles infection predisposes to the development of metastatic abscesses and other complications. This is suggested to occur because of decreased stimulation of cell-mediated immunity, secondary to decreased bacterial protein synthesis. Despite the frequent suggestion that antimicrobials are contraindicated, there are no substantial experimental or case-based data to support the assertion. In fact, outbreaks have been reported in the literature with substantial frequency of complications and no use of antimicrobials among the cases.[7,10,18]

Immunologic Complications

The most frequent type of immunologic complication is PH, an immune-mediated type III hypersensitivity reaction that results in vasculitis. Like all type III hypersensitivities, vasculitis occurs secondary to deposition of immune complexes within the vascular intima and results in substantial ventral edema and necrosis. This manifestation is most frequently seen 3 to 4 weeks after strangles infection or after administration of strangles vaccine. Animals that are already hypersensitized to *S equi* subsp *equi* surface antigens are at increased risk of developing purpura, as identified by SeM titers greater than 1:1600.[4] It has been suggested that increased IgA antibodies are specifically related to purpura severity and that IgG antibodies may have a protective effect.[20,21] Although *S equi* infection is among the more common causes of PH, there are other possible bacterial, viral, and neoplastic causes.

The hallmark sign of purpura is substantial subcutaneous pitting edema, frequently including the distal limbs, ventral part of the head/neck, and ventral midline. Skin necrosis and sloughing may occur, often in the most edematous areas. Petechial and ecchymotic hemorrhages are present on many mucosal surfaces, and non-affected mucosal areas may seem hyperemic. Vasculitis and subsequent edema may also occur on interior surfaces, including the gastrointestinal tract and lungs, and any routine clinical sign of vasculitis can be seen as part of the purpura complex.

Immune complex deposition on specific tissue surfaces can also result in local inflammatory effects. Myositis is a relatively rare localized immunologic complication that presents as various syndromes. Acute rhabdomyolysis is reported primarily in Quarter horses less than 7 years old.[22] Most reported cases became recumbent soon after development of clinical signs and were subsequently euthanized, with findings of severe muscle necrosis on postmortem examination. An association with exotoxin and a toxic shock-like syndrome has been suggested for these cases.[22,23] Focal muscle infarction is also reported secondary to classic PH.[22] Affected horses present for muscle stiffness or colic. Subsequent examination typically reveals focal areas of apparent rhabdomyolysis and generally other clinical signs consistent with systemic inflammation and purpura.[23] This form of myositis is also associated with a high fatality rate. Finally, an immune-mediated polymyositis syndrome is reported secondary to several causes, including *S equi* infection. Quarter horses were overrepresented in the population of affected horses, and cases were primarily younger than 8 years or older than 17 years.[24] Presenting signs varied but typically included rapid muscle atrophy and depression. Histopathologic evaluation of muscle tissue revealed widespread lymphocytic inflammatory infiltrate, with marked change most evident in atrophied muscle samples. Additional work exploring all the various forms of strep-associated myositis is ongoing because these forms of disease have received more attention. Immunologically mediated glomerulonephritis and myocarditis are also theoretically possible with streptococcal antigen in patients of many species and thus may be seen with *S equi* subsp *equi* infection.

DIAGNOSIS

Significant work has been completed over the past several years focused on sensitive and accurate diagnosis of clinical *S equi* subsp *equi* infection. This effort is in part due to additional attention paid to identification and isolation of nonclinical shedders as a means of controlling disease.[7,25] Classic diagnosis has relied on culture of various samples, ideally purulent discharge collected from an abscess. This methodology relies on adequate infectious material being present to flourish in culture media. Furthermore, for samples collected from the upper respiratory tract, *S equi* subsp *equi* must outcompete other normal respiratory flora in order to be readily identified in culture. While still cited by some as the gold standard of diagnosis, culture results must be carefully interpreted, especially when used to screen samples collected from the upper respiratory tract. PCR testing has more recently become important for the diagnosis of strangles, particularly for inapparent shedders and horses without the usual external lymphadenopathy. The inherent issues of PCR testing are still present; even dead bacteria are positively identified by PCR testing, so a recently recovered horse may be yield positive result with this test. Nonetheless, PCR is sensitive and key for identification of infected animals.[26–28] Serologic testing is also available and useful for a few specific subsets of affected horses. Unfortunately, serology is not adequate for diagnosis of routine cases or inapparent shedders in the equine population.[29]

The most typical presentation is for evaluation of a horse with submandibular or retropharyngeal lymphadenopathy and/or purulent nasal discharge. If temperature has been monitored, there will commonly be a history of fever. Physical examination is generally unremarkable beyond the lymphadenopathy. Multiple lymph nodes may be involved, and the abscesses can become quite substantial in size (over 10 cm in some cases) before rupture. Complications seen secondary to large lymph nodes can include occlusion of the airway or esophagus, yielding respiratory distress or difficulty in swallowing. Infections of the GPs can result in inflammation and subsequent deficits of local cranial nerve function, but this clinical presentation is fairly rare. Moderate fevers are typically present until rupture of the abscessed lymph nodes, but this finding is variable. Mucous membranes may seem slightly injected. Careful thoracic auscultation is indicated, because secondary *S equi* subsp *equi* pneumonia is also a reported complication. In cases with purulent nasal discharge and no outward lymphadenopathy, endoscopy of the upper airway is indicated and may reveal enlarged/abscessed nodes that have expanded into the floor of the GP instead of an externally visible location (**Figs. 1–4** for endoscopic images of GP infections).

In the acute clinical case, samples for testing should be collected from the specific site of infection. This typically would be an abscessed lymph node or material from the GP (in cases of empyema). If purulent debris is present, it should be collected for submission via GP lavage, percutaneous lymph node puncture with a large-gauge needle, or direct collection of accessible debris. Ideally, samples should be submitted for both routine culture and PCR testing. Many laboratories that perform PCR testing routinely complete both these tests on all submitted samples. If finances dictate the submission of only one diagnostic test, PCR testing provides the most sensitive result and can allow the practitioner to more accurately rule out *S equi*.[26,27]

The management of outbreak situations often requires the evaluation and testing of many horses that may be in various stages of infection. Separation of potential cases based on the presence or absence of fever and lymphadenopathy is recommended. Further division may be made in animals with no clinical signs, based on potential

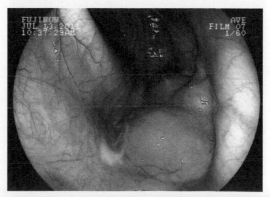

Fig. 1. Retropharyngeal lymphadenopathy impinging into the guttural pouch floor in acute strangles case. The horse had no outward evidence of lymphadenopathy.

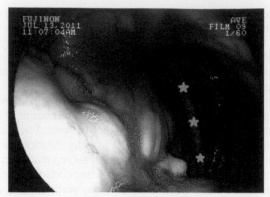

Fig. 2. Profound lymphadenopathy, with small amount of purulent debris, filling the entire medial guttural pouch. For perspective, the stylohyoid bone is starred. The 2-year-old horse had nasal discharge and minimal palpable submandibular lymphadenopathy.

for exposure to clinical cases. Starting with animals that have no clinical signs and minimal possible exposure, all horses on the farm can be evaluated and tested, working from least to most likely infected animals. Physical examination should focus on the common clinical signs and presence or absence of a fever, but typically diagnostic testing is also used to assist in identifying infected horses and managing the outbreak.

Various sampling methods have been critically evaluated in routine outbreaks and have indicated that nasopharyngeal or GP lavage samples (as opposed to nasal swab) are the most sensitive means of testing horses.[4,26] Again, samples should be submitted for both PCR testing and culture. Nasopharyngeal lavage is straightforward to perform and easy to do in a farm setting. A uterine insemination pipette, 5F 22-in polypropylene catheter, or red rubber catheter can be used to lavage 120 mL of sterile saline into the nasopharynx. The lavage fluid is then collected as it exits the nares (a clean plastic bag or plastic boot should be used for collection and the fluid should be transferred into a submission cup). Alternatively, the GP can be examined and sampled with endoscopy or blindly sampled using a Chambers catheter. When performing serial examinations and sample collections on several horses, it is of utmost

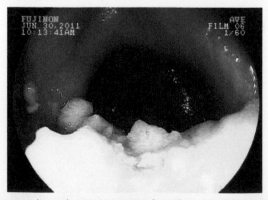

Fig. 3. Significant guttural pouch empyema seen in a chronic strangles case. Purulent debris fills the pouch to the extent that the stylohyoid bone cannot be seen, and the endoscope is held at the absolute outer opening of the pouch.

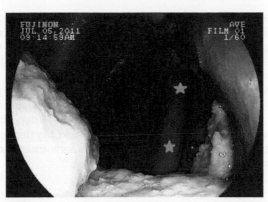

Fig. 4. Reevalution of the case seen in **Fig. 3**, after 5 days of guttural pouch lavage. Some normal anatomic structures are visible (stylohyoid bone is starred), but the pouch is still quite full of debris. The infection was resolved with 5 additional days of medical treatment.

importance that all equipment be disinfected between animals, examination gloves be worn, and attention be paid to avoiding cross-contamination. This effort yields the most useful diagnostic results.

Diagnostics: Disease Complications

Complications of strangles infection can be broadly divided into direct and immunologic effects. In cases of direct complications of infection, horses often have a recent or ongoing case of strangles and subsequently develop additional problems. Many of these horses already have a diagnosis of *S equi* subsp *equi* infection, but require investigation to clarify the extent of their secondary issue. Identification of metastatic abscesses typically relies on diagnostic imaging (radiography, ultrasonography, or both) to determine the extent of infection. Direct sampling of the abscess is frequently feasible, and samples obtained can be tested with PCR and culture analogous to testing for routine infections. In addition, serology can assist in diagnosing cases that are more chronic in nature. SeM titers greater than 1:12,800 are most associated with metastatic strangles infection, and values of 1:3200 to 1:6400 are found with recent infection and recovery.[4,30]

A subset of affected horses become persistent shedders of *S equi* after resolution of their primary disease. The infectious material is typically found within the GP, although it is also rarely reported to occur in the sinuses.[25] For this reason, it is of utmost importance to confirm the clearance of infection before returning cases to normal management. Although there is no single validated screening method for persistent shedders, research suggests that samples collected from washing the GPs and/or the pharyngeal area of the upper airway are the most sensitive. These samples should be tested by both PCR and culture.[26,27] Visual inspection of the GP via endoscopy is an excellent means to further ensure that chronic cases are identified. The combination of endoscopy and pharyngeal sample collection have been used successfully in outbreak investigations as a means of finding the outbreak's index case or chronic shedder.[9] Investigators have examined the use of serology to identify chronic shedders of *S equi* subsp *equi*, but results do not support adequate sensitivity and specificity for this method to be used as a screening tool.[29]

Immunologic complications, including PH and myositis, occur separately from the original strangles infection and generally are not associated with shedding of *S equi* subsp *equi* or classic clinical signs of infection. Complete blood cell count of PH cases yields leukocytosis, mature neutrophilia, mild anemia, and increased fibrinogen levels.[31,32] Serologic testing assists to confirm purpura, with cases having SeM titers of greater than 1:12,800.[4] Ideally, confirmation of PH also requires a full-thickness skin biopsy, revealing a leucocytoclastic vasculitis.[32]

Conversely, SeM titers do not reliably increase in association with myositis cases.[22] Myositis and myolysis is typically responsible for increased muscle enzymes seen on biochemistry and possibly azotemia secondary to pigment nephropathy. For acute rhabdomyolysis, levels of muscle enzymes and evidence of systemic disease become profoundly increased. Horses suspected of having immune-mediated myositis should also undergo biopsy of epaxial and/or gluteal muscles.[22]

TREATMENT

Treatment of the vast majority of strangles cases is straightforward and primarily focused toward helping horses to resolve the infection on their own.

When managing an outbreak situation, it has been suggested that immediate treatment with antimicrobials at the first evidence of fever (and before the development of lymphadenopathy) prevents lymph node abscesses from developing. This tactic has been used successfully to slow outbreaks and decrease morbidity. It is important to remember that horses treated as such do not develop protective immunity from the infection and remain very susceptible should they be reexposed to the infection.

Uncomplicated cases of strangles primarily require good nursing care to speed resolution. The combination of fever and lymphadenopathy often results in anorexia. Treating with nonsteroidal antiinflammatories, such as phenylbutazone or flunixin meglumine, helps in addressing this issue and boost appetite. In addition, soft, palatable foods and easily accessible water should be offered. Encouraging the development and maturation of any abscesses present speeds resolution. Hot packing and topical application of a drawing or softening agent (eg, ichthammol ointment) have been recommended. Occasional abscesses are not adequately mature and rupture, thus requiring surgical intervention. It is important to still wait until the abscess is sufficiently mature and soft so that the drainage established is successful. After drainage has commenced, daily lavage of the abscess with dilute povidone iodine solution should be instituted.

Horses that develop respiratory distress because of the severity of lymphadenopathy may require placement of a temporary tracheostomy. Rarely, severe cases may also require intravenous fluids or nasogastric feedings to provide additional support. It is generally recommended that cases with lymphadenopathy of this severity should also be treated with antimicrobials.

As discussed previously, there is substantial contention regarding the use of antimicrobial therapy in clinical cases of strangles. Cases in which they are indicated include horses with internal abscesses, pneumonia, young foals with profound lymphadenopathy, and myositis.

When required, the overwhelming antimicrobial of choice for *S equi* subsp *equi* is penicillin. Reasonable alternatives based on sensitivity data may include cephalosporins or macrolides (where age appropriate). Although sensitivity patterns may suggest in vitro success with trimethoprim sulfadiazine, there is often in vivo resistance to the medication in equine streptococcal isolates. Local application of penicillin gel compounds is also used in efforts to clear the GP of chronically infected cases, although there is minimal evidence to confirm the efficacy of this therapy.[8,33]

Metastatic abscessation typically requires a combination of long-term antimicrobial therapy and local drainage/lavage when feasible. The occasional metastatic site may be amenable to surgical debridement or removal of the abscess in toto.

PH is primarily treated with antiinflammatory doses of corticosteroids. The typical choice is dexamethasone (at an initial dose of 0.1 mg/kg every 24 h), given as a tapering course of medication. Supportive care is required for many of these horses, with fluid therapy and ensuring adequate feed intake being important components. In cases with active infection or risk of secondary infections, antimicrobial treatment with penicillin is also appropriate.[31]

The acute forms of strangles-associated myopathy require aggressive treatment with corticosteroids, antimicrobials, and vascular support. Even with early intervention, many of these cases do not respond to treatment. The more subacute myositis syndrome that results in muscle atrophy also requires treatment with tapering antiinflammatory doses of corticosteroids. Antimicrobials are indicated if there is evidence of active infection. These horses are typically systemically stable and do not require the same extent of systemic care.[12,22] Recurrence is reported in some cases and requires additional courses of corticosteroid treatment.[22,24]

There are various approaches to disease localized to the GP. Treatment selection depends on the type of infection found (empyema vs chondroids) and the extent of involvement. Although there is some evidence-based data to guide treatment selection, anecdotal experiences are often used by clinicians to guide therapy.[8,33] Simple empyema, particularly when the diseases is localized to less than one-third to one-half of the GP in volume, often responds to repeated GP lavage. Cases with a few chondroids present can be further addressed with endoscopic snare for retrieval, in combination with lavage.[12,33] These procedures require the use of an endoscope and/or Chambers catheter to access the GP for repeated instillations of saline solution. The patient should be sedated, so that all lavage fluid drains away from the pharynx. Saline lavage fluid is instilled via gravity flow tubing or with a pressure bag or arthroscopic pump device to allow faster delivery. When using high-pressure delivery devices, lavage under endoscopic guidance helps to avoid complications associated with rupture of the GP or aspiration of the lavage fluid. Some clinicians have applied 20% acetylcysteine solution to the purulent material, attempting to speed clearance of the empyema from the GP, but this preparation can be irritating to mucosa and should be used with caution. After removal of GP empyema and chondroids, topical application of penicillin gel may speed resolution of the bacterial infection.[4,8,33]

An alternative approach to emptying the GP is surgical removal via a modified Whitehouse approach. A surgical approach is ideal in cases in which nonsurgical removal has failed or is expected to fail (because of the amount of chondroids or empyema present).[33] Surgery can be performed under standing sedation or under general anesthesia. There are several benefits specific to the standing approach: contamination of the surgical suite and the risks of general anesthesia can be avoided.[8,34] However, there are risks involved in the surgical approach, regardless of whether it is performed under sedation or under general anesthesia, because of the large and sensitive neurovascular structures found in the GP.[35,36]

PREVENTION

Most horses develop a durable immunity to disease for around 5 years after recovery. This immunity can be measured indirectly by evaluation of SeM titers with a proprietary enzyme-linked immunosorbent assay assay. Titers greater than 1:1600 are considered high enough such that vaccination may trigger immunologic reactions and likely reflect adequate immunity to disease.[4,30]

Vaccination

At this time, development of a truly protective vaccine for strangles is considered feasible but has not been fully achieved with the available products. There is significant research in this arena, and some characteristics of the routine microbe-host interaction suggest that vaccination can be successful.[37] In the interim, vaccines are available, but none can be considered fully protective against disease. It is essential to avoid vaccination of horses with clinical signs of strangles or recent exposure to the disease. Vaccination in the face of an outbreak does not reduce severity, and the proximity to exposure increases the risk of immunologic complications. In addition, horses that have recently recovered from clinical infection are likely to have a high, protective titer and can develop immunologic complications to vaccination. In situations in which there is a history of strangles infection, SeM titers should be measured before vaccinating recovered horses. Previous recommendations suggested administration of vaccine with a titer less than 1:1600, but more recent data suggest that this cut-point may be too low. Additional research is required to better guide practitioners regarding vaccination.[4,30]

Extract Vaccines

The currently available bacterial extract vaccine in the United States is Strepvax II. This vaccine contains purified M protein antigen extracted from *S equi* subsp *equi*. This vaccine is administered intramuscularly. There are reports of vaccine site abscess formation at a higher rate than for other vaccines. The primary vaccine series in a naive horse is 2 to 3 doses given 2 weeks apart, followed by an annual booster. Pregnant mares can be vaccinated 1 month before foaling to yield colostral immunity to *S equi* subsp *equi*. Available research suggests that this category of vaccine can reduce the amount and severity of clinical cases, but is not able to completely prevent cases from occurring.[38]

Modified Live Vaccine

The modified live vaccine is administered intranasally to result in contact with the pharyngeal and lingual tonsilar tissue, designed to elicit local mucosal and innate immunity.[39] As with all modified live products, it should only be administered to healthy, afebrile animals and never during an outbreak of strangles. The product available in the United States is Pinnacle I.N. Primary vaccination series for this product is 2 doses, given 2 to 3 weeks apart. Revaccination should be on an annual basis. Reported complications of vaccination include abscesses, fever, depression, and PH.[40] Young horses also seem more susceptible to potentially serious side effects of vaccination.[41]

There are no data available regarding colostral antibody production after intranasal vaccination. In addition, the immune response to *S equi* subsp *equi* in young foals seems primarily mediated by IgGb found in both mucosal secretions and milk, instead of IgA. In Europe, a mucosally administered modified live vaccine has been used with the same goal of eliciting local immunity and with some of the same challenges with complications.[42–44]

Biosecurity

From an infection control perspective, it is important to consider cases with appropriate clinical signs to be strangles until proven otherwise. The most common scenario for a practitioner is to be presented with one or a few horses with lymphadenopathy and/or significant purulent nasal discharge. These presenting signs, especially in conjunction with documented fevers and appropriate history, should suggest to the examining veterinarian that biosecurity precautions are in order. Those horses presenting with appropriate clinical signs should be isolated from the remainder of the equids on their property or farm until diagnostic testing results are available. In addition, all equine movement on and off the farm should be halted.

After confirmation of *S equi* subsp *equi* infection, all infected horses should be isolated into a dirty area until resolution of their infection and confirmation that they are free from shedding. In addition, the remaining horses on the property should be clustered into 2 groups: exposed horses with no clinical signs and unexposed horses. These 2 groups should be isolated from one another. It is important to interview the farm manager to gather relevant historical information and understand the traffic flow and geography of the farm in order to best categorize all horses.

There is often tremendous pressure placed on the veterinarian and farm manager to avoid a lengthy quarantine for strangles infection. Despite this public attention, it is important to follow responsible biosecurity precautions in order to prevent further spread of disease. Halting horse movement off the property is likely to be an unpopular rule, but one that should be strictly enforced. In some states and provinces, strangles is considered a reportable disease and the state veterinarian may assist with enforcement of quarantine.

Practically, each separate isolated group should be housed in different barns or pastures, with no opportunity to contact noses, transmit nasal secretions, or share buckets/troughs/feeders. Equipment and personnel are the most common fomites responsible for spread of infection between horses. If feasible, specific personnel should only care for 1 of the 3 groups of horses, avoiding any contact with the other 2 populations. If crossover of equipment or staff is required, disinfection of tools, shoes, hands, and clothing between areas is essential. Coveralls and shoe covers will help to keep personnel clean. Disinfectant footbaths and handwashing stations should be used at the exit of each population's farm area.

After division into the 3 separate populations, rectal temperatures should be monitored at a minimum of once daily on all horses. Horses that develop a fever can be further removed from their group until infection can be confirmed or ruled out. Subsequent confirmed cases are moved to the infected group. After the institution of appropriate biosecurity precautions, identification of new cases will likely continue for about 2 weeks. Nonetheless, it is prudent to wait a full 3 weeks from the onset of clinical signs in the final case before releasing uninfected horses from quarantine.

Procedures for releasing horses from various quarantine groups should be set by the treating veterinarian at the outset of the outbreak. There is always a cost-benefit decision to set the extent of diagnostic testing that will be required. Ideally, standards are set for clearing each of the 3 groups that were initially created: clinical cases, animals exposed (but no evidence of disease), and unexposed animals. At a minimum, all clinical cases should be free of any signs (ie, fever, discharge, lymphadenopathy) for 3 weeks. In addition, testing between 1 and 3 times to ensure resolution of bacterial shedding is most appropriate. The most conservative approach requires 3 negative test results. If minimal diagnostic testing is used to release animals from quarantine, a longer waiting period after resolution of clinical signs is prudent, because there is recent work suggesting that prolonged shedding is more common than previously thought.[6]

In the other 2 categories (exposed with no signs of disease and unexposed), the standard for exiting quarantine may be lower. For example, remaining free of fever/signs for the 3-week period after resolution of all clinical cases at the farm may be adequate. Additional testing of the animals that were previously exposed (with no signs of disease) should be completed if the budget allows. For all horses being tested to ensure clearance of bacterial shedding, a nasopharyngeal wash sample can be collected. Ideally, the GPs should also be visually inspected and sampled.

In outbreaks with no clear originating source of infection, it can be useful to screen all resident horses to identify chronic shedders using the diagnostic testing described above.[7-9] Although this is a time-consuming and costly process, the peripheral costs of a persistent outbreak scenario may prove to be higher for a busy breeding or training facility.

After resolution of an outbreak, it is important to ensure adequate disinfection of all areas used to house clinical cases. Impervious surfaces amenable to disinfection should all be cleaned of organic debris and disinfected routinely—this includes water and feed containers, tools used to clean stalls, stall walls and floors, halters/leads, and any other items used in the isolated areas. Streptococcus equi subsp equi is not particularly resistant to disinfection, and routine use of dilute bleach or quaternary ammonium compounds is generally adequate. Although some older work cites very long periods of bacterial survival in the environment, a more recent study actually found survival of no more than 3 days on wood, rubber, or metal surfaces.[45] In this study, there was a significant effect of sunlight exposure, with survival of less than 24 hours for all samples in direct sunlight, but no significant effect of rain or surface on microbial survival time. Nonetheless, it is commonly recommended that pastures be left open for 4 weeks after resolution of the outbreak. Careful disinfection and quarantine of dirty areas is important to prevent any immediate recurrence of disease.

REFERENCES

1. Anzai T. In vivo pathogenicity and resistance to phagocytosis of Streptococcus equi strains with different levels of capsule expression. Vet Microbiol 1999; 67(4):277–86. http://dx.doi.org/10.1016/S0378-1135(99)00051-6.
2. Boschwitz JS, Timoney JF. Inhibition of C3 deposition on Streptococcus equi subsp. equi by M protein: a mechanism for survival in equine blood. Infect Immun 1994;62(8):3515–20.
3. Timoney JF, Kumar P. Early pathogenesis of equine Streptococcus equi infection (strangles). Equine Vet J 2008;40(7):637–42. http://dx.doi.org/10.2746/042516408X322120.
4. Sweeney CR, Timoney JF, Newton JR, et al. Streptococcus equi infections in horses: guidelines for treatment, control, and prevention of strangles. J Vet Intern Med 2005;19(1):123–34.
5. Evers WD. Effect of furaltadone on strangles in horses. J Am Vet Med Assoc 1968;152(9):1394–8.
6. Boyle AG. Retrospective analysis of Streptococcus equi subsp equi infections in 108 horses in the field (2005–2012). In: ACVIM Forum Proceedings. Nashville, TN, June 4-7, 2014.
7. Newton JR, Wood JL, Dunn KA, et al. Naturally occurring persistent and asymptomatic infection of the guttural pouches of horses with Streptococcus equi. Vet Rec 1997;140(4):84–90.
8. Verheyen K, Newton JR, Talbot NC, et al. Elimination of guttural pouch infection and inflammation in asymptomatic carriers of Streptococcus equi. Equine Vet J 2010;32(6):527–32. http://dx.doi.org/10.2746/042516400777584703.

9. Newton JR, Verheyen K, Talbot NC, et al. Control of strangles outbreaks by isolation of guttural pouch carriers identified using PCR and culture of *Streptococcus equi*. Equine Vet J 2010;32(6):515–26. http://dx.doi.org/10.2746/042516400777584721.

10. Sweeney CR, Whitlock RH, Meirs DA, et al. Complications associated with *Streptococcus equi* infection on a horse farm. J Am Vet Med Assoc 1987;191(11): 1446–8.

11. Mair TS, Sherlock CE. Surgical drainage and post operative lavage of large abdominal abscesses in six mature horses: drainage of abdominal abscesses. Equine Vet J 2011;43:123–7. http://dx.doi.org/10.1111/j.2042-3306.2011.00405.x.

12. Whelchel DD, Chaffin MK. Sequelae and complications of *Streptococcus equi* subspecies *equi* infections in the horse. Equine Vet Educ 2009;21(3):135–41. http://dx.doi.org/10.2746/095777309X386600.

13. Sweeney CR. Strangles: *Streptococcus equi* infection in horses. Equine Vet Educ 1996;8(6):317–22. http://dx.doi.org/10.1111/j.2042-3292.1996.tb01713.x.

14. Whelchel DD, Arnold CE, Chaffin MK. Subscapular lymph node abscessation as a result of metastatic *Streptococcus equi* subspecies *equi* infection: an atypical presentation of bastard strangles in a mare. Equine Vet Educ 2009;21(3): 131–4. http://dx.doi.org/10.2746/095777309X386619.

15. Finno C, Pusterla N, Aleman M, et al. *Streptococcus equi* meningoencephalo-myelitis in a foal. J Am Vet Med Assoc 2006;229(5):721–4. http://dx.doi.org/10.2460/javma.229.5.721.

16. Kaplan NA, Moore BR. *Streptococcus equi* endocarditis, meningitis and panophthalmitis in a mature horse. Equine Vet Educ 1996;8(6):313–6. http://dx.doi.org/10.1111/j.2042-3292.1996.tb01712.x.

17. Meijer MC, Weeren PR, Rijkenhuizen AB. *Streptococcus equi* in the fetlock joint of a mature horse. Equine Vet Educ 2001;13(2):72–4. http://dx.doi.org/10.1111/j.2042-3292.2001.tb01889.x.

18. Spoormakers TJ, Ensink JM, Goehring LS, et al. Brain abscesses as a metastatic manifestation of strangles: symptomatology and the use of magnetic resonance imaging as a diagnostic aid. Equine Vet J 2003;35(2):146–51.

19. Caniglia CJ, Davis JL, Schott HC, et al. Septic funiculitis caused by *Streptococcus equi* subspecies *equi* infection with associated immune-mediated haemolytic anaemia: septic funiculitis with secondary IMHA. Equine Vet Educ 2014;26(5):227–33. http://dx.doi.org/10.1111/eve.12116.

20. Galan JE, Timoney JF. Immune complexes in purpura hemorrhagica of the horse contain IgA and M antigen of *Streptococcus equi*. J Immunol 1985;135(5): 3134–7.

21. Heath SE, Geor RJ, Tabel H, et al. Unusual patterns of serum antibodies to *Streptococcus equi* in two horses with purpura hemorrhagica. J Vet Intern Med 1991; 5(5):263–7.

22. Valberg SJ. Immune mediated myopathies. In: AAEP Proceedings, San Antonio, TX. vol. 52. 2006. p. 354–8.

23. Sponseller BT, Valberg SJ, Tennent-Brown BS, et al. Severe acute rhabdomyolysis associated with *Streptococcus equi* infection in four horses. J Am Vet Med Assoc 2005;227(11):1800–7. http://dx.doi.org/10.2460/javma.2005.227.1800.

24. Lewis SS, Valberg SJ, Nielsen IL. Suspected immune-mediated myositis in horses. J Vet Intern Med 2007;21(3):495–503. http://dx.doi.org/10.1892/0891-6640(2007)21 [495:SIMIH]2.0.CO;2.

25. Newton JR, Wood JL, Chanter N. Strangles: long term carriage of *Streptococcus equi* in horses. Equine Vet Educ 1997;9(2):98–102. http://dx.doi.org/10.1111/j.2042-3292.1997.tb01285.x.

26. Lindahl S, Båverud V, Egenvall A, et al. Comparison of sampling sites and laboratory diagnostic tests for *S. equi* subsp. *equi* in horses from confirmed strangles outbreaks. J Vet Intern Med 2013;27(3):542–7. http://dx.doi.org/10.1111/jvim.12063.

27. Grønbaek LM, Angen O, Vigre H, et al. Evaluation of a nested PCR test and bacterial culture of swabs from the nasal passages and from abscesses in relation to diagnosis of *Streptococcus equi* infection (strangles). Equine Vet J 2010;38(1):59–63. http://dx.doi.org/10.2746/042516406775374324.

28. Boyle AG, Boston RC, O'Shea K, et al. Optimization of an in vitro assay to detect *Streptococcus equi* subsp. *equi*. Vet Microbiol 2012;159(3–4):406–10. http://dx.doi.org/10.1016/j.vetmic.2012.04.014.

29. Knowles EJ, Mair TS, Butcher N, et al. Use of a novel serological test for exposure to *Streptococcus equi* subspecies equi in hospitalised horses. Vet Rec 2010;166(10):294–7. http://dx.doi.org/10.1136/vr.b4753.

30. Boyle AG, Sweeney CR, Kristula M, et al. Factors associated with likelihood of horses having a high serum *Streptococcus equi* SeM-specific antibody titer. J Am Vet Med Assoc 2009;235(8):973–7. http://dx.doi.org/10.2460/javma.235.8.973.

31. Pusterla N, Watson JL, Affolter VK, et al. Purpura haemorrhagica in 53 horses. Vet Rec 2003;153(4):118–21.

32. Morris DD. Cutaneous vasculitis in horses: 19 cases (1978–1985). J Am Vet Med Assoc 1987;191(4):460–4.

33. Judy CE, Chaffin MK, Cohen ND. Empyema of the guttural pouch (auditory tube diverticulum) in horses: 91 cases (1977–1997). J Am Vet Med Assoc 1999;215(11):1666–70.

34. Perkins JD, Schumacher J, Kelly G, et al. Standing surgical removal of inspissated guttural pouch exudate (chondroids) in ten horses. Vet Surg 2006;35(7):658–62. http://dx.doi.org/10.1111/j.1532-950X.2006.00204.x.

35. Perkins JD, Schumacher J. Complications incurred during treatment of horses for empyema of the guttural pouch. Equine Vet Educ 2007;19(7):356–8. http://dx.doi.org/10.2746/095777307X220443.

36. Freeman DE. Complications of surgery for diseases of the guttural pouch. Vet Clin North Am Equine Pract 2008;24(3):485–97. http://dx.doi.org/10.1016/j.cveq.2008.10.003, vii.

37. Sheoran AS, Sponseller BT, Holmes MA, et al. Serum and mucosal antibody isotype responses to M-like protein (SeM) of *Streptococcus equi* in convalescent and vaccinated horses. Vet Immunol Immunopathol 1997;59(3–4):239–51. http://dx.doi.org/10.1016/S0165-2427(97)00074-3.

38. Hoffman AM, Staempfli HR, Prescott JF, et al. Field evaluation of a commercial M-protein vaccine against *Streptococcus equi* infection in foals. Am J Vet Res 1991;52(4):589–92.

39. Walker JA, Timoney JF. Construction of a stable non-mucoid deletion mutant of the *Streptococcus equi* Pinnacle vaccine strain. Vet Microbiol 2002;89(4):311–21.

40. Al-Ghamdi GM. Characterization of strangles-episodes in horses experiencing post-vaccinal reaction. J Anim Vet Adv 2012;11(19):3600–3. http://dx.doi.org/10.3923/javaa.2012.3600.3603.

41. Borst LB, Patterson SK, Lanka S, et al. Evaluation of a commercially available modified-live *Streptococcus equi* subsp *equi* vaccine in ponies. Am J Vet Res 2011;72(8):1130–8. http://dx.doi.org/10.2460/ajvr.72.8.1130.

42. Jacobs AA, Goovaerts D, Nuijten PJ, et al. Investigations towards an efficacious and safe strangles vaccine: submucosal vaccination with a live attenuated *Streptococcus equi*. Vet Rec 2000;147(20):563–7.

43. Kemp-Symonds J, Kemble T, Waller A. Modified live *Streptococcus equi* ("strangles") vaccination followed by clinically adverse reactions associated with bacterial replication. Equine Vet J 2007;39(3):284–6. http://dx.doi.org/10.2746/042516407X195961.
44. Reinhold B, Venner M. Safety of multiple, submucosal inoculations of a live attenuated strangles vaccine in pregnant mares: safety of inoculations of live strangles vaccine in pregnant mares. Equine Vet Educ 2010;22(1):40–2. http://dx.doi.org/10.2746/095777309X479.
45. Weese JS, Jarlot C, Morley PS. Survival of *Streptococcus equi* on surfaces in an outdoor environment. Can Vet J 2009;50(9):968–70.

Update on Fungal Respiratory Disease in Horses

Allison J. Stewart, BVSc, MS*, Rosemary S. Cuming, BVSc, MANZCVS

KEYWORDS

- Fungus • Horse • Pneumonia • Aspergillosis • Cryptococcosis
- Conidiobolomycosis • Coccidioides • Blastomycosis

KEY POINTS

- Fungal respiratory disease is rare in horses, although more common in certain geographic locations.
- Several fungal organisms are capable of causing respiratory disease in horses. Some are primary pathogens and others cause disease only in immunocompromised hosts.
- Treatment consists of various combinations of surgical debridement, topical and systemic antifungal medications, and supportive care.
- Prognosis is variable and may be influenced by lesion location, fungal organisms involved, treatment options available, and owner finances.

INTRODUCTION

Fungal respiratory disease is a rare, yet potentially life-threatening, occurrence in horses. Fungal infections have been reported to occur at all levels of the respiratory tract in horses but are most commonly observed in the paranasal sinuses, guttural pouches, and lungs. Diagnosis and treatment of fungal respiratory infections pose a challenge for the equine practitioner, and the prognosis for complete resolution of infection is often guarded. This article outlines the causes, clinical signs, diagnostic tests, and treatment options currently available for equine fungal respiratory disease.

ETIOLOGY

Fungi are eukaryotic organisms with a definitive cell wall made up of chitins, glucans, and mannans. Within the fungal cell wall, the plasma membrane contains ergosterol, a

---

J.T. Vaughan Large Animal Teaching Hospital, Department of Clinical Sciences, Auburn University College of Veterinary Medicine, 1500 Wire Road, Auburn, AL 36849, USA
* Corresponding author.
E-mail address: Stewaaj@gmail.com

Vet Clin Equine 31 (2015) 43–62
http://dx.doi.org/10.1016/j.cveq.2014.11.005
0749-0739/15/$ – see front matter © 2015 Elsevier Inc. All rights reserved.

Table 1 Fungal pathogens of the equine respiratory tract	
Primary Pathogenic Fungi	**Opportunistic Pathogenic Fungi**
Blastomyces dermatitidis	*Aspergillus* spp
Histoplasma capsulatum	*Candida* spp
Coccidioides immitis	*Fusarium* spp
Cryptococcus neoformans	*Emmonsia crescens*
Conidiobolus coronatus	*Pneumocystis carinii*

compound frequently targeted by antifungal agents. There are more than 70,000 species of fungi, but only 50 species are known to cause disease in mammals. Pathogenic fungi are divided into 3 groups: multinucleate septate filamentous fungi, nonseptate filamentous fungi, and yeasts. Dimorphic fungi are able to interchange between forms depending on environmental conditions, eg, *Blastomyces dermatitidis*, *Histoplasma capsulatum*, and *Coccioides immitis* exist in yeast form in vertebrate host tissue and in hyphal/mycelial form in vitro.

Fungi are ubiquitous in the equine environment (eg, in hay, soil, and bedding), and fungal infections have been reported in horses of all ages, breeds, and occupations. Fungal respiratory disease is considered rare in horses; however, geographic variability in frequency does exist. Pathogenic fungi can be primary pathogens, capable of infecting immunologically normal horses, or opportunistic pathogens, which are capable of infecting only horses that are immunocompromised, such as those undergoing treatment with corticosteroids or with a concurrent, unrelated disease, eg, colitis or neoplasia (**Table 1**). In most cases of upper respiratory tract fungal disease predisposing causes are not identified. By contrast, fungal pneumonia usually occurs in immunocompromised horses, although on occasion, the normal individual may be affected. Important predisposing factors for fungal pneumonia include qualitative and quantitative granulocyte abnormalities and the presence of devitalized tissue.

Respiratory fungal disease is most frequently acquired via inhalation of the causative organism; however, some cases of fungal pneumonia are thought to arise by penetration of fungi through a compromised gastrointestinal tract or open wound. After inhalation, the causative organisms are able to penetrate into the distal airways and alveoli because of their small sporular diameter. More than 90% of particles in stable air visible under a light microscope are spores of fungi or actinomycetes,[1] and one study showed that the concentration of respirable dust increases 6-fold during normal stable bedding down procedures.[2]

Cryptococcosis

Cryptococcosis is caused by *Cryptococcus neoformans* (var *neoformans* and var *gattii*). There is an epidemiologic relationship between *C neoformans* var *gattii* and the Australian river redgum tree (*Eucalyptus camaldulensis*), and *C neoformans* var *neoformans* has historically been associated with bird (particularly pigeon) excreta.[3] *Cryptococcus* is a ubiquitous, saprophytic, round, basidiomycetous, yeastlike fungus with a large heteropolysaccharide capsule. The capsule is both immunosuppressive and antiphagocytic and forms a clear halo when stained with India ink. This characteristic morphology allows for reliable diagnosis of cryptococcosis via cytology or histology (**Fig. 1**).[4] Serologic testing with latex agglutination to identify cryptococcal capsular antigen is also useful, with resolution of lesions correlated with declining serum titers.[5,6]

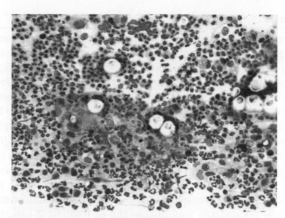

Fig. 1. *Cryptococcus neoformans* organisms with their characteristic wide nonstaining capsule and narrow-based budding obtained from a transtracheal wash specimen from a horse (Modified Wright stain, original magnification ×40). (*Courtesy of* Dr Elizabeth Welles, Auburn University, Auburn, AL.)

Cryptococcosis in horses is associated primarily with pneumonia, rhinitis (**Fig. 2**), meningitis, and abortion. Treatment success was rarely reported until the advent of financially viable and effective antifungal medications. A pony with multiple *C gattii* pulmonary cryptococcomas was treated successfully with amphotericin B for 1 month. One year after cessation of treatment, clinical signs had resolved and the cryptococcal antigen titer decreased from 4096 to 256.[6] Sinonasal cryptococcosis was successfully treated in 2 horses after extensive surgical debridement and long-term treatment with oral fluconazole.[5,7]

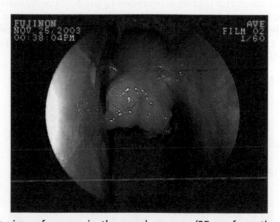

Fig. 2. Endoscopic view of a mass in the nasal passage (25 cm from the nares) in a horse with sinonasal cryptococcal granulomas that was evaluated because of bilateral mucosanguinous nasal discharge, intermittent right-sided epistaxis, and worsening dyspnea of 9 months' duration. (*From* Stewart AJ. Fungal infections of the equine respiratory tract. In: Smith, editor. Large animal internal medicine. 5th edition. Elsevier; 2014. p. 499; with permission.)

Conidiobolomycosis

Conidiobolus coronatus is a saprophytic fungus that causes granulomatous lesions of the nasal passages, trachea, or soft palate in horses. *C coronatus* hyphae are thin walled and highly septate and have irregular branches.[8] The histologic appearance of conidiobolomycosis is similar to that of pythiosis and basidiobolomycosis, and *Conidiobolus* granulomas typically contain large numbers of eosinophils and fewer macrophages, neutrophils, plasma cells, and lymphocytes surrounding the hyphae (**Fig. 3**). Definitive diagnosis is based on microbiological culture, immunodiffusion, or polymerase chain reaction (PCR).[9] Detection of serum antibodies by immunodiffusion is considered highly sensitive and specific and is used to monitor response to treatment.[10–12]

Conidiobolomycosis lesions can be treated with surgical excision, laser or cryotherapy, or long-term administration of iodides or antifungals.[9,10] Amphotericin B has been administered intralesionally or topically in combination with dimethyl sulfoxide,[12–15] and oral fluconazole was successful in treating 2 pregnant mares with nasal conidiobolomycosis[16] and numerous cases by the authors (**Fig. 4**). A vaccine

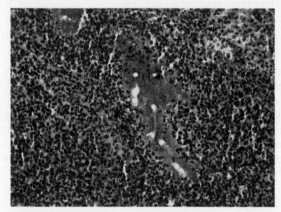

Fig. 3. *Conidiobolus coronatus* hyphae surrounded by predominantly neutrophils and fewer macrophages, eosinophils, plasma cells, and lymphocytes. *C coronatus* has broad, thin-walled hyphae. The hyphae are shown surrounded by acidophilic staining glycoprotein antigen-antibody complexes, known as Splendore-Hoeppli material (hematoxylin-eosin, original magnification ×40).

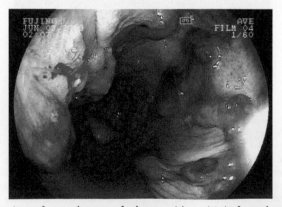

Fig. 4. Endoscopic view of nasopharynx of a horse with multiple fungal granulomas caused by *Conidiobolus coronatus*. The horse presented with bilateral serosanguinous nasal discharge and recovered uneventfully after 3 months of treatment with oral fluconazole.

using *C coronatus* antigen was unsuccessful in treating 7 horses with conidiobolomy-cosis.[9] Fluconazole would be considered the drug of choice for the treatment of con-idiobolomycosis, with treatment lengths varying between 4 and 16 weeks based on endoscopic reevaluation. Long-term therapy and reevaluation are essential as recur-rence can occur.[15]

Pseudallescheriosis

Pseudallescheria boydii is a saprophytic ascomycete. Its hyphae cannot be differen-tiated from *Fusarium* spp or *Aspergillus* spp unless cultured. *P boydii* cultured from the nasal cavity and sinus of a horse with chronic, malodorous nasal discharge was susceptible in vitro to miconazole, ketaconazole, natamycin, and clotrimazole.[17] After debriding and flushing the plaque, miconazole cream was infused twice daily for 4 weeks through lavage tubing that had been passed into the nasal passage through a hole in the sinuses. Adjunctive iodide therapy was also administered and the lesions resolved.[17] Nasal mycosis caused by *P boydii* has been reported in 2 other horses, both of which were euthanized.[18,19] *P boydii* has also been isolated from the pharynx of 2 of 60 normal donkeys and from horses with chronic uterine infection.[20,21]

Aspergillosis

Aspergillus spp are common in the equine environment, especially in moldy feed and bedding.[22] *Aspergillus* spp are opportunistic pathogens and often cause disease in horses that are immunosuppressed from debilitating disease or that have been treated with immunosuppressive drugs.[23–27] They have broad septate hyphae with parallel sides and acute right-angled branching on cytologic or histopathologic examination (**Fig. 5**). Definitive diagnosis of aspergillosis is by culture or staining by immunohisto-chemistry or immunofluorescence.

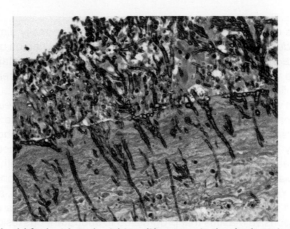

Fig. 5. A 1-month-old foal with *Escherichia coli* bacteremia that had received corticosteroids and developed secondary *Aspergillus* pneumonia. Photomicrograph of the pleural surface of the lung with extensive superficial and deep fungal growth. *Aspergillus* spp characteristically have parallel-sided, regular septate hyphae with acute-angled dichotomous branching (he-matoxylin-eosin, original magnification ×400). (*Courtesy of* Calvin Johnson, DVM, PhD, DACVP, Department of Pathobiology, College of Veterinary Medicine, Auburn University, Auburn, AL; and *From* Stewart AJ. Fungal infections of the equine respiratory tract. In: Smith, editor. Large animal internal medicine. 5th edition. Elsevier; 2014. p. 502; with permission.)

Infection is by inhalation of an overwhelming number of spores resulting in fungal proliferation and invasion of the small airways or by translocation of organisms across an inflamed gastrointestinal tract. Lesions center on large blood vessels, then develop after hematogenous spread. In 2 retrospective studies of invasive pulmonary aspergillosis, 41 of 49 cases were associated with enterocolitis.[23,27] *Aspergillus* spp pneumonia is almost uniformly fatal, often with no or mild respiratory signs, and antemortem diagnosis is made rarely. In a retrospective study of 29 cases of *Aspergillus* spp pneumonia, only 2 cases were diagnosed or suspected antemortem.[27] Transtracheal aspirates or bronchoalveolar lavages may not be helpful because hyphae and spores are often present extracellularly or within macrophages in aspirates and lavages from healthy animals,[23] and false-negative results also can occur. Serologic diagnosis may be useful[28] but is often unreliable because many horses have titers to *Aspergillus* spp. Development of a commercially available enzyme-linked immunosorbent assay (ELISA) is promising.[22,24]

There are limited reports of horses surviving pulmonary aspergillosis, comparable with human medicine, in which 50% to 90% of patients with invasive aspergillosis die despite treatment.[29] Amphotericin B has traditionally been the mainstay of treatment but is associated with nephrotoxicity in about 50% of human patients. Voriconazole, a new azole antifungal, is now considered the drug of choice, whereas caspofungin (in the new class of echinocandin antifungals) shows promising results in patients with refractory infections.[29] Oral voriconazole or itraconazole is currently the treatment of choice in horses. A neonatal foal with pulmonary aspergillosis was successfully treated by lung lobe resection followed by treatment with systemic voriconazole.[30] *Aspergillus* spp are usually resistant to fluconazole.

Treatment of aspergillus rhinitis and sinusitis in horses has been more successful. Oral itraconazole,[31] topical natamycin (flushed via an endoscope or indwelling sinus catheter), nystatin powder (insufflated up the nostril), and topical enilconazole have been curative.[32,33]

Blastomycosis

Blastomycosis is caused by inhalation of conidiae of the thermally dimorphic, saprophytic fungus *B dermatitidis*. *Blastomyces* yeasts can be identified on cytologic examination. They are spherical with a basophilic protoplasm and unstained, uniformly shaped refractile walls; are often seen within multinucleated giant cells; and display characteristic unilateral, broad-based budding.

Blastomycosis was reported to cause pyogranulomatous pleuropneumonia, pulmonary abscessation, peritonitis, and abscesses in a 5-year-old horse. *B dermatitidis* was positively identified from transtracheal wash fluid via a DNA probe, and serology showed strongly positive results. The horse was euthanized without treatment.[34] Disseminated blastomycosis was diagnosed in a miniature horse with subcutaneous infections associated with a chronic pectoral wound, pulmonary consolidation, and pleural effusion. Yeasts were observed histologically in many tissues, and *B dermatitidis* was cultured after 6 weeks.[35] Disseminated blastomycosis was diagnosed in a mare with unresponsive mastitis that progressed to subcutaneous lesions on the ventrum.[36] Treatment with amphotericin B, itraconazole, or fluconazole is recommended.

Histoplasmosis

Histoplasmosis is caused by the saprophytic, dimorphic fungus *H capsulatum*, which is most prevalent in moist soil containing bird or bat waste. Yeast organisms are 2 to 4 μm in diameter, with a thin clear halo surrounding a round or crescent-shaped basophilic cytoplasm. *H capsulatum* may occur in an enteric, pulmonary (**Fig. 6**), or

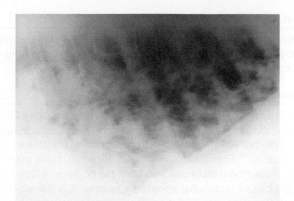

Fig. 6. Disseminated histoplasmosis in an 11-year-old quarter horse stallion that presented for severe weight loss. *Histoplasma* organisms were observed on the peripheral blood smear. Severe respiratory distress developed and thoracic radiographs showed a coalescing alveolar pattern around the hilar region, with air-filled cavitary lesions in the caudodorsal lung fields. The disease progressed rapidly and the stallion was euthanized. (*Courtesy of* Peggy Marsh, DVM, DACVIM, DACVECC, Lexington, KY.)

disseminated form, but horses are considered resistant to infection.[37] *H capsulatum* was identified in pulmonary granulomas in a horse dying of chronic *Yersinia* colitis[38] and has also been associated with severe granulomatous pneumonia in neonatal foals and a yearling and abortions in mares.[39] Successful treatment with amphotericin B was reported in a filly with pulmonary histoplasmosis diagnosed by cytologic identification on smears from a tracheal wash and a lung aspirate.[37] Treatment with amphotericin B or itraconazole is recommended.

Coccidiomycosis

Coccidioides immitis is a soil saprophyte that grows in semiarid areas with sandy, alkaline soils.[40] Inhaled arthroconidia enlarge to form nonbudding spherules, which incite an inflammatory reaction in the lungs and lymph nodes.[41] *C immitis* is difficult to culture, and spherules may not be observed histologically from antemortem lung biopsies; however, serology is useful to diagnose infection, as antibodies are rarely detected in healthy horses.[42] Decreasing titers are associated with clinical improvement,[40,43] and higher titers are associated with a poorer prognosis.[44] Horses with coccidiomycosis may display weight loss, fever, abdominal pain, and signs of respiratory disease or localized, reoccurring nasal granulomas.[41] Diffuse infections, with granulomas in the lungs, liver, kidney, or spleen, have a grave prognosis.[41] Horses with disseminated disease and pneumonia with thoracic effusion usually have severe clinical disease and frequently die.[44] Antifungal agents successful in the treatment of infected horses include itraconazole[45] and fluconazole.[43]

Scopulariopsis

Scopulariopsis pneumonia was diagnosed in a 2-year-old quarter horse filly with pleuropneumonia by culture of bronchoalveolar lavage fluid. The infection was treated successfully with a combination of systemic ketaconazole and aerosolized enilconazole,[46] although newer azole antifungals are likely to be just as efficacious with improved bioavailability.

Adiaspiromycosis

Adiaspiromycotic miliary fungal pneumonia caused by the saprophytic soil mold *Emmonsia crescens* was diagnosed in a horse by percutaneous lung biopsy. Euthanasia was performed without treatment.[47]

Acremonium strictum

A diagnosis of interstitial fungal pneumonia due to *Acremonium strictum* was made based on cytology, culture, and PCR testing of bronchoalveolar lavage fluid in a 10-year-old horse. The horse recovered with supportive treatment, which included 1 month of fluconazole.[48] Fluconazole has been shown to have poor activity against *A strictum* in vitro,[49] and the isolate cultured from the horse was later found to be resistant to fluconazole based on in vitro sensitivity testing. It is therefore uncertain if the fluconazole assisted in disease resolution.[48]

Candidiasis

In human medicine, candidemia is the most common fungal infection diagnosed in patients with burns, patients undergoing complex abdominal surgery, neutropenic patients with malignancies, and patients receiving total parenteral nutrition and long-term corticosteroid therapy.[29] *Candida albicans* is identified in 60% of cases, and the mortality rate is 40% to 75%.[29] Fluconazole is generally considered the drug of choice against *Candida* spp, although *Candida krusei* is resistant to fluconazole. Itraconazole, amphotericin B, caspofungin, or voriconazole are alternative antifungal agents.[29]

Systemic candidiasis was diagnosed and successfully treated in 4 neonatal foals.[50] Two of the foals were treated with intravenous amphotericin B and 2 with oral fluconazole. Each foal had prior sepsis attributable to gram-negative bacteria that had been aggressively treated with numerous antibiotics and parenteral nutrition. *C albicans* was cultured from a transtracheal wash from one of the foals. Three of the foals had *Candida* glossitis and one had panophthalmitis and fungal keratitis.[50] Superficial *Candida* spp infections of the mucous membranes (thrush) can occur in isolation or as part of a systemic infection.[51] Oral candidiasis can be treated by rinsing the mouth either with potassium permanganate (0.025% every 24 hours) or with nystatin (0.3 g in 10 mL water, every 8 hours). Fluconazole is effective against most candida species, otherwise voriconazole or amphotericin B would be recommended.

Pneumocystosis

Pneumocystis carinii has been reclassified from a protozoan to a saprophytic fungus based on the DNA sequence of its 16S-like RNA subunit. It exists as ameboid yeast or as cystic sporangia. *P carinii* cannot be cultured, and diagnosis is based on cytologic identification of characteristic morphologic features using specimens obtained by bronchoalveolar lavage. A fluorescent in situ hybridization method that targets the 18S ribosomal RNA is available to detect *P carinii* in histologic sections.[52] Immunohistochemistry can also be used.[53]

Pneumocystis carinii infection causes diffuse interstitial pneumonia. It is commonly reported in patients with AIDS and people undergoing immunosuppressive therapy after organ transplantation. It has been reported in immunocompromised equine patients,[54,55] such as Arabian foals with severe combined immunodeficiency,[56] and in 1 immunocompetent foal.[53] Trimethoprim-sulfamethozazole (TMS) (25–30 mg/kg by mouth every 12 hours) is the treatment of choice.[57] Dapsone (3 mg/kg by mouth daily for 2 months) was used to successfully treat a foal that developed *Salmonella* enterocolitis after treatment with TMS.[58]

Table 2	
Clinical signs associated with fungal respiratory infections in horses	
Upper Respiratory Tract Disease	**Lower Respiratory Tract Disease**
Unilateral or bilateral nasal discharge (serosanguinous, mucopurulent, epistaxis)	Cough
	Bilateral nasal discharge
Inspiratory or expiratory respiratory noise	Tachypnea
Coughing	Dyspnea
Facial deformation	Respiratory distress
Dyspnea	Hemoptysis
Protuberant granuloma from the nostrils	Lethargy
Dysphagia	Weight loss

PATIENT EVALUATION

Diagnosis of equine fungal respiratory infections can be made based on the history and clinical signs of the patient, diagnostic imaging results and histopathology, cytology, fungal culture, and/or molecular examination of collected tissue or fluid samples.

Clinical Signs

The clinical signs observed on presentation (**Table 2**) depend on the location of the infection within the respiratory tract, its nature, and its chronicity. Mycotic granulomas have been found in the nasal passages, paranasal sinuses, nasopharynx, guttural pouch, trachea, bronchioles, lungs, and mediastinum of infected horses. Mycotic plaques in the guttural pouch are often associated with the arterial blood supply and may progress to cause fatal epistaxis. Pulmonary fungal infections causing granulomas, diffuse pneumonia, or pleuropneumonia can present with signs similar to bacterial infection.

Diagnostic Imaging

Endoscopic examination may allow for direct visualization of fungal plaques or granulomas located in the nasal passages, nasopharynx, paranasal sinuses, guttural pouches (**Fig. 7**), trachea, or bronchioles. An 8- to 20-mm trephine is drilled into the nasal or maxillary sinus through which a sterile rigid arthroscope or flexible endoscope

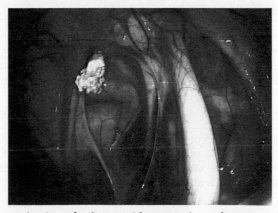

Fig. 7. Endoscopic evaluation of a horse with guttural pouch mycosis that presented for dysphagia and aspiration pneumonia. Medical treatment was attempted via guttural pouch lavage and topical treatment with enilconazole (Imaveral). (*Courtesy of* Marta Barba Recreo, LV, Department of Clinical Sciences, College of Veterinary Medicine, Auburn University, AL.)

is passed to directly view some lesions within the paranasal sinuses. Ultrasound imaging of the thorax in horses with fungal pneumonia or pleuropneumonia may reveal the presence of cavitary lung lesions, comet tail artifacts, lung consolidation, or free pleural fluid. Thoracic radiographs may result in virtually any infiltrative pattern in horses with fungal pneumonia. Although miliary patterns are occasionally seen, the most common initial finding is a patchy bronchopneumonia. Multiple focal sites are common, and lesions tend to be peripheral in distribution. Computed tomography or magnetic resonance imaging provides detailed imaging of the equine skull and is used to determine the extent of lesions and bony invasion.

Sample Collection

For nasal and nasopharyngeal lesions, specimens are obtained by use of an endoscopically guided biopsy instrument; however, these samples tend to be small, superficial, and often nondiagnostic. Larger biopsy samples can often be obtained by use of a uterine biopsy instrument passed nasally with visual guidance from a flexible endoscope. Excisional biopsy or surgical debulking may be performed through a sinus flap or via laryngotomy. Fungal pneumonia may be diagnosed via transtracheal wash, bronchoalveolar lavage, or lung biopsy. Lung biopsy is associated with significant risk if a pulmonary vessel is accidentally biopsied, and postbiopsy ultrasonographic monitoring for hemothorax should be performed. The biopsy should be performed after radiographic evaluation or with concurrent ultrasound guidance and should be obtained from the periphery of the lung. Spring-loaded biopsy needles are safer for lung biopsy compared with Tru-Cut biopsy instruments.[59]

Cytology

Fungal hyphae may be identified in airway fluid or in impression smears obtained from biopsied masses. Clinicians must take care in attributing significance to the presence of fungal elements, free or in large mononuclear cells, in transtracheal aspirate fluid, as they are commonly identified in healthy horses.[60] A study of healthy Thoroughbred racehorses demonstrated the presence of fungal elements in 70% of tracheal aspirates.[61] Barn fungi, such as *Alternaria* spp are nonpathogenic and rarely incite an inflammatory response in the host. These organisms often have a blocklike appearance and should be accompanied by a normal predominance of macrophages, lymphocytes, and nondegenerate neutrophils (<5%–10%).

To be significant cytologically, large numbers of fungi should be visualized. With fungal pneumonia, aspirates may contain predominately neutrophils that often are degenerate and may contain intracellular fungal hyphae. If processing of the sample is delayed, extracellular fungi may be phagocytized, confusing interpretation. Some fungi have characteristic morphologic features that can aid in a presumptive identification (**Table 3**).

Histopathology

Hyphae of certain fungi may be poorly visualized using routine hematoxylin and eosin stains; therefore, special stains such as periodic acid Schiff, Gridley fungus stain, and Grocott-Gomori methenamine silver nitrate are useful to stain histopathologic specimens. With chronicity, there is often evidence of extensive fibrosis.

Microbiologic Culture

Fungal organisms are difficult and slow to grow because of their fastidious growth requirements. Samples should be placed in a prepared culture media and transported at room temperature immediately after sample collection. Culture media such as

Sabouraund dextrose agar, inhibitory mold agar, or mycobiotic containing cyclo-heximide and chloramphenicol may improve the chances of a positive culture. As with cytology, culture results should be interpreted with caution, as 16% of healthy horses are reported to have fungal growth on tracheal aspirate bacterial culture plates.[62]

Molecular Techniques

Serologic tests that use immunodiffusion, radioimmunoassays, complement fixation, and ELISA can detect circulating antibodies against fungal organisms (see **Table 3**). These titers often decrease with diseased resolution; therefore, repeated measure-ments are used to monitor treatment response. Immunohistochemistry,[26,53,63] fluores-cent in situ hybridization,[52] and DNA probes[34] are used to diagnose fungal organisms in histopathology sections. A panfungal real-time PCR assay is used to detect fungal organisms in body fluids and fungal isolates, followed by species-specific real-time PCR to positively identify the organism.[48]

Immune Function Testing

Immunoglobulin quantification of blood by radial immunodiffusion and lymphocyte subpopulation phenotyping via flow cytometry[55,58] should be considered, given the association between immunocompromise and fungal disease in some patients.[54–56]

TREATMENT

Treatment of fungal respiratory disease is challenging in the horse, and in addition, prevention of fungal infections is nigh on impossible because of the ubiquitous nature of fungal spores in the environment. At present, the most important methods of dis-ease prevention are treating predisposing illnesses promptly and effectively and judi-ciously avoiding overuse of corticosteroids and broad-spectrum antimicrobials. Improving ventilation and minimizing exposure to inspired spores are most beneficial for immunocompromised patients.

Treatment of fungal granulomas of the upper respiratory tract typically comprises surgical therapy alone or in combination with medical therapy. Treatment of *Asper-gillus* spp pneumonia is associated with minimal success because of the rarity of early diagnosis and a concurrent severe underlying illness that is commonly present. How-ever, successful therapy has been reported for other causes of fungal pneu-monia.[6,37,43,46,48] Several pharmacokinetic studies on antifungal drugs have been performed,[64–69] and as these medications become more affordable, the success rate of therapy is likely to increase. In addition, fungal susceptibility testing is becoming more readily available, with the minimum inhibitory concentrations (MICs) for common fungal organisms against some antifungal drugs recently determined.[70] The drug of choice depends on the site of infection, the fungus involved, and the finan-cial resources of the owner (**Table 4**). In some cases, therapy may not be attempted because of the severity of the primary disease, expense, or the poor prognosis for dis-ease resolution.

Amphotericin B

Amphotericin B deoxycholate is a polyene antibiotic that combines with ergosterol in the fungal cell membrane to increase cell permeability. Intravenous amphotericin B should be used with caution, as it can cause nephrotoxicity and phlebitis. Other possible side effects include anorexia, anemia, cardiac arrhythmias, hepatic dysfunc-tion, and hypersensitivity reactions.[71] Liposomal amphotericin B has been associated

Table 3
Characteristic morphologic features and availability of serologic tests for fungal organisms reported to cause fungal granulomas in horses

Agent	Cytologic Appearance	Serologic Test	
	Tissue Form	Method	Veterinary Laboratory
Cryptococcus neoformans	Round, thin-walled, yeastlike fungus (5–10 μm) with a large heteropolysaccharide capsule (1–30 μm diameter) that does not take up common cytologic stains. Capsule is best stained using Mayer mucicarmine stain. Organisms show narrow-based budding and lack endospores	Capsular antigen ELISA (antigen) or Latex agglutination (antigen)[6]	$35.00 UT $21.50 CU $21.00 CSU $16.00 UGA $24.00 NMDA $33 MDL
Conidiobolus coronatus	Broad, thin-walled, highly septate, irregularly branched hyphae (5–13 μm in diameter).[8] Often surrounded by acidophilic staining glycoprotein antigen-antibody complex known as Splendore-Hoeppli material	Immunodiffusion is highly sensitive and specific. Decreasing titer correlated to disease resolution in horses[10,11]	Serologic testing not widely available
Pseudallescheria boydii	Hyaline, nonpigmented, septate, randomly branched hyphae (2–5 μm in diameter) with regular hyphal contours. Asexual form has nonbranching conidiophores with terminal conidia. Sexual form has cleistothecium (large round body) and ascospores[17]		
Coccidioides immitis	Spherules have a double-contoured wall, variable in size, can be large (20–80 μm, up to 200 μm). The mature spherules (sporangia) contain endospores (sporangiospores) 2–5 μm in diameter. In the environment, mycelium are thick-walled with barrel-shaped arthroconidia.	AGID (antibody) for IgM and IgG[40,42–44] MVista Quantitative EIA (antigen)	$22.00 UT $17.00 CSU $16.00 CU $17.00 NMDA $50.00 MDL
Aspergillus spp	Broad (2–4 μm diameter) septate hyphae with parallel sides and acute right-angled branching	Platelia Aspergillus galactomannan EIA (sandwich immunoassay) Some reactivity to Penicillium, Alternaria, and Paecilomyces AGID (antibody) A fumigatus only Aspergillus panel	$55.00 MDL $22.00 UT $17.00 CSU $16.00 CU $80.00 UT

Blastomyces dermatitidis	Yeasts are spherical (15–17 μm diameter) with basophilic protoplasm and unstained, uniformly shaped refractile walls. Unilateral, broad-based budding is characteristic. Yeasts are often located within multinucleated giant cells	AGID (antibody)[34] MVista Quantitative EIA (antigen)	$22.00 UT $17.00 CSU $16.00 CU $55.00 MDL
Histoplasma capsulatum	Yeasts (2–4 μm in diameter) have a thin clear halo surrounding a round or crescent-shaped basophilic cytoplasm	AGID (antibody)[39] MVista Quantitative EIA (antigen)	$22.00 UT $17.00 CSU $16.00 CU $55.00 MDL
Acremonium strictum	Mononuclear cells contain single, spherical, intracytoplasmic encapsulated spores 3–5 μm in diameter[48]		
Candida spp	Ovoid budding yeast cells (2–4 μm in diameter) with thin walls, or they can occur in chains that produce septate pseudohyphae when blastospores remain attached after budding division. Filamentous, regular, true hyphae also may be visible		
Pneumocystis carinii	Trophozoite (yeast form) is a 2- to 5-μm-diameter ameboid with filopodia that attach to the surface of type I pneumocytes. Sporangia (cystic form) are encapsulated spores (4–6 μm in diameter) containing 8 uninuclete spores (intracytic bodies)[53–55,81]		
Fungal serology panel	Antibody to *Histoplasma, Blastomyces, Coccidioides, Aspergillus* (AGID) The CU panel also includes *Cryptococcus* antigen		$54.00 CSU $62.75 CU $46.00 NMDA

Abbreviations: Ag (EIA), sandwich enzyme immunoassay; AGID, agar gel immunodiffusion; CF, complement fixation; CSU, Colorado State University. P (970) 297-1281, F (970) 297-0320, http://csu-cvmbs.colostate.edu/vdl/Pages/default.aspx; CU, Cornell University, Animal Health Diagnostic Center. P (607) 253-3900, F (607) 253 3943, http://ahdc.vet.cornell.edu/; ELISA, enzyme-linked immunosorbant assay; MDL, Miravista Diagnostics Laboratory. P (317) 856-2681, F (317)-856-3685, www.miravistalabs.com; NMDA, New Mexico Department of Agriculture Veterinary Diagnostic Services. P (505) 383- 9299, http://www.nmda.nmsu.edu/vds/; UGA, University of Georgia, College of Veterinary Medicine. P (706) 542-5812, F (706) 583-0843, http://www.vet.uga edu/idl/tests; UT, University of Tennessee, College of Veterinary Medicine. P (865) 974-5639 (mycology) or -5643 (serology), http://www.vet.utk.edu/diagnostic/index.php; UTHSCSA, The University of Texas Health Science Center at San Antonio, Center for Medical Mycology. P (210) 567-4131, F (210) 567-4076, http://www.sacmm.org/index.html.

Table 4
Treatment of common fungal infections in humans and horses

Infectious Condition	Recommended Treatment in Humans	Treatments Tried Successfully in Horses	Comments
Cryptococcosis	Amphotericin B: 0.7–1 mg/kg, plus 5-fluorocytosine 100 mg/kg/d Duration: 2 wk, then Fluconazole: 400 mg/d Duration: >10 wk	Amphotericin B: 0.35 mg/kg IV q 24 h, increasing over 8 d to 0.5 mg/kg IV q 24 h Dilute in 1 L 5% dextrose Duration: 1 mo[6] Fluconazole: Single loading dose of 14 mg/kg po followed by 5 mg/kg po q 24 h Duration: 1–8 mo after debulking of sinonasal granulomas[5,7]	Reported dosages range from 0.3 to 0.9 mg/kg in 1 L saline or 5% dextrose given slow IV over 1 h Long-term oral fluconazole is recommended as sole treatment or after 2 wk of IV amphotericin B.
Histoplasmosis	Amphotericin B: 0.7–1.0 mg/kg/d Duration: 2 wk, then Itraconazole: 200–400 mg/d Duration: 4–18 mo	Amphotericin B: 0.3–0.6 mg/kg q 48 h IV Duration: 1 mo; total cumulative dose was 6.75 mg/kg Filly became lethargic for 18–24 h after each treatment. Polyuria and polydipsia occurred in the fourth week, but filly was nonazotemic and had normal urine specific gravity (USGs)[37]	Dilute amphotericin B in 1 L saline or 5% dextrose and give over 1 h In vitro susceptibility to fluconazole is poor
Blastomycosis	Amphotericin B: 0.7–1.0 mg/kg/d to 0.5–2.5 g total, then Itraconazole: 200–400 mg/d		

Aspergillus (invasive pulmonary)	Voriconazole: 200–400 mg po q 12 h or 3–6 mg/kg IV q 12 h Amphotericin B: 1.0–1.5 mg/kg/d Duration: until response, then Itraconazole: 400 mg/d	Voriconazole: 4 mg/kg po q 24 h Duration: 24 d Amphotericin B: Treatment of a neonatal foal with pulmonary aspergillosis after lung lobe resection[30]	Oral itraconazole or voriconazole would be the drugs of choice, alone or after 2 wk of IV amphotericin B Fluconazole has limited efficacy
Candidiasis	Amphotericin B: 0.7–1.0 mg/kg/d or Fluconazole: 6 mg/kg po q 24 h or Caspofungin: 70 mg single loading dose, then 50 mg/d or Voriconazole: 200–400 mg po Duration: 2 wk	Amphotericin B: i. Total dose 2.6 mg/kg IV Duration: 8 d ii. Total dose 10.3 mg/kg IV Duration: 29 d Fluconazole: i. 5.5 mg/kg po q 24 h Duration: 6 wk ii. 4 mg/kg po q 24 h Duration: 4 wk Case series of 4 foals[50]	Fluconazole is generally considered the drug of choice against *Candida* spp, although *C krusei* is resistant to fluconazole
Pneumocystis	Trimethoprim-sulfamethoxazole Pentamidine isethionate Trimetrexate	Trimethoprim-sulfamethoxazole 25–30 mg/kg po q 12 h[57] Dapsone: 3 mg/kg po q 24 h Duration: 2 mo Used in 1 foal that developed enterocolitis after treatment with TMS[58]	Lacks ergosterol, therefore antifungals are not effective

with lower nephrotoxicity in human studies.[72] Amphotericin B has been used success-fully to treat histoplasmosis and pulmonary aspergillosis and cryptococcosis.[6,22,37] A high dose of oral amphotericin B successfully treated mucormycosis caused by *Absidia corymbifera*.[73] Topical amphotericin B has been successful in the treatment of nasopharyngeal *C coronatus*.[12–15]

Azoles

Benzimidazole derivatives in the class azoles destroy fungi by inhibition of ergosterol biosynthesis in the fungal cell membrane. Topical 2% miconazole was used in the res-olution of 4 cases of guttural pouch mycosis[74] and as part of successful multimodal therapy against nasopharyngeal *P boydii*.[17] Enilconazole has been used topically in the successful treatment of guttural pouch mycosis[75–77] and via nebulization for res-olution of *Scopulariopsis* pneumonia.[46] Ketoconazole is absorbed poorly in the nona-cidified form[64] but can be acidified for better absorption (30 mg/kg via nasogastric tube every 12 hours mixed with 0.2 N HCl).[46]

Itraconazole (Sporanox solution) is absorbed well orally. A dose of 5 mg/kg by mouth every 24 hours maintains concentrations more than the MIC for susceptible yeasts (*Histoplasma* spp and *Blastomyces* spp) and *Aspergillus* sp, with no detectable side effects.[66] The use of compounded itraconazole is not recommended because of its poor stability and highly lipophilic nature.

Oral fluconazole, at a loading dose of 14 mg/kg followed by 5 mg/kg every 24 hours, yields concentrations in plasma, cerebrospinal fluid, synovial fluid, aqueous humor, and urine more than the MIC reported for several equine fungal pathogens.[65] Fluconazole, however, reportedly has minimal activity against filamentous fungi (*Aspergillus* spp and *Fusarium* spp). Compounded fluconazole formulations are stable.

Voriconazole, a new broad-spectrum triazole antifungal agent, was approved for use in human medicine in 2002. It is now considered the drug of choice for initial treat-ment of invasive aspergillosis, candidiasis, cryptococcosis, and serious fungal infec-tions caused by *Scedosporium apiospermum* and *Fusarium* spp in patients that are unable to tolerate or are refractory to other therapeutic agents.[78] An initial single-dose pharmacokinetic study in horses recommended a dose of 4 mg/kg by mouth every 24 hours.[67] At this dose, therapeutic concentrations were reached in peritoneal, synovial, and cerebrospinal fluids; aqueous humor; periocular tear film; epithelial lining fluid; and urine.[68,69]

Systemic Iodide Therapy

Iodides have little, if any, direct in vitro antibiotic effects[79]; however, they seem to have a beneficial effect on the granulomatous inflammatory process. Although several successful cases are reported in which iodides were used as primary or adjunctive therapy, overall efficacy is considered limited. Treatment is inexpensive, but toxicity and resistance can occur. Iodide toxicity is characterized by excessive lacrimation, nonproductive cough, increased respiratory secretions, and derma-titis.[79] The recommended dose of 20% sodium iodide is 20 to 40 mg/kg/day intra-venous administration for 7 to 10 days.[10,12,15,80] Orally administered iodine is available in 2 forms. Inorganic potassium iodide (10–40 mg/kg/day) is available only as a chemical grade and is unstable in the presence of light, heat, and exces-sive humidity.[15,80] Organic ethylenediamine dihydriodide (0.86–1.72 mg/kg/day) is commercially available.[80] Administration of iodine to pregnant mares may cause congenital hypothyroidism in foals and should be avoided.

Surgical Intervention

Fungal granulomas of the nasal passages and paranasal sinuses may be resected or debulked surgically via sharp dissection or laser dissection. Guttural pouch mycosis responds well to arterial occlusion of the vessel beneath the fungal plaque. Cryotherapy may be performed on small masses or on surgical margins after excision.

REFERENCES

1. Clarke A. Air hygiene and equine respiratory disease. In Pract 1987;9:196–201.
2. Webster AJ, Clarke AF, Madelin TM, et al. Air hygiene in stables. I. Effects of stable design, ventilation and management on the concentration of respirable dust. Equine Vet J 1987;19:448–53.
3. Riley CB, Bolton JR, Mills JN, et al. Cryptococcus in seven horses. Aust Vet J 1992;69(6):135–9.
4. Jubb KV, Kennedy PC, Palmer N. Pathology of domestic animals. 3rd edition. Orlando (FL): Academic Press; 1985.
5. Stewart AJ, Salazar T, Waldridge BM, et al. Multimodal treatment of recurrent sinonasal cryptococcal granulomas in a horse. J Am Vet Med Assoc 2009;235(6): 723–30.
6. Begg LM, Hughes KJ, Kessell A, et al. Successful treatment of cryptococcal pneumonia in a pony mare. Aust Vet J 2004;82(11):686–92.
7. Cruz VC, Sommardahl CS, Chapman EA, et al. Successful treatment of a sinonasal cryptococcal granuloma in a horse. J Am Vet Med Assoc 2009;234(4): 509–13.
8. Miller RI, Campbell RS. The comparative pathology of equine cutaneous phycomycosis. Vet Pathol 1984;21:325–32.
9. Taintor J, Schumacher J, Newton J. Conidiobolomycosis in horses. Comp Cont Educ Pract 2003;25(11):872–6.
10. Steiger RR, Williams MA. Granulomatous tracheitis caused by *Conidiobolus coronatus* in a horse. J Vet Intern Med 2000;14:311–4.
11. Kaufman L, Mendoza L, Standard PG. Immunodiffusion test for serodiagnosing subcutaneous zygomycosis. J Clin Microbiol 1990;28(9):1887–90.
12. French DD, Haynes PF, Miller RI. Surgical and medical management of rhinophycomycosis (conidiobolomycosis) in a horse. J Am Vet Med Assoc 1985;186:1105–7.
13. McMullan WC, Joyce JR, Hanselka DV, et al. Amphotericin-B for treatment of localized subcutaneous phycomycosis in horses. J Am Vet Med Assoc 1977; 170:1293–8.
14. Hanselka DV. Equine nasal phycomycosis. Vet Med Small Anim Clin 1977;72: 251–3.
15. Zamos DT, Schumacher J, Loy JK. Naspharyngeal conidiobolomycosis in a horse. J Am Vet Med Assoc 1996;208:100–1.
16. Taintor J, Crowe C, Hancock S, et al. Treatment of conidiobolomycosis with fluconazole in two pregnant mares. J Vet Intern Med 2004;18:363–4.
17. Davis PR, Meyer GA, Hanson RR, et al. *Pseudallescheria boydii* infection of the nasal cavity of a horse. J Am Vet Med Assoc 2000;217(5):707–9.
18. Johnson GR, Schiefer B, Pantekoek JF. Maduromycosis in a horse in Western Canada. Can Vet J 1975;16(11):341–4.
19. Brealey JC, McCandlish IA, Sullivan M, et al. Nasal granuloma caused by *Pseudallescheria boydii*. Equine Vet J 1986;18(2):151–2.
20. El-Allawy T, Atria M, Amer M. Mycoflora of the pharyngeotonsillar portions of clinically healthy donkeys in Assuit. Assiut Vet Med J 1977;4:63–9.

21. Carter ME, di Menna ME. Letter: *Petriellidium boydii* from the reproductive tracts of mares. N Z Vet J 1975;23(1–2):13.
22. Guillot J, Sarfati J, de Barros M, et al. Comparative study of serological tests for the diagnosis of equine aspergillosis. Vet Rec 1999;145(12):348–9.
23. Slocombe RF, Slauson DO. Invasive pulmonary aspergillosis of horses: an association with acute enteritis. Vet Pathol 1988;25(4):277–81.
24. Blomme E, Del Piero F, La Perle KM, et al. Aspergillosis in horses: a review. Equine Vet Educ 1998;10(2):86–93.
25. Johnson PJ, Moore LA, Mrad DR, et al. Sudden death of two horses associated with pulmonary aspergillosis. Vet Rec 1999;145:16–20.
26. Tunev SS. Necrotizing mycotic vasculitis with cerebral infarction caused by *Aspergillus niger* in a horse with acute typholocolitis. Vet Pathol 1999;36(4):347–51.
27. Sweeney CR, Habecker PL. Pulmonary aspergillosis in horses: 29 cases (1974-1997). J Am Vet Med Assoc 1999;214:808–11.
28. Moore BR, Reed SM, Kowalski JJ, et al. Aspergillosis granuloma in the mediastinum of a non-immunocompromised horse. Cornell Vet 1993;83(2):97–104.
29. Chandrasekar P. Riches usher dilemmas: antifungal therapy in invasive aspergillosis. Biol Blood Marrow Transplant 2005;11(2):77–84.
30. Hilton H, Galuppo L, Puchalski SM, et al. Successful treatment of invasive pulmonary aspergillosis in a neonatal foal. J Vet Intern Med 2009;23:375–8.
31. Korenek NL, Legendre AM, Andrews FM. Treatment of mycotic rhinitis with itraconazole in three horses. J Vet Intern Med 1994;8:224–7.
32. Kendall A, Brojer J, Karlstam E, et al. Enilconazole treatment of horses with superficial *Aspergillus* spp. rhinitis. J Vet Intern Med 2008;22(5):1239–42.
33. Greet TR. Nasal aspergillosis in 3 horses. Vet Rec 1981;109:487–9.
34. Toribio RE, Kohn CW, Lawrence AE, et al. Thoracic and abdominal blastomycosis in a horse. J Am Vet Med Assoc 1999;214(9):1357–60.
35. Dolente BA, Habecker P, Chope K, et al. Disseminated blastomycosis in a miniature horse. Equine Vet Educ 2003;15(3):139–42.
36. Wilson JH, Olson EJ, Haugen EW, et al. Systemic blastomycosis in a horse. J Vet Diagn Invest 2006;18(6):615–9.
37. Cornick JL. Diagnosis and treatment of pulmonary histoplasmosis in a horse. Cornell Vet 1990;80:97.
38. Katayama Y, Kuwano A, Yoshihara T. Histoplasmosis in the lung of a race horse with yersiniosis. J Vet Med Sci 2001;63(11):1229–31.
39. Rezabek GB, Donahue JM, Giles RC, et al. Histoplasmosis in horses. J Comp Pathol 1993;109:47–55.
40. Ziemer EL, Pappagianis D, Madigan JE, et al. Coccidioidomycosis in horses: 15 cases (1975-1984). J Am Vet Med Assoc 1992;201(6):910–6.
41. Hodgin EC, Conaway H, Ortenburger AI. Recurrence of obstructive nasal coccidiodal granuloma in a horse. J Am Vet Med Assoc 1984;184:339–40.
42. Higgins JC, Leith GS, Voss ED, et al. Seroprevalence of antibodies against *Coccidioides immitis* in healthy horses. J Am Vet Med Assoc 2005;226(11):1888–92.
43. Higgins JC, Leith GS, Pappagianis D, et al. Successful treatment of *Coccidioides immitis* pneumonia with fluconazole in two horses. J Vet Intern Med 2005;19:482–3.
44. Higgins JC, Pusterla N, Pappagianis D. Comparison of *Coccidioides immitis* serological antibody titres between forms of clinical coccidioidomycosis in horses. Vet J 2007;173(1):118–23.
45. Foley JP, Legendre AM. Treatment of coccidioidomycosis osteomyelitis with itraconazole in a horse: a brief report. J Vet Intern Med 1992;6:333.

46. Nappert G, Van Dyck T, Papich M, et al. Successful treatment of a fever associated with consistent pulmonary isolation of *Scopulariopsis* sp. in a mare. Equine Vet J 1996;28(5):421–4.
47. Pusterla N, Pesavento PA, Leutenegger CM, et al. Disseminated pulmonary adiaspiromycosis caused by *Emmonsia crescens* in a horse. Equine Vet J 2002;34(7):749–52.
48. Pusterla N, Holmberg T, Lorenzo-Figueras M, et al. *Acremonium strictum* pulmonary infection in a horse. Vet Clin Pathol 2005;34(4):413–6.
49. Guarro J, Gams W, Pujol I, et al. Acremonium species: new emerging fungal opportunists - in vitro antifungal susceptibilities and review. Clin Infect Dis 1997;25:1222–9.
50. Reilly LK, Palmer JE. Systemic candidiasis in four foals. J Am Vet Med Assoc 1994;205:464–6.
51. McClure JJ, Addison JD, Miller RI. Immunodeficiency manifested by oral candidiasis and bacterial septicemia in foals. J Am Vet Med Assoc 1985; 186:1195–7.
52. Jensen TK, Boye M, Bille-Hansen V. Application of fluorescent in situ hybridization for specific diagnosis of *Pneumocystis carinii* pneumonia in foals and pigs. Vet Pathol 2001;38(3):269–74.
53. Perron Lepage MF. A case of interstitial pneumonia associated with *Pneumocystis carinii* in a foal. Vet Pathol 1999;36(6):621–4.
54. Franklin RP, Long MT, MacNeill A, et al. Proliferative interstitial pneumonia, *Pneumocystis carinii* infection and immunodeficiency in an adult Paso Fino horse. J Vet Intern Med 2002;16:607–11.
55. MacNeill A, Alleman R, Franklin RP, et al. Pneumonia in a Paso Fino mare. Vet Clin Pathol 2003;32(2):73–6.
56. Perryman LE, McGuire TC, Crawford TB. Maintenance of foals with severe combined immunodeficiency: causes and control of secondary infections. Am J Vet Res 1978;39:1043–7.
57. Flaminio MJ, Rush BR, Cox JH, et al. CD4+ and CD8+ T-lymphocytopaenia in a filly with *Pneumocystis carinii* pneumonia. Aust Vet J 1998;76(6):399–402.
58. Clarke-Price SC, Cox JH, Bartoe JT, et al. Use of dapsone in the treatment of *Pneumocystis carinii* pneumonia in a foal. J Am Vet Med Assoc 2004;224(3): 407–10.
59. Venner M, Schmidbauer S, Drommer W, et al. Percutaneous lung biopsy in the horse: comparison of two instruments and repeated biopsy in horses with induced acute interstitial pneumopathy. J Vet Intern Med 2006;20:968–73.
60. Beech J. Cytology of tracheobronchial aspirates in horses. Vet Pathol 1975;12: 157–64.
61. Sweeney CR, Humber KA, Roby KA. Cytologic findings of tracheobronchial aspirates from 66 thoroughbred racehorses. Am J Vet Res 1992;53:1172–5.
62. Sweeney CR, Beech J, Roby KA. Bacterial isolates from tracheal bronchial aspirates from healthy horses. Am J Vet Res 1985;46:2562–5.
63. Thirion-Delalande C, Guillot J, Jensen HE, et al. Disseminated acute concomitant aspergillosis and murcomycosis in a pony. J Vet Med A Physiol Pathol Clin Med 2005;52:121–4.
64. Prades M, Brown MP, Gronwell R, et al. Body fluid and endometrial concentrations of ketoconazole in mares after intravenous injection or repeated gavage. Equine Vet J 1989;21(3):211–4.
65. Latimer FG, Colitz CM, Campbell NB, et al. Pharmacokinetics of fluconazole following intravenous and oral administration and body fluid concentrations of

fluconazole following repeated oral dosing in horses. Am J Vet Res 2001;62(10): 1606–11.

66. Davis JL, Gilger BC, Papich MG. The pharmacokinetics of itraconazole in the horse. J Vet Intern Med 2004;18:458.

67. Davis JL, Salmon JH, Papich MG. Pharmacokinetics of voriconazole after oral and intravenous administration to horses. Am J Vet Res 2006;67(6):1070–5.

68. Colitz CM, Latimer FG, Cheng H, et al. Pharmacokinetics of voriconazole following intravenous and oral administration and body fluid concentrations of voriconazole following repeated oral administration in horses. Am J Vet Res 2007;68(10):1115–21.

69. Passler NH, Chan HM, Stewart AJ, et al. Distribution of voriconazole in seven body fluids of adult horses after repeated oral dosing. J Vet Pharmacol Ther 2010;33(1):35–41.

70. Weiderhold NP. Antifungal susceptibility testing: what does the MIC mean and how do I apply this information? Paper presented at American College of Veterinary Internal Medicine. Nashville (TN), June 2014.

71. Chandna VK, Morris E, Gliatto JM, et al. Localised subcutaneous cryptococcal granuloma in a horse. Equine Vet J 1993;25(2):166–8.

72. Loo AS, Muhsin SA, Walsh TJ. Toxicokinetic and mechanistic basis for the safety and tolerability of liposomal amphotericin B. Expert Opin Drug Saf 2013;12(6): 881–95.

73. Guillot J, Coolobert C, Jensen HE, et al. Two cases of equine mucormycosis caused by *Absidia corymbifera*. Equine Vet J 2000;32(5):453–6.

74. Giraudet AJ. Medical treatment with miconazole in four cases of guttural pouch mycosis. J Vet Intern Med 2005;19:485.

75. Davis EW, Legendre AM. Successful treatment of guttural pouch mycosis with itraconazole and topical enilconazole in a horse. J Vet Intern Med 1994;8:304–5.

76. Vannieuwstadt RA, Kalsbeek HC. Guttural pouch mycosis - local treatment with an indwelling through-the-nose catheter with enilconazole. Tijdschr Diergeneeskd 1994;119:3–5.

77. Carmalt JL, Baptiste KE. Atypical guttural pouch mycosis in three horses. Pferdeheilkunde 2004;20(6):542–8.

78. Jeu L, Piacenti FJ, Lyakhovetskiy AG, et al. Voriconazole. Clin Ther 2003;25: 1321–81.

79. Plumb D. Veterinary drug handbook. 4th edition. Ames (IA): Iowa State University Press; 2002.

80. Scott DW, Miller WH Jr. Fungal skin diseases. In: Equine dermatology, ed 2. St Louis (MO): Saunders-Elsevier; 2003. p. 311–2.

81. Ewing PJ, Cowell RL, Tyler RD, et al. *Pneumocystis carinii* pneumonia in foals. J Am Vet Med Assoc 1994;204(6):929–33.

Update on Disorders and Treatment of the Guttural Pouch

David E. Freeman, MVB, PhD

KEYWORDS

- Guttural pouch • Tympany • Mycosis • Temporohyoid osteoarthropathy
- Ceratohyoidectomy • Arterial occlusion

KEY POINTS

- The most common diseases of the guttural pouch are empyema, tympany, mycosis, and temporohyoid osteoarthropathy.
- The challenge in diagnosis and treatment of the guttural pouch lies in the complex anatomy of the guttural pouch and its close relationship with other important structures in the skull.
- Endoscopy of the guttural pouch interior remains the gold standard for identifying most guttural pouch diseases.
- Surgical approaches to the guttural pouch include hyovertebrotomy, Viborg triangle approach, Whitehouse approach, and modified Whitehouse approach.
- Arterial occlusion for guttural pouch mycosis can be performed with balloon catheters, microcoils, and nitinol plugs.
- Ceratohyoidectomy is the preferred surgical procedure for temporohyoid osteoarthropathy.

The most common diseases of the guttural pouches are empyema, tympany, mycosis, and temporohyoid osteoarthropathy (THO), and updates on these diseases and their treatments are the focus of this review. Related to guttural pouch tympany is a form of nasopharyngeal obstruction in adult horses that also is addressed. A variety of other diseases have been documented, but these are rare and include neoplasia, fractured stylohyoid bone (with or without abscessation), foreign bodies, cysts, and rupture of the ventral straight muscles of the head.

The challenge in diagnosis and treatment of all these diseases lies in the complex anatomy of the guttural pouch, its close relationship with other important structures

Disclosures: None.
Large Animal Clinical Sciences, College of Veterinary Medicine, University of Florida, 2015 SW. 16th Avenue, PO Box 100136, Gainesville, FL 32610, USA
E-mail address: freemand@ufl.edu

Vet Clin Equine 31 (2015) 63–89
http://dx.doi.org/10.1016/j.cveq.2014.11.010
0749-0739/15/$ – see front matter © 2015 Elsevier Inc. All rights reserved.

at the base of the skull, easy confusion with diseases in other sites with similar clinical signs, and difficulty in safe surgical access to the affected structures within or in close contact to the guttural pouch. Improvements in diagnostic methods have considerably facilitated diagnosis, understanding, and treatment of guttural pouch diseases; however, endoscopy of the guttural pouch interior remains the gold standard for identifying most guttural pouch diseases.

MRI can provide useful information about the extent of soft tissue involvement in areas that cannot be examined by endoscopy, especially those deep to the mucosal lining, but is used only in select cases, and high-powered equipment requires general anesthesia. Examples of lesions suitable for MRI include melanomas and other tumors of the lateral compartment and parotid gland (**Fig. 1**). Whereas conventional angiography of the equine head requires surgical exposure of an artery and can be technically challenging, time-of-flight magnetic resonance angiography (TOF-MRA) uses signal intensity changes related to differences in saturation between tissues that are flowing and stationary, and does not require contrast agents (**Fig. 2**).[1] This technique can demonstrate all major intracranial vessels to approximately 2 mm in diameter so that third to fourth branches of ramification can be identified.[1] By contrast, veins have lower signal intensity, so the arteries are more visible. This method can be used to demonstrate a defect caused by guttural pouch mycosis and arteriovenous fistulas and thromboses, and to plan preoperatively for mass removals, so that critical vessels in the area can be identified beforehand.

GUTTURAL POUCH TYMPANY IN FOALS

Tympany is a unilateral or bilateral distention of the guttural pouches with air, with or without some fluid accumulation, in an otherwise healthy foal. Possible causes include a mucosal flap (or plica salpingopharyngea) acting as a one-way valve that traps air and fluid in the pouch, inflammation from an upper airway infection, persistent coughing, and muscle dysfunction.[2] Genetic studies have provided new information on

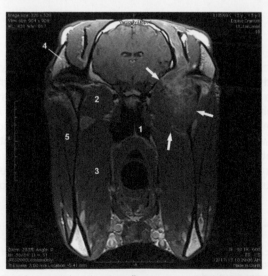

Fig. 1. MRI of horse with parotid melanoma (between *arrows*) extending rostrally from the left guttural pouch (1). 2, pterygoideus lateralis muscle; 3, pterygoideus medialis muscle; 4, squamous part of temporal bone; 5, masseter muscle. *Courtesy of* Dr. Carter Judy, Alamo Pintado Equine Medical Center.

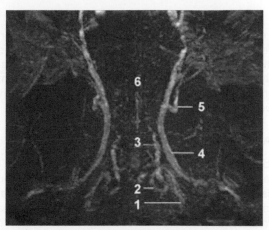

Fig. 2. MRA of the equine cerebral vasculature as viewed from the dorsal aspect. 1, ICA; 2, sigmoid flexure of the ICA; 3, middle cerebral artery; 4, ECA; 5, external ophthalmic artery; 6, corpus callosum artery.

breed and gender risks for this disease, such as the 3 to 1 greater prevalence in fillies than colts[3–6] and a breed predisposition in Arabian and Paint horse foals.[3] In one study, many of the Arabian purebred foals affected with guttural pouch tympany were from the same stud farm and some were full or half siblings.[4] Complex segregation analysis demonstrated a recessive major gene for German warmblood horses and that a polygenic or mixed monogenic-polygenic inheritance was most likely for Arabian horses.[5–7] Whole genome scan for guttural pouch tympany in Arabian and German warmblood horses has indicated a sex-specific quantitative trait locus, in agreement with the higher prevalence of this disease in fillies.[8] More recent work was able to identify linked and associated regions for a major gene causing guttural pouch tympany in Arabian and warmblood horses.[7]

Diagnosis

Clinical signs become evident in foals between birth and 1 year of age, with the most obvious being a nonpainful elastic swelling in the parotid region caused by entrapped air in the affected guttural pouch. In most cases, no gross anatomic abnormality can be identified at the guttural pouch opening to explain failure of air egress from the affected side.[3] Distention in the affected pouch can be severe enough to encroach on the opposite side of the neck, giving the impression of bilateral involvement. Dyspnea, dysphagia, secondary empyema, and inhalation pneumonia are rare complications of this disease. Distinction between unilateral and bilateral tympany can be made on direct endoscopy of each pouch,[9] and is important in selecting treatment.

Treatment

Temporary relief can be achieved by catheterizing the affected guttural pouch or pouches.[10] Surgical treatment is required for permanent resolution and should be performed promptly to prevent complications, such as empyema and bronchopneumonia.[11] The goal of surgery is to create a permanent means of evacuating air, either through the unaffected guttural pouch (fenestration of median septum), through the guttural pouch opening (removal of obstructing membrane), or through an artificially created opening into the pharynx (salpingopharyngeal fistula).

Prognosis

The prognosis for complete recovery and a successful racing career is favorable after median septum fenestration by any method,[9,11,12] although surgery is not always straightforward and repeat surgery is not uncommon.[3,13] Secondary empyema and pneumonia usually resolve spontaneously after successful treatment of tympany, although the prognosis is guarded for foals with aspiration pneumonia and dysphagia secondary to nerve damage induced at surgery.[10,12]

NASOPHARYNGEAL OBSTRUCTION CAUSED BY HEAD FLEXION

A recently described form of nasopharyngeal obstruction in adult horses has been attributed to impaired egress of air from one or both guttural pouches during poll flexion, possibly caused by an anatomic or functional defect in the salpingopharyngeal fold.[14] The proposed pathogenesis of this condition is similar to that responsible for guttural pouch tympany, and affected horses might have a form of guttural pouch tympany that is not manifested in the typical presentation in the foal.[14] These horses present with a history of respiratory noise and appear unwilling to perform in a sport that requires the head be held in a flexed position. For example, the flexed poll position that produces the desired head carriage for dressage could interfere with the normal escape of air from the guttural pouch induced by swallowing.[14] A standing procedure was used for laser fenestration of the median septum in a group of affected horses, followed by use of a high-frequency wire snare to resect the salpingopharyngeal fold in the more severely affected guttural pouch.[14] The response to treatment is generally very good, with an increased nasopharyngeal diameter evident during flexion on endoscopy and radiographs 3 days after surgical treatment, and improved performance then and subsequently.[14]

EMPYEMA

Empyema of the guttural pouches is an accumulation of purulent material in one or both guttural pouches, which can become inspissated or form chondroids, independent of duration of infection.[15] Upper respiratory tract infections (especially those caused by *Streptococcus equi* subspecies *equi*; see article by Mallicote, elsewhere in this issue) can cause abscessation and rupture of retropharyngeal lymph nodes into the guttural pouch. Less common causes are infusion of irritant drugs, fracture of the stylohyoid bone, congenital or acquired stenosis of the pharyngeal orifice, and pharyngeal perforation by a nasogastric tube.[2,16]

Diagnosis

Clinical signs include intermittent nasal discharge, swelling of submandibular and pharyngeal lymph nodes, parotid swelling and pain, extended head carriage, loud respiratory noise, and difficulties in swallowing and breathing. Signs of cranial neuropathy are rare. Although most horses with guttural pouch chondroids will present with the typical history and clinical signs described previously, chondroids have been found in horses that had no external swelling or other obvious signs.

On endoscopic examination, a purulent discharge can be seen at the pharyngeal orifice of the affected side, with pharyngeal collapse in some horses (**Fig. 3**). On standing lateral radiographs, fluid lines within the guttural pouch are suggestive of liquid or inspissated contents, and discrete round masses indicate chondroids. Aspirates or saline washings from the guttural pouch are submitted for culture and sensitivity testing and for polymerase chain reaction analysis for *S equi* subspecies *equi* as

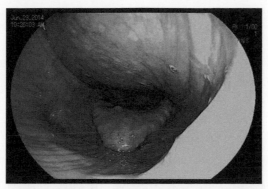

Fig. 3. Pronounced collapse of the roof of the pharynx of a horse with severe guttural pouch empyema. Such cases can be candidates for a tracheotomy.

period after procedures. Ultrasonographic examination of tissues lateral and ventral to the guttural pouch can be used to assess lymph node involvement.

Treatment

Treatment of this condition usually includes combinations of lavage and systemic antibiotics. Aggressive use of large volumes of fluid under pressure through large-bore tubes is not recommended because this can rupture the guttural pouch lining,[17] and spread the infection into dissecting tracts from which it cannot be readily removed.[18] Noninvasive methods for chondroid removal can be slow and tedious,[15] and include maceration, endoscopically guided grasping forceps, basket snare, diathermic snare, a wire loop, and retrieval basket.[19] The cost and potential complications of protracted medical treatment should be weighed against the benefits of surgery if a slow response seems likely, especially if contents are inspissated or chondroids have formed (surgical approaches are discussed later).

Prognosis

Response to medical treatment and surgery is usually satisfactory and residual nerve damage is rare.

GUTTURAL POUCH MYCOSIS

Guttural pouch mycosis affects the roof of one (or rarely both) guttural pouch without any apparent age, sex, breed, or geographic predisposition. The cause is unknown and different fungi have been isolated, although *Aspergillus (Emericella) fumigatus* is the most common isolate, and is more likely to be found by direct examination of biopsies than by culture.[20] Guttural pouch mycosis typically forms a diphtheritic membrane of variable size, composed of necrotic tissue, cell debris, different bacteria, and fungal mycelia.[2] Although mostly reported in stabled horses in the northern hemisphere, it also has been reported in nonstabled horses in New Zealand.[21]

Diagnosis

The most common clinical sign is moderate-to-severe epistaxis caused by fungal erosion of the internal carotid artery (ICA) in most cases and of the maxillary artery (MA) in approximately one-third of cases (**Fig. 4**).[22–27] However, the external carotid artery (ECA) and any of its other branches could be affected. Several bouts of hemorrhage usually precede a fatal episode. Aneurysm formation rarely precedes or follows

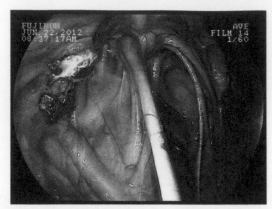

Fig. 4. Endoscopic image of a mycotic plaque on the MA of the right guttural pouch.

arterial invasion[28] and, therefore, is not essential to the pathogenesis of arterial rupture. Mucus and dark blood continue to drain from the nostril on the affected side for days after acute hemorrhage ceases.

The second most common clinical sign is dysphagia caused by damage to the pharyngeal branches of the vagus and glossopharyngeal nerves, which can lead to aspiration pneumonia. Even a focal lesion on the pharyngeal branch of the vagus nerve can cause irreversible dysphagia, evidence of the importance of this nerve for motor innervation of the pharynx.[29] Abnormal respiratory noise can be caused by pharyngeal paresis or laryngeal hemiplegia, the latter caused by recurrent laryngeal nerve damage.[24] Horner syndrome from damage to the cranial cervical ganglion and postganglionic sympathetic fibers causes ptosis, miosis, and enophthalmos, patchy sweating, and congestion of the nasal mucosa. Ptosis is caused by decreased tone of the superior tarsus muscle,[30] and is assessed by observing eyelash angles from a frontal view (**Fig. 5**). Pupillary response to decreased sympathetic tone in horses is variable.[30] Less common signs are parotid pain, mucopurulent nasal discharge, abnormal head posture, head shyness, sweating and shivering, corneal ulcers, colic, blindness, locomotion disturbances, facial nerve paralysis, paralysis of the tongue, and septic arthritis of the atlanto-occipital joint.[19]

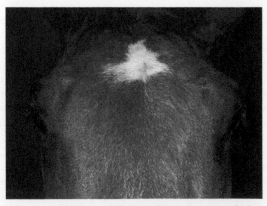

Fig. 5. Horse with left-sided Horner syndrome. Note downward direction of the upper eyelid compared with the normal right side.

Endoscopy, combined with history and clinical signs, is critical for diagnosis. Endoscopy can demonstrate blood draining from the pharyngeal orifice in horses with epistaxis (**Fig. 6**), and pharyngeal collapse, displaced soft palate, and food material in the nasopharynx and nasal passages in horses with dysphagia. When the guttural pouch interior is not obscured by blood clots, the typical lesion can be seen as a diphtheritic membrane on the roof (see **Fig. 4**), without any apparent relationship between size and the severity of clinical signs. The stylohyoid bone can be thickened and coated with a diphtheritic membrane, but these changes do not appear to cause clinical signs. Fistulas can form between the opposite guttural pouch and into the pharynx.[22] True bilateral involvement was described in 19% in a report on 31 horses.[28]

Medical Treatment

Little progress has been made in finding a safe, effective, and inexpensive antifungal agent for use in horses. Also, the response to medical treatment is generally slow and inconsistent, so that clinical signs can progress to death or euthanasia before the infection or its effects have resolved. Care must be given when attributing success to any treatment method of this disease because of its ability to resolve spontaneously, sometimes within short periods after diagnosis.[19] The current status of antifungal agents in horses is as follows:

- Amphotericin B at 0.38 to 1.47 mg/kg diluted in 1 L of 5% dextrose has been given intravenously (IV) daily for up to 40 days to treat phycomycosis.[31] Concerns about potential irreversible nephrotoxicity limit its use[32] and there are no reports on its efficacy for guttural pouch mycosis.
- Itraconazole at 5 mg/kg orally every 24 hours can achieve plasma concentrations that are inhibitory against fungi that infect horses.[33] Itraconazole has a similar spectrum of activity as fluconazole, except that it is effective against *Aspergillus* spp.[32]
- A combination of itraconazole (5 mg/kg body weight orally) and topical enilconazole (60 mL of 33.3 mg/mL solution per daily flush) was used successfully in a horse with guttural pouch mycosis.[34]
- Itraconazole at 3 mg/kg twice a day in the feed was effective against *Aspergillus* and other fungi in the nasal passage of horses, but 4 months or so of treatment may be required.[35]

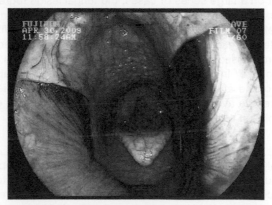

Fig. 6. Hemorrhage from the left guttural pouch in a horse with guttural pouch mycosis. Blood is also draining from the right guttural pouch to a lesser extent because the mycosis eroded the septum between the 2 guttural pouches.

- Topical infusion of 30 to 60 mL of 10 mg/mL itraconazole through the biopsy channel of the endoscope every other day for 10 days and the oral paste at 5 mg/kg orally once daily for 3 months was used successfully by the author in a horse with guttural pouch mycosis.
- Fluconazole is another triazole antifungal agent that could be used to treat fungal infections in horses, based on bioavailability data after oral and IV administration.[36] However, it has poor activity against *Aspergillus* spp.[32]
- Ketoconazole has poor efficacy against *Aspergillus* spp, and, because it is insoluble in the equine stomach, it is not absorbed after oral administration.[33]
- Daily guttural pouch irrigations with a 0.08% clotrimazole emulsion in 500 mL water for 14 days prevented recurrence of a discrete lesion in one horse.[29] A 3-day depot preparation of clotrimazole is available and might be more suitable for treatment of guttural pouch mycosis.[29] Advantages of this drug are its availability in preparations specifically intended for mucosal fungal infections, its ability to adhere to mucosal surfaces, and the lack of inflammation at sites of application.

Horses with blood loss should be treated with polyionic fluids and blood transfusions if necessary, and horses with dysphagia should be fed by nasogastric tube or by esophagostomy and should receive nonsteroidal anti-inflammatory drugs to reduce neuritis.[19]

Surgical Treatment

Surgical removal of the diphtheritic membrane can be considered when dysphagia or persistent mucopurulent nasal discharge or both are the predominant clinical signs. However, the fungal invasion can persist postoperatively in submucosal structures deep to the diphtheritic membrane and proteinaceous material that can be safely removed with instruments, gentle swabbing, and lavage. Also, surgery carries the risk of iatrogenic nerve damage and hemorrhage and probably should be reserved for horses in which the arteries in the guttural pouch have been occluded.

Surgical occlusion of the affected artery (see later in this article) has been credited with hastening spontaneous resolution of the mycotic lesion and thereby rendering medical therapy unnecessary.[37] However, none of the studies that make this claim[28,37] have demonstrated a more rapid resolution of the lesion than the rate of spontaneous resolution documented in horses that did not undergo arterial occlusion.[24] In a report on a large series of cases, the fungal lesion regressed completely on endoscopic examination between 30 and 180 days and incompletely between 51 to 269 days after transarterial coil embolization.[28] Such time frames cannot be regarded as hastened resolution. Also, the author has experienced cases in which fungal invasion progressed after similar arterial occlusion methods as those associated with resolution.[28,37] In one horse in which fungal invasion actually progressed after embolization of the affected ICA, neurologic signs accompanied growth of the lesion.[38] Therefore, the available evidence would suggest that the effects of arterial occlusion on resolution of the mycosis are unresolved.

Prognosis

The approximately 50% mortality rate reported in horses with epistaxis[24] can be considerably reduced by the occlusion procedures described later in this article. Although the mycotic lesion disappears with time regardless of treatment, this is a very slow process and neurologic signs can persist after the lesion has disappeared.[29] Laryngeal hemiplegia is one of the more common clinical signs[28] and is typically permanent, although recovery has been reported.[26] Some horses with dysphagia can eventually recover, although incompletely, and sometimes 6 to 18 months may be required.[24,26] Most horses recover from Horner syndrome and facial nerve paralysis.[28]

TEMPOROHYOID OSTEOARTHROPATHY (MIDDLE EAR DISEASE)

THO is considered to be a sequela of an inner or middle ear infection of hematogenous origin that spreads to and thickens the stylohyoid bone, the cartilaginous tympano-hyoid, and squamous portion of the temporal bone. These changes are progressive, and fusion of the temporohyoid joint follows.[39] Although guttural pouch mycosis can involve the same area as is affected with THO, it rarely if ever causes this disease.[19,24] However, the 2 diseases have been reported concurrently in the same horse, one in each guttural pouch.[38] Recent computed tomographic and histopathological studies have demonstrated a bilateral, age-related increase in severity of degenerative changes in the normal equine temporohyoid joint, although milder than changes in horses with THO.[40] This would suggest a degenerative, rather than infectious, underlying cause,[40] consistent with increasing development of neurologic signs with increasing age.[41]

Although the average age of onset of clinical signs is 10.8 years,[42] the disease has been reported over a wide age range (6 months–23.5 years).[41–45] Quarter Horse–types accounted for 62.8% of horses with THO in 4 hospitals with diverse breed populations.[41] Quarter Horses are uncommon in the United Kingdom, which could explain why THO is less commonly diagnosed in that country compared with the United States.[43]

The bony changes associated with THO can be exacerbated by forces generated through movement of the tongue and larynx during swallowing, vocalizing, combined head and neck movements, oral or dental examinations, and teeth floating. These forces can be transmitted through the fused temporohyoid joint to fracture the petrous part of the temporal bone, thereby injuring the adjacent facial nerve (cranial nerve [CN] VII) and vestibulocochlear nerve (CN VIII).[46–49] Caudal extension of the fracture with associated bone production and inflammation could damage the glossopharyngeal and vagus nerves where they leave the medulla through the jugular foramen, caudal to the vestibulocochlear nerve.[50] After fracture of the petrous temporal bone, middle or inner ear infection could extend around the brain stem and involve additional cranial nerves and hindbrain structures. Fractures also can extend into the bones of the calvarium and cause seizures and meningitis.[42]

A recent study demonstrated crib-biting in 31.3% of horses with THO, and a significant association between this behavior and being afflicted with the disease.[41] Compared with the general population, horses with neurologic disease associated with THO were 8 times more likely to be crib-biters.[41] The act of crib-biting could be a response to pain from THO, but a more likely explanation is that the repeated pressure on the hyoid apparatus during cribbing could exacerbate neurologic signs in horses with existing osteoarthropathy.[41] However, experiences with another case suggest that pain from THO could prevent cribbing.[51]

Diagnosis

Early signs include head tossing or shaking, ear rubbing, refusing to take the bit, refusing to position the head properly when under saddle, resistance to digital pressure around the base of the ears or on the basihyoid bone, facial hyperesthesia, compulsive circling to one side, and other nonspecific behavioral changes.[39,43,52] Signs referable to the vestibulotrochlear nerve can develop acutely and without apparent warning, such as asymmetrical ataxia, head tilt (**Fig. 7**), and spontaneous

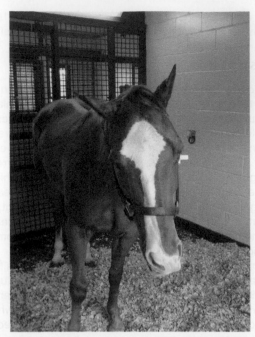

Fig. 7. Horse with right-sided temperohyoid osteoarthropathy. Note head tilt to the affected side, with ear droop, and muzzle deviation.

nystagmus with the slow component to the affected side.[39] These signs can be revealed or exacerbated by blindfolding. Pain on periauricular palpation and reduced mobility of the hyoid apparatus can be supportive findings.[51] In one horse, the clinical signs of headshaking were diminished by infusion of 2% lidocaine into the ear canals, and this response was attributed to blocking an inflammatory response in the ear canal or inner ear.[52]

In one study of 33 horses with THO, 29 had facial nerve deficits and 23 had vestibulocochlear nerve deficits.[42] Signs of facial nerve damage include paresis or paralysis of the ear on the affected side and deviation of the upper lip away from the affected side (see **Fig. 7**).[49,50] Decreased tear production and inability to close the eyes also are common sequelae to facial nerve damage and may cause corneal ulcers, keratoconjunctivitis sicca, and exposure keratitis.[49,50] Dysphagia could be caused by pain associated with tongue movement[43] or by glossopharyngeal or vagal nerve dysfunction.[50] Seizures and sudden death are reported rarely.[42]

Endoscopy of the guttural pouches is the most reliable procedure for diagnosis of THO, because it can clearly demonstrate the bony proliferation and irregular shaping of the proximal aspect of the stylohyoid bone (**Fig. 8**). Serous exudate from the temporohyoid joint has been reported but is a rare finding.[43] In one study, 22.6% of horses with unilateral clinical signs actually had bilateral disease, with only the more severely affected side showing obvious clinical signs.[42] Therefore, both guttural pouches always should be examined. Although some minor individual variations in the anatomy of the normal stylohyoid bone are possible,[41] the high frequency of bilateral involvement should be considered when comparing the side with clinical signs with the contralateral side.[51]

Dorsoventral radiographs of the skull demonstrate proliferation and osteitis of the affected bones; however, the extent of bony, articular, and soft tissue changes can

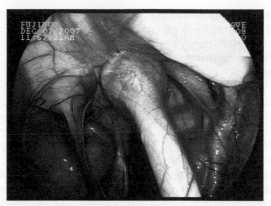

Fig. 8. Endoscopic evidence of thickening of the stylohyoid bone typical of THO.

be more completely demonstrated by computed tomography (CT).[43,44,53] Also, CT can identify thickening of the ceratohyoid bone, proliferation of its articulation with the stylohyoid bone, and subclinical bilateral disease in horses considered clinically to be affected on one side.[44] In those horses with bilateral changes, the stylohyoid bone is significantly wider on the side with obvious neurologic deficits.[44] The standing CT units available in some practices are well suited for horses with THO because they eliminate risks associated with anesthetic recovery in horses with acute vestibular signs (**Fig. 9**). Scintigraphy has been used for diagnosis of THO,[54] but was helpful in only 1 of 2 affected horses in one study.[43] Brainstem auditory-evoked response (BAER) can be completely or partially lost on the affected side, and therefore BAER testing might have diagnostic value in horses with THO.[55]

Treatment

Medical treatment includes broad-spectrum antibiotics for infection and nonsteroidal anti-inflammatory drugs to relieve pain and inflammation.[51] Antimicrobial drugs with activity against *Staphylococcus aureus* have been recommended (ampicillin, trimethoprim-sulfa, enrofloxacin, and chloramphenicol).[51] Tympanocentesis is technically demanding, but could be used to identify specific bacterial pathogens and thereby determine antimicrobial therapy.[56] Gabapentin to control neuropathic pain

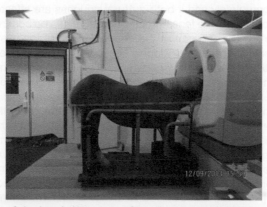

Fig. 9. Standing CT of the head. (*Courtesy of* Dr. Tim Mair, Bell Equine Veterinary Clinic.)

associated with the affected nerves reduced head shaking in one reported case.[45] Multifocal split-lid tarsorrhaphy is recommended for horses with corneal ulceration to improve patient comfort, corneal protection, and corneal repair.[51] Permanent tarsorrhaphies are not recommended because facial nerve function could recover in 3 weeks to 18 months.[51]

Prognosis

Medical and surgical treatments can be partially or totally effective for horses with THO, but little information is available to guide treatment selection.[41,43] Neurologic signs can persist to some degree in most horses, especially if treatment is delayed.[42,46,57] In most horses treated medically, a year or longer can be required for maximal improvement, and prognosis for return to some type of athletic function is fair.[42] A favorable response to medical treatment might be more likely in mildly affected cases. In one study, substantial improvement was recorded in 89% of horses at 1 year after ceratohyoidectomy (see later in this article) and in 87% that had a partial stylohyoid ostectomy, with most of the improvement within the first 6 months.[58] In another study, ceratohyoidectomy resolved clinical signs in 2 of 5 cases and improved the remainder.[43] Information about the response to combined medical and surgical treatment is currently lacking.

SURGICAL TREATMENT OF GUTTURAL POUCH DISEASES

Recent developments in guttural pouch surgery reflect a progressive migration away from the traditional direct approaches, and their replacement with minimally invasive techniques.[19] The advantages of the latter are avoidance of a difficult surgery in an anatomically complicated structure and reduced risk of damage to vital structures under the guttural pouch mucosa. However, occasions do arise when the guttural pouches have to be opened surgically, which requires considerable care to avoid life-threatening complications.

SURGICAL TREATMENT OF GUTTURAL POUCH TYMPANY

The traditional method for median septum fenestration in unilateral cases involves entering the affected guttural pouch through the Viborg triangle or a modified Whitehouse approach and then removing a segment of median septum (**Fig. 10**).[19] This allows trapped air to egress from the tympanitic pouch through the normal side. The fenestration procedure can fail if both opposing mucosal surfaces of the septum are not resected completely and if both guttural pouches are affected.

For bilateral involvement, the fenestration procedure can be combined with removal of a small segment (1.5 × 2.5 cm) of the medial lamina of the eustachian tube and associated mucosal fold (plica salpingopharyngea) on the floor of the tubular entryway into the guttural pouch to form a larger pharyngeal opening.[9,12] The main problem with this approach is the wide variation in descriptions of the tissues resected and a failure to understand the role of the resected tissue in the disease process. Satisfactory outcomes have been described after partial resection of only the plica salpingopharyngea,[59] resection of the cartilaginous lamina of the eustachian tube and plica salpingopharyngea,[11,60] combined fenestration of the septum with partial resection of the plica salpingopharyngea,[3] and resection of only the cartilaginous flap.[61] Premature closure of the guttural pouch opening can cause recurrence and empyema.[11,13]

Transendoscopic electrocautery[2,62] or a laser (diode or a neodymium:yttrium-aluminum-garnet [Nd:YAG]) can be used to create a fenestration in the septum as a standing procedure or with the horse anesthetized.[9,63] A simpler method is to create

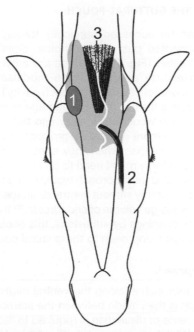

Fig. 10. Method of elevating the median septum for resection through a Viborg triangle approach (1), using the tip of the endoscope (2) in the opposite guttural pouch for elevation and illumination of the membrane. 3, ventral straight muscles of the head. A Chamber mare catheter can be used instead of the endoscope, although illumination will be lost.

a salpingopharyngeal fistula in the wall of the pharynx, caudal to the guttural pouch opening, with the laser under videoendoscopic control.[63,64] A Foley catheter placed through the fistula for 7 to 10 days acts as a stent and as a route for lavage of the guttural pouch.[63] If the salpingopharyngeal fistula is placed too far rostrally or ventrally, it could fail to bypass the defective pharyngeal ostium or it could become sealed by inflammation.[11] The major advantage of these approaches is that they avoid the risk of nerve damage that can follow open approaches.[65]

In the absence of overwhelming evidence of bilateral involvement, the author recommends entering the affected guttural pouch through the Viborg triangle and then resecting a 2-cm^2 segment of median septum elevated by an endoscope in the opposite side (see **Fig. 10**). The Viborg triangle is defined by the sternocephalicus muscle, vertical ramus of the mandible, and linguofacial vein, and is selected because the distended guttural pouch is near that site and submucosal nerves can be identified. To avoid cranial nerve damage, blunt entry with a hemostat is preferred to opening the guttural pouch by elevating a segment of mucosa and incising it with scissors.[60,61] Complete resection of both mucosal surfaces of the septum can be confirmed by passing the endoscope through the fenestration. The incision through the Viborg triangle can be left open to heal by second intention. The owner should be warned that recurrence is possible and probably indicates bilateral involvement with need for a more extensive surgery. Most cases are unilateral and this method for fenestration is a considerably simpler procedure with a lower complication rate than those intended to enlarge the pharyngeal ostium. A standing laser technique can accomplish the same, if preferred.[63]

SURGICAL DRAINAGE OF THE GUTTURAL POUCH

The guttural pouches can be accessed surgically through 4 well-described approaches to remove inspissated pus or chondroids, diphtheritic plaques, foreign bodies, and other abnormalities (**Fig. 11**).[19] These are a hyovertebrotomy, a Viborg triangle approach, a Whitehouse approach, or a modified Whitehouse approach (see **Fig. 11**). Because all approaches enter the pouch cavity in the same approximate area on the floor, none reduces the risk of nerve damage more than others. However, the hyovertebrotomy approach would allow entry into the guttural pouch at a point where the nerves and ICA are more compactly grouped in a fold of membrane that could be identified more readily than when they spread out onto the floor. If used for empyema, the hyovertebrotomy might need to be combined with a Viborg triangle approach to obtain drainage, and this approach would place nerves on the floor at risk of injury. However, hyovertebrotomy without ventral drainage has been reported to be very effective for removal of a large volume of chondroids.[66] If empyema is the result of occlusion of guttural pouch openings by adhesions, this occlusion can be relieved by blunt division through a surgical approach to the guttural pouch.[67]

Modified Whitehouse Approach

The original Whitehouse approach is along the ventral midline at the junction of the head and neck. An incision is then made between the sternohyoideus and omohyoideus muscles and a long route of dissection is required to reach the affected guttural pouch. With the modified Whitehouse approach (**Fig. 12**), a 12- to 16-cm skin incision is made over the sternocephalicus muscle and along the ventral edge of the linguofacial vein, as if for a laryngoplasty, and extended onto the medial aspect of the caudal ramus of the mandible, axial to the linguofacial vein. Because the guttural pouch can be so deep to any approach, a generous incision is required to improve access through dissection to the floor. Careful dissection divides the fascia between the linguofacial vein and omohyoideus muscle, and this plane of dissection can be followed to the floor of the guttural pouch. The ventral edge of the stylohyoid bone can be used

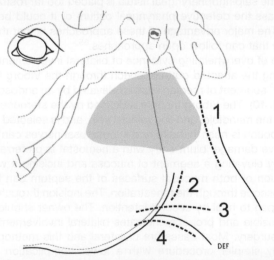

Fig. 11. Surgical approaches to the guttural pouch. 1, hyovertebrotomy; 2, Viborg triangle; 3, modified Whitehouse; 4, Whitehouse. Shading is the guttural pouch.

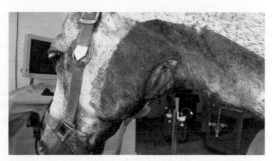

Fig. 12. Modified Whitehouse approach used as a standing procedure to empty a guttural pouch of 2 kg of inspissated pus. The most dorsal part of the incision was partly closed to cover the exposed segment of sternocephalicus muscle. The incision was made long enough so that a surgeon with a small hand could manually remove contents from the guttural pouch.

to guide dissection toward the medial compartment, taking care to avoid confusion with the thyrohyoid bone. Large arteries are avoided by palpating their tubular shapes and obvious pulses.

The major advantage of the modified Whitehouse approach over the original Whitehouse method is that blunt dissection through a natural fascial plane allows access to the floor of the guttural pouch, which is closer to the incision (see **Fig. 11**). It allows good access to all parts of the guttural pouch, excellent ventral drainage, and simultaneous access through the septum to both pouches. It is also well suited as a standing procedure.[17]

If the guttural pouch is distended, the floor is prominent and more easily recognized. In the absence of distention and mucosal thickening, identifiation of the lining and underlying nerves (or their absence) can be improved by illumination though an endoscope in the medial compartment. The lining of the guttural pouch must be penetrated with great care, and sharp instruments, including scissors, should not be used. A Kelly hemostat, a straight Carmalt forceps, or a Rochester-Pean forceps can be used to bluntly penetrate the lining of the floor of the guttural pouch, which is confirmed by purulent material on the instrument in horses with empyema or collapse in foals with tympany.

The instrument should not be withdrawn until it has been opened repeatedly to establish an incision of sufficient size to be easily located. Failure to mark the point of penetration until an obvious opening is made will necessitate repeating the process, each time with risk of nerve damage. The size of the opening can be expanded by carefully spreading its edges digitally, ideally creating sufficient room to accommodate a small hand, if the horse is large enough. After this step, a curved or straight sponge forceps can be used to remove the contents and a small hand can manually direct inspissated material from the lateral compartment into the rostral aspect of the medial compartment, from where it can be more readily removed. The amount of inspissated pus or chondroids that can be removed surgically can far exceed what would be estimated based on the maximum capacity of the guttural pouch.[66] Copious lavage with a sterile physiologic solution follows to dislodge any remaining material, and this can be confirmed by endoscopy. A 28-French Foley catheter can be inserted through a stab incision in the skin and guided into the guttural pouch for subsequent lavage. The most caudal 5 cm of the skin incision can be closed with interrupted suture material to cover the exposed segment of sternocephalicus muscle.

In horses with empyema, immediate postoperative improvement should be evident as an empty guttural pouch and reduced collapse of the dorsal pharyngeal wall, if the latter were evident beforehand. After surgery, the incision should be left open to drain and to allow repeated lavage and endoscopy of the pouch.

Modified Garm Technique

A modified Garm technique allows access to the lateral compartment of the guttural pouch and can be performed as a standing procedure for lavage and drainage in horses with mild empyema.[68] For this approach, a 6-cm skin incision is made 4 cm more rostrally than in the Garm original technique, between the ramus of the mandible and the submandibular lymph nodes.[68] Blind digital dissection is continued to the rostroventral aspect of the lateral compartment, where the mucosa can be perforated without risk to important vessels or nerves.[68] Because of the depth of dissection and tight path created, little can be accomplished through this route except to insert a tube for lavage.[68] Also, the hypoglossal nerve and the lingual artery are skirted along the route of dissection to the guttural pouch, making it even less attractive.

Standing Surgical Removal of Inspissated Pus and Chondroids

Many cases of guttural pouch empyema are caused by *S equi* subspecies *equi*, and can develop inspissated exudate and chondroids. Surgery in such cases preferably should be done as a standing procedure in an isolation facility, so the horse does not move through other parts of the hospital and contaminate surgery suites and anesthetic equipment with a highly contagious organism. Standing surgery also avoids the expense and risks of general anesthesia, although it does lose the only major advantage of general anesthesia, a more comfortable position for the surgeon and assistants. However, access to the guttural pouch is difficult by any method and is not greatly facilitated by anesthetizing the horse.

A modified Whitehouse approach (see **Fig. 12**) is used because this gives the best access and allows ventral drainage. Horses can be sedated with detomidine HCl (0.005–0.01 mg/kg IV) or xylazine HCl (0.2 mg/kg IV), plus/minus butorphanol tartrate (0.03 mg/kg IV). A constant rate infusion of detomidine IV (0.6 μg/kg/min) also can be used. Preferably, horses should be placed in stocks with the lower jaw on a solid support.

The surgical site is infiltrated with approximately 30 mL of 2% mepivacaine HCl. Some of the local anesthetic can be infiltrated in deeper tissues toward the floor of the guttural pouch, but care must be taken to prevent puncture of major vessels in this area. If problems are anticipated during deep dissection because of the horse's temperament, a sterile syringe loaded with local anesthetic can be placed on the surgery tray and used as needed to provide deeper anesthesia.

Horses with chondroids are more likely to have retropharyngeal and pharyngeal swelling than those without this complication,[15] and this facilitates surgical access. If the guttural pouch is not distended, an assistant can insert a Chambers catheter into the nasal cavity and guide it with the endoscope through the nasopharyngeal ostium of the guttural pouch.[17] Before insertion, this catheter should be bent into a smooth curve at approximately one-third the length of the catheter from the tip, or at the approximate level of the medial canthus of the eye, with the tip at the angle of the vertical ramus of the mandible. When the tip of the catheter is in the medial compartment, the surgeon should be able to palpate it through the floor of the guttural pouch and thereby help the assistant push it through the mucosal lining at this point.[17] Once the catheter has penetrated the floor of the guttural pouch, a size 2 suture material can be tied above the bulbous end of the catheter and this can be used to identify the opening, once the catheter has been withdrawn.[17] Alternatively, the tip of a hemostatic forceps can be placed in the open end of the catheter tip to guide the forceps into the guttural pouch, where it can then be used to expand the opening.[17]

Aftercare

Open incisions in the guttural pouch are cleaned daily, and the guttural pouch cavity should be flushed daily with a nonirritating solution. Open incisions close spontaneously in approximately 14 days. Perioperative antibiotics can be given, usually penicillin and gentamicin.

LASER PROCEDURES FOR GUTTURAL POUCH DRAINAGE

Chronic empyema of the guttural pouches that is unresponsive to medical therapy because of poor drainage through the pharyngeal ostia, can be successfully treated by using the laser to make a permanent pharyngeal fistula into the guttural pouch.[69] In a pony with chondroids and occlusion of the pharyngeal ostium by deformity and a fibrotic adhesion, the median septum was fenestrated from the healthy guttural pouch with the Nd:YAG laser as a standing procedure.[70] The fenestration allowed purulent material to drain through the healthy side and also allowed repeated access for endoscopic snare or basket removal of all the chondroids.[70] This approach was used because a catheter could not be inserted into the diseased pouch to guide safe and effective laser penetration from the pharynx to create a drainage fistula.[70]

ARTERIAL OCCLUSION FOR GUTTURAL POUCH MYCOSIS

Once the limitations of ligation methods in preventing fatal hemorrhage from guttural pouch mycosis were recognized, the challenge of safely occluding the complex terminal vasculature of the equine carotid arterial system prompted an evolution of methods, such as balloon catheters, detachable balloons, microcoils, and nitinol plugs.[19] The last 2 transcatheter methods have emerged as the methods of choice in university veterinary hospitals, where the necessary equipment, inventory, and expertise can be provided by veterinary cardiologists and interventional radiologists.[19]

Occlusion procedures must be performed as soon as possible after the first bout of hemorrhage to prevent subsequent bouts that could be fatal or render the horse a poor candidate for anesthesia and surgery. The vessel to be occluded is determined by endoscopy. If accurate identification is impossible because landmarks are obscured by blood and diphtheritic membrane, all major branches of the carotid artery in the guttural pouch should be occluded, and this is well tolerated.[17,25] TOF-MRA is a noninvasive technique to examine the carotid arterial system (see **Fig. 2**), and could be used to identify vascular changes caused by guttural pouch mycosis.[1] Because contrast arteriography is integral to transcatheter methods of arterial embolization and can accurately identify the relevant vessels and lesions, TOF-MRA would appear to offer little advantage in such cases, and the time in the MRI unit would only prolong the anesthetic period unnecessarily.

Balloon Catheter Occlusion

The nondetachable balloon catheter method is the forerunner of other methods and continues to be used in many hospitals that lack the specialized equipment for coil or plug delivery.[21] It is also a simple, inexpensive, and highly effective method. The balloon catheter technique allows immediate intravascular occlusion of the artery and prevents retrograde flow to the site of hemorrhage from the cerebral arterial circle (circle of Willis) for the ICA[22,71] and from the major palatine artery for the MA.[25]

To occlude the ICA, the artery is ligated close to its origin, and a size 6 French venous thrombectomy catheter (Fogarty-Edwards Laboratories, distributed by American V. Mueller, Chicago, IL) is inserted through an arteriotomy for a distance of approximately 13 cm (**Fig. 13**).[71] At this distance, the balloon tip of the catheter is arrested at the sigmoid flexure of the ICA, within the venous sinuses and distal to the site of infection (see **Fig. 13**). The balloon is inflated with sterile saline and the redundant portion is buried as the incision is closed (see **Fig. 13**). Removal is not essential, but infection can develop along the catheter, which should then be removed promptly to prevent rare but fatal consequences.[19]

Complications associated with this procedure are rare and manageable.[19,22,71] The most serious complication arises because this procedure is typically performed without angiography, and so any deviations from normal anatomy are not identified. For this reason, a small number of horses would be at risk of failed occlusion of the affected artery if an aberrant branch diverts the catheter away from the affected segment.[72–74] However, the balloon catheter has an advantage over embolization methods, because it is more rigid than catheters used in these systems and is inserted closer to the site of arterial invasion, 2 attributes that allow the balloon tip to be more easily advanced beyond arterial obstruction or narrowing distal to the lesion. Unfortunately, the same attributes could be blamed for accidental penetration of the catheter through the eroded segment of artery at surgery or subsequently.[19]

If the MA is involved, the ECA is ligated after the linguofacial trunk or is occluded with a balloon inserted in retrograde fashion through the transverse facial artery.[25] To reduce retrograde flow, a size 6 French Fogarty venous thrombectomy catheter is advanced through the major palatine artery to place the balloon in the MA cranial to the lesion.[19,25] Although the MA has many collateral branches in the segment between the balloons, this procedure has been effective to date and does not cause blindness, even when combined with occlusion of the ICA.[25] However, systolic pressure in the segment closed off by balloons on the cardiac and cephalic sides of the typical site of fungal erosion remains at approximately 58% of control values in

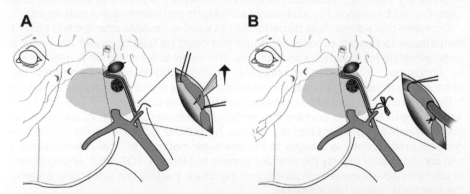

Fig. 13. (*A*) Insertion of a balloon catheter into the left ICA so the balloon is inflated between the first and second flexures of the sigmoid bend in the artery and distal to the lesion (*black with white highlights*). Insert shows method of making an arteriotomy with a number 11 scalpel blade, inserting the blade halfway across the width of the artery between a ligature tied proximally and a preplaced ligature distally and cutting upward (*arrow*) to produce an opening sufficient to accommodate the catheter. (*B*) Balloon catheter secured in the artery by tightening the preplaced ligature around it and then tying the long ends to the folded redundant portion of the catheter. This portion of the catheter is then buried in the incision.

standing horses.[75] This would suggest that any methods designed to close off this segment of the MA could allow substantial retrograde blood flow from contralateral vessels into the occluded arterial segment. Although ligation of the major palatine artery at its rostral end could prevent retrograde flow, a combination of this procedure with ligation of the ECA and ICA can cause ischemic optic neuropathy and permanent blindness.[76] This can be attributed to the "steal phenomenon" **(Fig. 14)**.

Detachable Balloon Catheter Systems

Although a detachable, self-sealing, latex balloon has been described to successfully occlude the ICA and aberrant vessels under angiographic control,[74,77] recent reports on this method are lacking. Possibly this could be explained by a trend that favors other embolization methods in human and small animal medicine.

Transarterial Coil Embolization

The transarterial coil embolization (TACE) technique uses angiographic studies to image the affected vessels and identify any unusual branches and sites of bleeding, and then places an embolization coil in the selected portion of the affected artery.[28,78,79] A stainless steel coil of appropriate size is delivered to the target artery through a catheter inserted in the common carotid artery (CCA), and expands as it emerges from the catheter to lodge within the artery. The Dacron fibers on the surface of the coil induce rapid thrombosis in the occluded segment. After coil placement, the catheter and introducer system are removed and the CCA puncture is closed with 5-0 suture in a cruciate pattern, preferably with absorbable synthetic monofilament material.[79] The muscle layers and skin are closed in routine fashion.

The TACE technique is superior to the balloon catheter technique because it uses fluoroscopic guidance, is less invasive (all arteries in the guttural pouch are accessed through a single incision in the CCA), and does not require removal of an implant. The disadvantages of this technique are the need for fluoroscopy, radiation-shielding apparel and equipment, a well-maintained inventory of coils and insertion catheters, and expertise with their use.

The original procedure was described with the horse under general anesthesia with the head and neck supported to allow intraoperative fluoroscopy.[28,78] The same procedure has been used successfully in 5 standing horses with guttural pouch mycosis.[79] The standing approach was developed in 8 normal horses to demonstrate that accurate placement of the coils was possible by this method and that it was well tolerated.[79] The standing procedure avoids general anesthesia and associated complications (especially in a horse suffering from hemorrhagic shock or anemia), decreases the total time for the procedure, and reduces the cost of the procedure. The main concern is the possibility of an adverse reaction to the contrast material (a bolus of 5 to 10 mL of meglumine ioxithalamate); this was an isolated but manageable problem in one horse.[79] Special care is taken during this step, such as warming the material to body temperature and injecting slowly initially to assess the response.[79]

Transarterial Nitinol Vascular Occlusion Plug Embolization

Transarterial occlusion with nitinol plugs[80] is the method of choice in the author's hospital. A nitinol vascular plug is a nickel-titanium wire mesh that expands into a dumbbell configuration when delivered at the target segment of artery to be occluded **(Fig. 15)**.[80] Both ends are marked with radiopaque platinum marker bands (see **Fig. 15**) and one end is attached to a flexible delivery cable from which the plug can be detached by counterclockwise rotation. The procedure is performed under

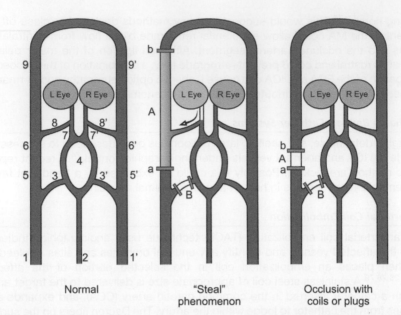

Normal   "Steal"   Occlusion with
                      phenomenon   coils or plugs

Fig. 14. Anatomy of the "steal" phenomenon as a cause of blindness after certain ligation procedures. Normal anatomy (structures on the right side are designated by the prime symbol): 1, left CCA; 2, vertebral artery; 3, ICA; 4, circle of Willis; 5, ECA; 6, MA; 7, internal ophthalmic artery (from circle of Willis); 8, external ophthalmic artery (from the MA); 9, major palatine artery. The major blood supply to the horse's eye is through the external ophthalmic artery (8), which anastomoses inconsistently with the internal ophthalmic artery (7). The MA joins with the same artery from the other side to form an arterial loop around the upper jaw. The middle diagram shows how the "steal" phenomenon develops when the external carotid is ligated at "a" and the major palatine artery is ligated at "b" to reduce or eliminate blood flow through the intervening segment (A) and prevent bleeding through an erosion in the MA. The ICA can be occluded at the same time if there is doubt about the source of hemorrhage (inconclusive endoscopic examination, other). These combinations of ligations can divert blood flowing into the external ophthalmic artery from remaining collateral sources, such as the internal ophthalmic artery, to drain back to A through the external ophthalmic artery (*arrow*). A drop in blood pressure in A, which is the goal of the surgery, would favor such diversion of blood flow from the external ophthalmic artery in the direction of the arrow. In this way, segment A "steals" blood from the eye, which denies the eye a source of retrograde flow when its normal blood supply is occluded. The role of the ICA occlusion is unknown in this scheme, except that it could reduce blood flow through the internal ophthalmic artery, thereby jeopardizing blood flow to the eye even more. Blindness is considerably less likely after balloon catheter occlusion of segment A, presumably because the physical presence of the catheter in that segment reduces its intravascular volume and hence its capacity to "steal" blood from the eye. If the affected arterial segments are selectively occluded by embolization with coils or plugs, blood flow to the eye should be preserved, possibly through an intact retrograde flow through the major palatine artery. L, left; R, right.

fluoroscopic guidance using an approach and equipment similar to that used for coil embolization.

The nitinol plug has all the advantages of the transarterial coils in achieving complete interruption of blood flow to the site of hemorrhage with a minimally invasive approach.[80] However, only a single plug is required at each site, whereas at least 2

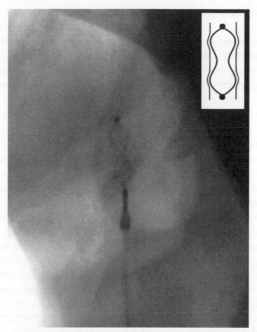

Fig. 15. Nitinol plug in the ICA while still attached to the delivery catheter. Note the dumbbell shape of the plug with 2 radiopaque markers at each end, also illustrated in the inset.

transarterial coils are typically used at each site to stop blood flow. The nitinol plug also can be retracted into the delivery cable to correct an unsatisfactory placement, and migration or dislodgement from the target vessel is very unlikely because the expanded plug is held securely by radial tension from the arterial wall.[80] There is little difference in cost between the 2 methods, and both have the same disadvantages, such as need for specialized equipment and expertise.

Failures after transcatheter embolization methods are rare. Hemorrhage from a failed occlusion typically happens in the recovery stall, and leads to death or euthanasia.[28,72] Hemorrhage after occlusion with a nondetachable balloon catheter is usually caused by failure to recognize or avoid an aberrant branch that would allow persistent retrograde flow to the site of hemorrhage.[72] Arterial occlusion of only one side in bilateral cases can be followed by fatal hemorrhage from the side that was not occluded,[28] but this is rare.

With nitinol plugs and embolization coils, failure to advance catheters rostral to eroded portions of arteries has been attributed to a thrombosis or to narrowing of the artery rostral to the site of hemorrhage.[28,78,80] This is likely with embolization methods, because the catheters are flexible and the catheter tip is too far from the site of insertion to allow the necessary pressure to force it through the obstruction. Nonetheless, the transcatheter embolization systems (coils and nitinol plugs) remain the methods of choice when the necessary equipment is available.

CERATOHYOIDECTOMY

Portions of the hyoid apparatus can be surgically removed on the affected side to decrease forces on the ankylosed temporohyoid joint and thereby reduce recurrent fractures of the callus and skull that exacerbate nerve compression.[81] Problems with unilateral partial ostectomy of the stylohyoid bone are transient dysphagia, injury to the hypoglossal nerve,[81] and regrowth of the stylohyoid bone with recurrence of clinical signs.[50] To prevent injury to the hypoglossal nerve and lingual vessels, periosteum is not removed during partial stylohyoidectomy[81] and therefore remains to form the framework for repair of the resected portion of bone.[50] This has prompted development of ceratohyoidectomy as a safer, easier, and more permanent surgical alternative (**Fig. 16**).[50]

For ceratohyoidectomy, with the horse in dorsal recumbency, a 10- to 15-cm skin incision is made medial to the linguofacial vein on the affected side and centered from cranial to caudal on the basihyoid bone, approximately 2 cm from the midline.[50] The fibers of the sternohyoideus muscle and geniohyoid muscle are separated bluntly until the basihyoid bone is exposed. The ceratohyoid–basihyoid synovial joint is identified and disarticulated with cartilage scissors (see **Fig. 16**). The freed end of the ceratohyoid bone is grasped and the ceratohyoid bone dissected from its attachments to the ceratohyoideus, the hyoideus transversus, and the genioglossus muscles (see **Fig. 16**). The hypoglossal nerve (**Fig. 17**) and lingual branches of the mandibular and glossopharyngeal nerves are lateral to the ceratohyoid bone and can be avoided by gently retracting them, although this is not essential. Alternatively, the ceratohyoid bone can be bluntly separated from its soft tissue attachments with a narrow osteotome or periosteal elevator. The cartilaginous articulation between the ceratohyoid bone and the stylohyoid bone is cut by cartilage scissors or continued elevation with the osteotome, taking care to avoid tension on the stylohyoid bone and temporohyoid joint. Also, the lingual artery must be avoided where it lies close to the ceratohyoid bone (see **Fig. 17**).

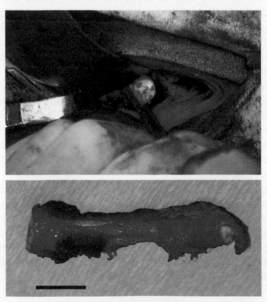

Fig. 16. Top shows a ceratohyoidectomy at point where the ceratohyoid bone has been disarticulated from the basihyoid bone and its articular surface is displayed. Some of the muscle attachments have been dissected off the ceratohyoid bone dorsally to expose the attachment to the stylohyoid bone. Bottom shows the removed ceratohyoid bone (scale bar = 1 cm).

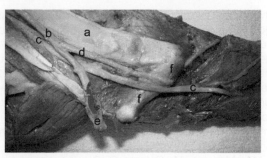

Fig. 17. Anatomy of the lateral aspect of the right stylohyoid and ceratohyoid bones, with dorsal uppermost. a, stylohyoid bone; b, linguofacial artery; c, hypoglossal nerve; d, lingual artery; e, facial artery; f, ceratohyoid bone. Note the close relationship between the lingual artery and the rostral edge of the ceratohyoid bone where the artery assumes a medial course toward the tongue.

The same procedure can be performed effectively with the horse standing and sedated, after local anesthetic solution has been infiltrated along the proposed line of incision.[82] The reason for using the standing approach is to avoid risks associated with recovery from general anesthesia in horses with severe vestibular disease.[82] However, this procedure has not been described to date in clinically affected horses.[82]

Bilateral partial stylohyoidectomy can cause permanent problems with prehension,[82] although it also reduced signs of dysphagia and unilateral facial nerve paralysis in one horse and allowed it to return to light pleasure riding.[50] In one reported case, clinical signs recurred approximately 2 years after unilateral ceratohyoidectomy and resolved after removal of the contralateral ceratohyoid bone.[52] The favorable short-term outcome in this case would seem to justify removal of the remaining ceratohyoid bone if clinical signs recurred on the same side as the original ceratohyoidectomy, especially when CT findings confirm absence of the ceratohyoid bone or any vestige of its recovery in the original surgery site.[52] However, based on available information, unilateral ceratohyoidectomy should be the first option in most bilateral cases.

REFERENCES

1. Manso-Díaz G1, García-Real MI, Casteleyn C, et al. Time-of-flight magnetic resonance angiography (TOF-MRA) of the normal equine head. Equine Vet J 2013;45: 187–92.
2. Cook WR. Diseases of the ear, nose, and throat in the horse: part 1. The ear. In: Grunsell CS, editor. The veterinary annual. Bristol (United Kingdom): John Wright and Sons; 1971. p. 12–43.
3. Blazyczek I, Hamann H, Deegen E, et al. Retrospective analysis of 50 cases of guttural pouch tympany in foals. Vet Rec 2004;154:261.
4. Blazyczek I, Hamann H, Ohnesorge B, et al. Inheritance of guttural pouch tympany in the Arabian horse. J Hered 2004;95:195.
5. Blazyczek I, Hamann H, Ohnesorge B, et al. Population genetic analysis of the heritability of guttural pouch tympany in Arabian purebred foals. Dtsch Tierarztl Wochenschr 2003;110:417–9.
6. Blazyczek I, Hamann H, Ohnesorge B, et al. Guttural pouch tympany in German warmblood foals: influence of sex, inbreeding and blood proportions of founding breeds as well as estimation of heritability. Berl Munch Tierarztl Wochenschr 2003;116:346–51.

7. Metzger J, Ohnesorge B, Distl O. Genome-wide linkage and association analysis identifies major gene loci for guttural pouch tympany in Arabian and German warmblood horses. PLoS One 2012;7(7)):e41640.

8. Zeitz A, Spötter A, Blazyczek I, et al. Whole-genome scan for guttural pouch tympany in Arabian and German warmblood horses. Anim Genet 2009;40:917–24.

9. Tetens J, Tulleners EP, Ross MW, et al. Transendoscopic contact neodymium:yttrium aluminum garnet laser treatment of tympany of the auditory tube diverticulum in two foals. J Am Vet Med Assoc 1994;204:1927.

10. Bell C. Pharyngeal neuromuscular dysfunction associated with bilateral guttural pouch tympany in a foal. Can Vet J 2007;48:192–4.

11. Schambourg MA, Marcoux M, Céleste C. Salpingoscopy for the treatment of recurrent guttural pouch tympany in a filly. Equine Vet Educ 2006;8:231–4.

12. McCue PM, Freeman DE, Donawick WJ. Guttural pouch tympany: 15 cases (1977–1986). J Am Vet Med Assoc 1989;194:1761–3.

13. Milne DW, Fessler JR. Tympanitis of the guttural pouch in a foal. J Am Vet Med Assoc 1972;161:61.

14. Barton AK, Cehak A, Rohn K, et al. Transendoscopic laser surgery to correct nasopharyngeal obstruction caused by head flexion in horses. Vet Surg 2014; 43:418–24.

15. Judy CE, Chaffin MK, Cohen ND. Empyema of the guttural pouch (auditory tube diverticulum) in horses: 91 cases (1977–1997). J Am Vet Med Assoc 1999;215: 1666–70.

16. Rashmir-Raven AM, DeBowes RM, Gift LJ, et al. What is your diagnosis? Upper airway obstruction in a horse caused by pharyngeal perforation during nasogastric intubation. J Am Vet Med Assoc 1991;198:1991–2.

17. Perkins JD, Schumacher J, Kelly G, et al. Standing surgical removal of inspissated guttural pouch exudate (chondroids) in ten horses. Vet Surg 2006;35: 658–62.

18. Fogle CA, Gerard MP, Johansson AM, et al. Spontaneous rupture of the guttural pouch as complication of treatment for guttural pouch empyema. Equine Vet Educ 2007;19:351–5.

19. Freeman DF, Hardy J. Guttural pouch. In: Auer J, Stick J, editors. Equine surgery. 4th edition. St Louis (MO): Saunders; 2012. p. 623–42.

20. Ludwig A, Gatineau S, Reynaud MC, et al. Fungal isolation and identification in 21 cases of guttural pouch mycosis in horses (1998–2002). Vet J 2005;169:457–61.

21. Archer RM, Knight CG, Bishop WJ. Guttural pouch mycosis in six horses in New Zealand. N Z Vet J 2012;60:203–9.

22. Caron JP, Fretz PD, Bailey JV, et al. Balloon-tipped catheter arterial occlusion for prevention of hemorrhage caused by guttural pouch mycosis: 13 causes (1982–1985). J Am Vet Med Assoc 1987;191:345.

23. Church S, Wyn-Jones G, Park AH, et al. Treatment of guttural pouch mycosis. Equine Vet J 1986;18:362.

24. Cook WR. The clinical features of guttural pouch mycosis in the horse. Vet Rec 1968;83:336.

25. Freeman DE, Ross MW, Donawick WJ, et al. Occlusion of the external carotid and maxillary arteries in the horse to prevent hemorrhage from guttural pouch mycosis. Vet Surg 1989;18:39.

26. Greet TR. Outcome of treatment in 35 cases of guttural pouch mycosis. Equine Vet J 1987;19:483.

27. Smith DM, Barber SM. Guttural pouch hemorrhage associated with lesions of the maxillary artery in two horses. Can Vet J 1984;25:239.

28. Lepage OM, Piccot-Crézollet C. Transarterial coil embolisation in 31 horses (1999–2002) with guttural pouch mycosis: a 2-year follow-up. Equine Vet J 2005;37:430–4.
29. Eichentopf A, Snyder A, Recknagel S, et al. Dysphagia caused by focal guttural pouch mycosis: mononeuropathy of the pharyngeal ramus of the vagal nerve in a 20-year-old pony mare. Ir Vet J 2013;66:13–20.
30. Hahn CN. Horner's syndrome in horses. Equine Vet Educ 2003;15:86–90.
31. McMullan WC, Joyce RJ, Hanselka DV, et al. Amphotericin B for the treatment of localized subcutaneous phycomycosis in the horse. J Am Vet Med Assoc 1977; 170:1293.
32. Davis JL. The use of antifungals. Comp Equine 2008;3:128–33.
33. Davis JL, Salmon JH, Papich MG. Pharmacokinetics and tissue distribution of itraconazole after oral and intravenous administration to horses. Am J Vet Res 2005;66:1694–701.
34. Davis EW, Legendre AM. Successful treatment of guttural pouch mycosis with itraconazole and topical enilconazole in a horse. J Vet Intern Med 1994;8:304–5.
35. Korenek NL, Legendre AM, Andrews FM, et al. Treatment of mycotic rhinitis with itraconazole in three horses. J Vet Intern Med 1994;8:224–7.
36. Latimer FG, Colitz CM, Campbell NB, et al. Pharmacokinetics of fluconazole following intravenous and oral administration and body fluid concentrations of fluconazole following repeated oral administration in horses. Am J Vet Res 2001;62: 1606–11.
37. Speirs VC, Harrison IW, van Veenendaal JC, et al. Is specific antifungal therapy necessary for the treatment of guttural pouch mycosis? Equine Vet J 1995;27: 151–2.
38. Ernst NS, Freeman DE, MacKay RJ. Progression of mycosis of the auditory tube diverticulum (guttural pouch) after arterial occlusion in a horse with contralateral temporohyoid osteoarthropathy. J Am Vet Med Assoc 2006;229:1945–8.
39. Blythe LL. Otitis media and interna and temporohyoid osteoarthropathy. Vet Clin North Am Equine Pract 1997;13:21–42.
40. Naylor RJ, Perkins JD, Allen S, et al. Histopathology and computed tomography of age-associated degeneration of the equine temporohyoid joint. Equine Vet J 2010;42:425–30.
41. Grenager NS, Divers TJ, Mohammed HO, et al. Epidemiological features and association with crib-biting in horses with neurological disease associated with temporohyoid osteoarthropathy (1991–2008). Equine Vet Educ 2010;22:467–72.
42. Walker AM, Sellon DC, Cornelisse CJ, et al. Temporohyoid osteoarthropathy in 33 horses (1993–2000). J Vet Intern Med 2002;16:697–703.
43. Palus V, Bladon B, Brazil T, et al. Retrospective study of neurological signs and management of seven English horses with temporohyoid osteoarthropathy. Equine Vet Educ 2012;24:415–22.
44. Hilton H, Puchalski SM, Aleman M. The computed tomographic appearance of equine temporohyoid osteoarthropathy. Vet Radiol Ultrasound 2009;50:151–6.
45. Readford PK, Lester GD, Secombe CJ. Temporohyoid osteoarthropathy in two young horses. Aust Vet J 2013;91:209–12.
46. Blythe LL, Watrous BJ. Temperohyoid osteoarthropathy (middle ear disease). In: Robinson NE, editor. Current therapy in equine medicine. 4th edition. Philadelphia (PA): WB Saunders; 1997. p. 323–5.
47. Blythe LL, Watrous BJ, Schmitz JA, et al. Vestibular syndrome associated with temporohyoid joint fusion and temporal bone fracture in three horses. J Am Vet Med Assoc 1984;185:775.

48. Newton SA, Knottenbelt DC. Vestibular disease in two horses: a case of mycotic otitis media and a case of temporohyoid osteoarthropathy. Vet Rec 1999;145: 142–4.
49. Spurlock SL, Spurlock GH, Wise M. Keratoconjunctivitis sicca associated with fracture of the stylohyoid bone in a horse. J Am Vet Med Assoc 1989;194:258–9.
50. Pease AP, Van Biervliet J, Dykes NL, et al. Complication of partial stylohyoidectomy for treatment of temporohyoid osteoarthropathy and an alternative surgical technique in three cases. Equine Vet J 2004;36:546–50.
51. Divers TJ, Ducharme NG, deLahunta A, et al. Temporohyoid osteoarthropathy. Clin Tech Equine Pract 2006;5:17–23.
52. Bras JJ, Davis E, Beard WL. Bilateral ceratohyoidectomy for the resolution of clinical signs associated with temporohyoid osteoarthropathy. Equine Vet Educ 2014; 26:116–20.
53. Tucker RL, Farrell E. Computed tomography and magnetic resonance imaging of the equine head. Vet Clin North Am Equine Pract 2001;7:131–44.
54. Frame EM, Riihimaki M, Berger M, et al. Scintigraphic findings in a case of temporohyoid osteoarthropathy in a horse. Equine Vet Educ 2005;17:11–5.
55. Aleman M, Puchalski SM, Williams DC, et al. Brainstem auditory-evoked responses in horses with temporohyoid osteoarthropathy. J Vet Intern Med 2008; 22:1196–202.
56. Koch C, Witte T. Clinical Commentary. Temporohyoid osteoarthropathy in the horse. Equine Vet Educ 2014;26:121–5.
57. Hassel DM, Schott HC, Tucker RL, et al. Endoscopy of the auditory tube diverticula in four horses with otitis media/interna. J Am Vet Med Assoc 1995;207: 1081.
58. Maher O, MacDonald MH, Aleman M, et al. Surgical management of temporohyoid osteoarthropathy: 24 cases (1993–2008). Proc Amer Assoc Equine Pract 2008;54:44–5.
59. Sparks HD, Stick JA, Brakenhoff JE, et al. Partial resection of the plica salpingopharyngeus for the treatment of three foals with bilateral tympany of the auditory tube diverticulum (guttural pouch). J Am Vet Med Assoc 2009;235:731–3.
60. Adams S. Median septum fenestration and pharyngeal orifice enlargement for guttural pouch tympany. In: Adams SB, Fessler JF, editors. Atlas of equine surgery. Philadelphia: WB Saunders; 2000. p. 171–3.
61. McIlwraith CW, Robertson JT. In: McIlwraith W, Robertson JT, editors. McIlwraith and Turner's Equine Surgery Advanced Techniques. 2nd Edition. Baltimore (MD): Williams and Wilkins; 1998. p. 261.
62. Sullins KE. Endoscopic application of cutting current for upper respiratory surgery in the standing horse. Proc Am Assoc Equine Pract 1990;36:439–44.
63. Tate LP, Blikslager AT, Little ED. Transendoscopic laser treatment of guttural pouch tympanites in eight foals. Vet Surg 1995;24:367.
64. Krebs W, Schmotzer WB. Laser fenestrated salpingopharyngeal fistulas for treatment of bilateral guttural pouch tympany in a foal. Equine Vet Educ 2007;19:419–23.
65. Freeman DE. Complications of surgery for diseases of the guttural pouch. Vet Clin North Am Equine Pract 2008;24:485–97.
66. Schaaf KL, Kannegiete NJ, Lovell DK. Surgical treatment of extensive chondroid formation in the guttural pouch of a warmblood horse. Aust Vet J 2006;84: 297–300.
67. Verheyen K, Newton JR, Talbot NC, et al. Elimination of guttural pouch infection and inflammation in asymptomatic carriers of Streptococcus equi. Equine Vet J 2000;32:527.

68. Muñoz JA, Stephen J, Baptiste KE, et al. A surgical approach to the lateral compartment of the equine guttural pouch in the standing horse: modification of the forgotten "Garm technique." Vet J 2008;177:260–5.

69. Hawkins JF, Frank N, Sojka JE, et al. Fistulation of the auditory tube diverticulum (guttural pouch) with a neodymium:yttrium-aluminum-garnet laser for treatment of chronic empyema in two horses. J Am Vet Med Assoc 2001;218:405.

70. Gehlen H, Ohnesorge B. Laser fenestration of the mesial septum for treatment of guttural pouch chondroids in a pony. Vet Surg 2005;34:383–6.

71. Freeman DE, Donawick WJ. Occlusion of internal carotid artery in the horse by means of a balloon-tipped catheter: clinical use of a method to prevent epistaxis caused by guttural pouch mycosis. J Am Vet Med Assoc 1980;176:236.

72. Freeman DE, Staller GS, Maxson AD, et al. Unusual internal carotid artery branching that prevented arterial occlusion with a balloon-tipped catheter in a horse. Vet Surg 1993;22:531.

73. Bacon Miller C, Wilson DA, Martin DD, et al. Complications of balloon catheterization associated with aberrant cerebral arterial anatomy in a horse with guttural pouch mycosis. Vet Surg 1998;27:450.

74. Cheramie HS, Pleasant RS, Dabareiner RM, et al. Detachable latex balloon occlusion of an internal carotid artery with an aberrant branch in a horse with guttural pouch (auditory tube diverticulum) mycosis: evaluation of a technique to occlude the internal carotid artery of horses. J Am Vet Med Assoc 2000;216:888–91.

75. MacDonald DG, Fretz PB, Baptiste KE, et al. Anatomic, radiographic and physiologic comparisons of the internal carotid and maxillary artery in the horse. Vet J 1999;158:182–9.

76. Hardy J, Robertson JT, Wilkie DA. Ischemic optic neuropathy and blindness after arterial occlusion for treatment of guttural pouch mycosis in two horses. J Am Vet Med Assoc 1990;196:1631.

77. Cheramie HS, Pleasant RS, Robertson JL, et al. Evaluation of a technique to occlude the internal carotid artery of horses. Vet Surg 1999;28:83.

78. Lévéille R, Hardy J, Robertson JT, et al. Transarterial coil embolization of the internal and external carotid and maxillary arteries for prevention of hemorrhage from guttural pouch mycosis in horses. Vet Surg 2000;29:389–97.

79. Benredouane K, Lepage O. Trans-arterial coil embolization of the internal carotid artery in standing horses. Vet Surg 2012;41:404–9.

80. Delfs KC, Hawkins JF, Hogan DF. Treatment of acute epistaxis secondary to guttural pouch mycosis with transarterial nitinol vascular occlusion plugs in three equids. J Am Vet Med Assoc 2009;235:189–93.

81. Blythe LL, Watrous BJ, Shires GM, et al. Prophylactic partial stylohyoidostectomy for horses with osteoarthropathy of the temporohyoid joint. J Equine Vet Sci 1994; 14:32.

82. O'Brien T, Rodgerson D, Livesey M. Surgical excision of the equine ceratohyoid bone in conscious sedated horses. Vet Surg 2011;40:E40.

Update on Viral Diseases of the Equine Respiratory Tract

James R. Gilkerson, BVSc, BSc (Vet), PhD*,
Kirsten E. Bailey, BVSc (Hons), MANZCVSc,
Andrés Diaz-Méndez, MedVet, MSc, PhD,
Carol A. Hartley, BSc (Hons), PhD

KEYWORDS

- Equine • Herpesvirus • Influenza • Picornavirus • Rhinitis virus • Hendra virus
- Arteritis virus

KEY POINTS

- Viruses are an important cause of serious respiratory disease outbreaks in horses.
- Equine influenza and the equine alphaherpesviruses are the most common causes of viral respiratory disease of horses.
- The role and significance of the equine picornaviruses and the equine gammaherpesviruses are unclear and need further research.
- Hendra virus and African horse sickness virus, although geographically limited in their distribution, cause serious systemic disease in infected horses, which can manifest as respiratory disease.

INTRODUCTION

Respiratory disease is an important clinical manifestation in horses, especially in equine athletes. Respiratory disease has been identified as the second most important cause of lost training days in a survey of wastage in Australian racehorses.[1] In addition to loss of athletic performance, however, respiratory disease is a common cause of morbidity in foals and adult horses and in some cases can also cause death. The horse has several important physical barriers to infection that are important to remember when considering the pathogenesis of equine infectious respiratory diseases. The horse is an obligate nasal airway breather and has a long nasopharynx; thus, all inspired air passes the turbinates, and the turbulence this creates increases the likelihood of particulate matter contacting the upper respiratory mucosa and failing to access the respiratory tract. The epithelium of the upper respiratory tract is primarily

Centre for Equine Infectious Disease, The University of Melbourne, Victoria 3010, Australia
* Corresponding author.
E-mail address: jrgilk@unimelb.edu.au

Vet Clin Equine 31 (2015) 91–104
http://dx.doi.org/10.1016/j.cveq.2014.11.007
0749-0739/15/$ – see front matter © 2015 Elsevier Inc. All rights reserved.

pseudostratified ciliated columnar epithelium. Goblet cells among these epithelial cells secrete mucus into the lumen of the respiratory tract. The combined effect of the beating of the cilia toward the pharynx and mucus secretion onto the epithelial surface is the formation of a mucociliary escalator that serves to trap small particles and propel them back toward the pharynx, where they are swallowed. In addition to physically trapping these particles, the secreted mucus contains a significant concentration of immunoglobulin A if the horse has previously mounted a mucosal immune response; thus, the mucus can neutralize inspired pathogens and prevent infection. The cough reflex is the last physical defense mechanism of the lower respiratory tract. Once pathogens pass the carina and enter the lower respiratory tract, the horse relies on immunologic defenses, such as phagocytosis by alveolar macrophages and the innate and adaptive immune response.

Many viral agents have been associated with respiratory disease of the horse, although the level of evidence of causation for some of these agents is tenuous. Treatment of viral respiratory disease is often supportive. It is hoped that antimicrobial therapy is limited to treatment of bacterial infections. Although there are antiviral agents such as the nucleoside analogues (acyclovir and related agents) for treating herpesvirus infections and the neuraminidase receptor analogues (oseltamivir and zanamivir) for treating influenza infections, for the most part in equine medicine these agents are not widely used and are reserved for use in high-value individuals.

Equine Influenza

Equine influenza (EI) is a highly contagious disease of horses that is endemic in Europe, North and South America, North Africa, the Middle East, and Asia. The contagious nature of equine influenza is best seen when outbreaks occur in countries previously free from influenza. In the 2007 Australian EI outbreak, 76,000 horses were infected during an 18-week outbreak when a Florida Clade I lineage H3N8 EI strain was brought to Australia with a group of breeding stallions from Japan.[2,3] Equine influenza virus is a member of the family Orthomyxoviridae with a segmented, negative-sense, single-stranded RNA genome. The first reported isolate of influenza virus in horses was designated influenza virus A/Equine/Prague/1/56 (H7N7) in 1956[4]; however, another subtype of influenza was isolated from horses in the United States, A/Equine/Miami/1/63 (H3N8) in 1963.[5] Viruses from the H3N8 subtype have been the predominant influenza viruses isolated from horses in recent decades. Although there has been no evidence of any subsequent antigenic shift events (reassortment or recombination), there has been substantial antigenic drift (gradual accumulation of genetic mutations) reported in the currently circulating H3N8 viruses.[6,7] Sporadic outbreaks of disease occur frequently in endemic countries when local herd immunity levels wane, owing to increased numbers of unvaccinated or inadequately vaccinated horses. More serious epidemics occur in endemic regions when an antigenically different virus strain emerges or is introduced, such as occurred with the divergence of Eurasian and American sublineages of H3N8 equine influenza, or when the circulating field strains have undergone sufficient mutation to be different from the vaccine.[8]

Equine influenza is spread primarily by the respiratory route through aerosol and direct contact between infectious and susceptible horses in close proximity, although fomites and the movement of personnel can also contribute to virus spread.[9] The incubation period of EI is a short period, particularly during an outbreak, of between 1 and 3 days. In experimental studies, the incubation period varies between 18 hours and 5 days and is inversely proportional to the inoculating dose of challenge virus.[10] Among fully susceptible horses, the most common clinical signs are sudden onset of fever, serous nasal discharge that progresses to mucopurulent discharge, and coughing.[9] Onset of coughing has been associated with loss of ciliated epithelium of the upper airway of infected horses with consequential loss of mucociliary clearance and accumulation of mucus and bacteria in the airway.[11] Regeneration of this epithelium may take weeks, but horses generally recover from uncomplicated influenza.[9]

In a susceptible population, presumptive diagnosis of equine influenza may be made based on clinical signs, especially coughing, and the rapid spread of disease through the population[9]; however, vaccination may mask the clinical signs of disease. In fully vaccinated racehorses, the predominant clinical sign may be suboptimal performance,[12] and the reduced severity of clinical signs in a group of vaccinated horses delayed the diagnosis of influenza in the racing population in Hong Kong in 1992.[13] A definitive diagnosis can only be made by detection of EI virus in nasal or nasopharyngeal swabs or by demonstration of an increasing antibody titer in affected horses.[9] Although nasal swabs were used extensively during the 2007 Australian outbreak, a recent study comparing nasal and nasopharyngeal swabs found that nasopharyngeal swabs were more sensitive and therefore should be used in surveillance situations, such as in quarantine testing.[14] An antigen capture enzyme-linked immunosorbent assay developed at the Animal Health Trust in Newmarket[15] and reverse transcription polymerase chain reaction (RT-PCR) assays[16,17] are found to be effective and sensitive tools for the diagnosis of EI. Various "horse-side" kits are available, but the sensitivity of these tests is poor compared with either RT-PCR or antigen capture enzyme-linked immunosorbent assay.[14,17,18]

Although antiviral agents specific for influenza are available, they are not widely used in horses. Currently, prophylactic protection by vaccination remains the only effective means of controlling the spread of EI in endemic countries. Vaccination of highly mobile subpopulations, such as racehorses, is widely practiced in many endemic countries, and many racing authorities and other competition organizers have mandatory vaccination policies.[9] A variety of live attenuated, cold-adapted, inactivated and recombinant vector EI vaccines are available commercially. Much of the efficacy data supporting the use of influenza vaccines have been based on small-scale experimental challenge studies. Although limited in study population size, experimental challenge studies have repeatedly found a strong correlation between antibody levels and protective immunity against subsequent infection with antigenically homologous field isolates.[19] Studies from large-scale field outbreaks have confirmed the efficacy of influenza vaccines against antigenically similar strains.[19–21] During the 2007 Australian outbreak, the recombinant canarypox vector was used because of the rapid onset of immunity after one dose[22] and the potential DIVA (differentiation of infected and vaccinated animals) capacity that facilitated the subsequent declaration of freedom from disease.

Equine Alphaherpesviruses

Herpesviruses are enveloped double-stranded DNA viruses that infect an enormous diversity of animal species. Five equid herpesviruses (EHV) have been isolated from horses. Of these viruses, the alphaherpesviruses EHV-1 and EHV-4 are both respiratory tract pathogens that have been associated with outbreaks of respiratory disease, and EHV-1 also causes outbreaks of abortion and, less frequently, neurologic disease.[23]

EHV-1 and EHV-4 are well-recognized respiratory pathogens of horses. Both of these viruses are transmitted via the respiratory route and undergo primary replication in the upper respiratory tract epithelium. EHV-4 is predominantly a local pathogen of the respiratory tract and causes a rhinopharyngitis and tracheobronchitis. EHV-1 respiratory disease is clinically indistinguishable from that caused by EHV-4; however, EHV-1 spreads rapidly beyond the respiratory tract to become a systemic infection.[24,25] Abortion and neurologic disease associated with EHV-1 infection are direct sequelae of vasculitis in response to the systemic spread of this virus. The clinical signs of EHV-1 and EHV-4 respiratory disease are profuse serous nasal discharge that becomes mucopurulent in character with secondary bacterial infection, enlarged submandibular lymph nodes, and occasional ocular discharge. Microscopically, there is necrosis of the respiratory epithelium with inflammatory infiltration of the terminal bronchioles and the surrounding parenchyma. EHV-1/4 respiratory disease spreads rapidly from horse to horse, and few in-contact susceptible horses escape infection.[26,27] Clinical signs of EHV-1/4 respiratory disease are most severe in young horses, and outbreaks of rhinopneumonitis have been characteristically reported in young foals after weaning. EHV-4, not EHV-1, is more commonly isolated from horses during outbreaks of respiratory disease.[21,22] These viruses also cause disease in adult horses. In Japan, EHV-1 was isolated from racehorses with respiratory disease in the winter months, whereas in the same study, EHV-4 was isolated from horses of all ages with clinical signs of respiratory disease regardless of the season.[28]

As with all other herpesviruses, EHV-1 and EHV-4 establish latent infections in the horse,[29,30] and these horses then become carriers of these viruses for life. Latency is central to the epidemiology of these viruses, as this is the main mechanism by which herpesviruses evade the host's immune response and persist and propagate within the population. Latently infected horses can reactivate an EHV-1 or EHV-4 infection during periods of stress, and this recrudescent virus is then shed from the respiratory tract to infect other in-contact susceptible horses. The epidemiology of EHV-1 and EHV-4 is complicated and is probably best understood in the broodmare and foal population.[31,32] Early epidemiologic studies did not differentiate between EHV-1 and EHV-4; thus, their results should be interpreted with caution. Serologic evidence collected over several seasons (in vaccinated and unvaccinated horses) suggests that foals are infected with EHV-1 at an early age and that the most likely source is their dam.[31–33] EHV-1 infection spreads between foals within the mare and foal population before weaning and continues to spread among weanlings. These serologic studies are supported by detection of EHV-1 by PCR from nasal swab samples collected from suckling foals between 22 and 58 days of age.[34] These studies were designed to elaborate the epidemiology of EHV-1 and EHV-4 transmission within a mare and foal herd and thus did not make any attempt to show any association between EHV-1 or EHV-4 infection and clinical respiratory disease. However, previous studies found that EHV-4 was more likely to be isolated from the respiratory tract of weanling foals with signs of respiratory disease, such as copious serous or mucopurulent nasal discharge, than from weanling foals with no signs of disease.[35] Although there is little debate that EHV-1 and EHV-4 are serious pathogens of horses on breeding farms, their significance as pathogens of racing and other performance horses is not as completely understood as previously thought and remains a subject for future research. Inactivated and attenuated vaccines containing EHV-1 and EHV-4 have been released commercially and have been extensively used in racing stables and breeding herds. A widely used inactivated vaccine has been experimentally found to reduce the severity of EHV-1 respiratory disease[36] and is registered with this claim. Much of the evidence for the efficacy of EHV-1 and EHV-4 vaccines has been derived from experimental challenge studies rather than extensive field trials.[19] There is published evidence that inactivated vaccines reduce the likelihood of EHV-1 abortion and the severity and duration of EHV-1 and EHV-4 respiratory disease,[37] but little data are available to evaluate the efficacy of other EHV-1 vaccines.[19]

Equine Gammaherpesviruses

The equine gammaherpesviruses, EHV-2 and EHV-5, are closely related viruses that were first differentiated by genomic restriction profiles in 1987.[38] These viruses have been detected in horse populations worldwide, including from horses in Iceland where the horse population has been isolated for more than 1000 years.[39] Herpesviruses and their hosts have been coevolving for more than 200 million years, and gammaherpesviruses in particular have evolved many immune evasion strategies. After inhalation, the virus infects nasal mucosal cells of the upper respiratory tract and B lymphocytes[40–42] probably at the site of draining lymphoid tissue.[40] Virus is disseminated systemically after infected B lymphocytes enter the circulation. After infection, the immune system often fails to completely eliminate the infection, and the virus establishes a latent infection. Latency is a characteristic feature of all herpesviruses and enables virus to be shed throughout the lifetime of the host. EHV-2 is latent in B lymphocytes, macrophages, and possibly Langerhans cells,[41,43,44] whereas the sites of latency for EHV-5 are unknown. EHV-2 and likely EHV-5 contain a range of immunomodulatory genes that interact with the immune system of the host,[45] and this is suggested to compromise host immunity and increase susceptibility of the host to opportunistic infections.[40,46–50]

Epidemiologic studies of these viruses are complicated by the high rate of infection in the population and the range of clinical signs associated with detection of these viruses. Infection with EHV-2 seems to occur early in life, with evidence of infection in foals as young as 2 to 4 months of age.[51] Infection with EHV-5 seems to occur later in the life of the foal,[42,52] although EHV-5 DNA has been detected in nasal swabs from foals as young as 1 month.[51] Definitive diagnosis and establishment of a causal association between infection and disease remains challenging, as these viruses are readily detected in clinical samples collected from horses with and without clinical signs of respiratory disease. Infections of foals with EHV-2 have been more frequently associated with disease than those in adult horses. Infection of foals in natural and experimental field settings has been associated with mild to severe pharyngitis with or without lymphadenopathy and rhinitis or pyrexia.[50,53–56] Evidence from natural and experimental field settings is also consistent with a role for EHV-2 in the pathogenesis of keratoconjunctivitis in foals and yearlings following immunosuppressive doses of dexamethasone.[54,57] Few studies describe comparative investigations with normal/unaffected horses. EHV-2 and EHV-5 have been detected in cases of pneumonia, granulomatous dermatitis, dermatitis, and oral and esophageal ulcers and in horses with poor performance and aborted fetuses.[46,56,58–63]

More investigations are examining the role of EHV-5 (alone or in association with EHV-2 or asinine herpesvirus 5) in the development of equine multinodular pulmonary fibrosis (EMPF). Cases of EMPF have multiple coalescing nodules of fibrosis in the lung with histologic evidence of interstitial fibrosis and pneumonia with infiltrations of mixed inflammatory cells such as neutrophils and macrophages.[64–70] EHV-5 has been detected in bronchoalveolar lavage and postmortem tissue from these cases. The highest loads of EHV-5 were detected in the most severe EMPF lesions compared with moderate lesions and draining lymph nodes.[66] However, it is not yet clear whether EHV-5 caused the EMPF lesions or whether the environment in the lung caused by EMPF resulted in recruitment of cells infected with EHV-5. Careful comparison with equine gammaherpesvirus detection in unaffected horses is required. Recently, the experimental induction of EMPF has been described after inoculation with EHV-5 containing cultures derived from EMPF lesions.[71] Although this finding certainly adds evidence for a causal relationship, the low-level detection of EHV-5 in lesions compared with that in other studies, combined with the inability to detect EHV-5 sequences consistent with the EHV-5 inoculum (in all but one sample), suggest further work is required to clarify whether EHV-5 load is potentiated by the EMPF lesions rather than the direct cause.

There are few reports of vaccine development for these viruses, possibly because of their ubiquitous nature and the limitations of the evidence defining disease causation. A vaccine has been described for EHV2 as a cofactor in disease, in which vaccination with EHV2 either with or without *Rhodococcus equi* was reported to protect horses from *R equi* pneumonia.[46,72] Some nucleoside analogue therapy has ameliorated disease signs attributed to EHV2, such as conjunctivitis in young foals.[57,73,74] Successful treatments of EMPF with acyclovir and valacyclovir have also been reported.[70,75]

Equine Picornaviruses

The equine picornaviruses, equine rhinitis A virus (ERAV), and equine rhinitis B virus (ERBV), were formerly known as equine rhinoviruses. ERAV, (formerly equine rhinovirus 1) has been assigned to the genus *Aphthovirus*, ERBV1 (formerly equine rhinovirus 2), ERBV2 (formerly equine rhinovirus 3), and ERBV3 (formerly acid-stable picornavirus) have been included in the genus *Erbovirus*.[76–79] Both ERAV and ERBV have been implicated as a cause of respiratory disease in horses[80,81]; however, the true role of these viruses as a primary cause of disease in their own right remains to be fully described. Recent investigations found that these viruses are directly associated with respiratory disease[82] and, more importantly, associated with respiratory and urinary shedding and persistent infections.[83]

Equine picornaviruses have been detected not only from diseased horses, but also from clinically normal animals.[84,85] It has been hypothesized that horses are exposed to these viruses via aerosol or direct contact early in life. Generally, these viruses are isolated from the respiratory tract and in some occasions from other organs. Importantly, ERAV is shed in the urine of infected horses.[83,85,86] ERAV experimental intranasal infection induced clinical respiratory signs in the horse, characterized by nasal discharge, pyrexia, and viremia that lasted 4 to 5 days.[87] Additionally, in this study, the virus was isolated from the feces of infected horses. Only ERAV has been recovered from samples other than respiratory secretions, whereas ERBV1 and ERBV2 seem to be recovered exclusively from respiratory samples. In a more recent experimental study, it was confirmed that ERAV induces not only clinical upper respiratory disease but also induces changes in the lower airways.[82] Horses in these experiments showed increased body temperature for up to 6 days, submandibular lymphadenopathy, abnormal lung sounds, increased amounts of tracheal and bronchial mucoid secretions, increased nasal discharge, and hyperemia in the lower trachea and large bronchi. Additionally, increased tracheal and bronchial mucoid secretions were endoscopically detectable up to days 21 after infection. Equine picornavirus infection is diagnosed by detection of a serologic response or by detection of the virus by culture- or PCR-based testing. A serum antibody response is first detected 4 to 7 days after infection, and this response is commonly associated with a decrease in the severity of the clinical signs. Serum samples are collected at least 10 to 14 days apart and analyzed as paired sera using the viral neutralization test. A 4-fold increase in antibody titers in paired samples is considered significant; however, these changes are time dependent and should be carefully interpreted. Nasopharyngeal swabs are best collected from suspected infected horses within 24 to 36 hours of infection to detect or isolate the virus. Although virus isolation is considered highly sensitive, drawbacks such as price and turnaround time limit its reliability. The use of molecular techniques, such as PCR and RT-PCR has become more popular in the last decade because of high sensitivity, cost, and turnaround times.[86,88,89] Vaccination against ERAV or ERVB has not been performed in the past; however, recently a commercial ERAV vaccine became available in the United States.

Equine Arteritis

Equine arteritis virus (EAV) was first identified as the cause of abortion and respiratory disease, equine viral arteritis (EVA), in horses during an extensive outbreak of these diseases on a farm near Bucyrus, Ohio, in 1953.[90] Since then, serologic surveys have reported EAV infection in many countries worldwide. The only countries in which EAV has not been serologically detected are Iceland, Singapore, and Japan.[91] EAV is highly species specific, and infection is limited to species of the family *Equidae*, such as horses, donkeys, mules, and zebra.[92] EVA is a respiratory and reproductive disease, although the clinical signs can vary considerably, depending on host factors (such as age and reproductive status), route of infection, and the virulence of the challenge strain.[92] Respiratory infection occurs by inhalation of infectious aerosols or by contact with infected horses or aborted fetuses and membranes. Initial viral replication occurs in respiratory tract epithelium. EAV is spread within the lungs within days of infection and spreads via the bronchial lymph nodes to the bloodstream. Viremia is established rapidly, and viral replication in macrophages and in endothelium results in a high virus titer in the blood and this virus can cross the placenta. Replication in the endothelial cells results in segmental necrosis of small arteries throughout the body and is associated with the clinical signs of edema and abortion. The incubation period of EAV is 3 to 14 days (typically, 6–8 days after venereal infection).[93] Most EAV infections are subclinical; however, acutely diseased animals may exhibit clinical signs predominantly associated with edema or respiratory disease.[91] Outbreaks of abortion between 3 and 10 months of gestation follow EVA respiratory disease in groups of pregnant mares. Modified live and killed vaccines are available, but because disease occurrences are so uncommon, the need for vaccination is often doubtful. Identification of carrier stallions is the key to controlling the spread of EVA along with the isolation of any mares covered by these stallions for a period of 4 weeks. Carrier stallions should be prevented from mating or be restricted to covering seropositive or vaccinated mares. Vaccination has been used, particularly in the United States, to prevent infection of colts intended for breeding purposes and for prevention of abortion. The modified live vaccine has not been recommended for use in pregnant mares, especially in the last 2 months of gestation, although a recent study suggests that this practice may be safe.[94]

Hendra Virus

Hendra virus causes severe, peracute respiratory disease in some affected horses. Hendra virus (then called equine morbillivirus) was first recognized in 1994 as a cause of severe acute respiratory disease of horses with a high mortality rate.[95,96] Since then, there have been numerous further outbreaks reported in horses, in most of which only a single horse was affected. Hendra virus is the most important infectious disease of horses in Australia because of the high mortality rate in affected horses and the catastrophic consequence of zoonotic transmission of this virus to people. In total, 7 human cases of Hendra have been reported, 4 of them fatal.[97] Veterinarians and staff are the group that is most at risk from this virus. To date, 3 of the 7 human cases have been veterinarians (2 fatal) and another 2 cases involved people assisting veterinarians, (1 was a veterinary nurse working in an equine hospital and the other was assisting an equine postmortem examination).

The natural hosts of Hendra virus are the 4 mainland species of Australian pteropid fruit bats[98]; however, the exact mechanism of transmission of virus from bats to other mammalian species is unknown. Hendra virus circulates within bat populations, generally with no disease manifestations after experimental infection.[98] Hendra virus has been detected in fetal and neonatal lung and from uterine fluid and renal tissue of adult bats.[98–100] Collection of urine and feces from beneath flying fox roosting sites has found that Hendra virus is excreted in detectable titers in these body fluids[101] and is a likely source of virus for transmission to other animal species.

The exact mechanism of pathogenesis of Hendra virus disease in horses and the reasons why the clinical signs range from respiratory disease to neurologic disease, with some horses showing vague nonspecific signs of disease, are not clear, and studies in this area are hindered by the difficulties involved in working with horses under Biosecurity level 4 conditions. Experimental infection studies of horses have found that viral RNA is detectable in clinical samples before the onset of clinical signs, although no infectious virus was isolated at this time.[102] Horses in these studies had clinical signs and were euthanized. Importantly, samples collected during postmortem investigations yielded high titers of infectious virus from a wide range of tissue types, which reinforces the need for extreme caution and the use of effective personal protective equipment when conducting a necropsy examination on horses suspected of being infected with Hendra. To date, there have been no reported bat-to-human cases of Hendra virus infection; all of the known cases of Hendra in humans have been associated with equine clinical cases.[97] A vaccine that contains recombinant Hendra virus glycoprotein G, which induces virus-neutralizing antibodies that were protective in a laboratory animal model of Hendra virus infection, has been recently released.[103,104] In experimental challenge trials of the vaccine in horses, 2 doses of commercially formulated recombinant glycoprotein G prevented infection in 7 of 7 horses exposed to an otherwise lethal dose of Hendra virus.[105] Currently, vaccination is the single most effective way of reducing the risk of Hendra virus infection in horses, with the corollary that it is also the single most effective way to reduce the risk of Hendra virus infection in humans.

African Horse Sickness

From a global perspective, African horse sickness (AHS) is a serious threat to the horse industry. Historically, AHS is associated with sub-Saharan Africa; however, outbreaks in the Middle East and India in the late 1950s[100] and as far afield as Spain in the 1980s[101,102] clearly found that this disease is not geographically restricted. Although outbreaks outside of southern Africa can be generally traced back to movement of infected horses, several outbreaks in North Africa have occurred in which this link was not established.[103] AHS is an infectious, but not contagious, disease that is transmitted by biting midges, of which Culicoides imicola and bolitinos are the most important vector species. Spread of AHS can occur as a result of wind-borne spread of infected vectors.[104] Nine serotypes of AHS virus have been reported, and there is little or no serologic cross-protection between serotypes. African horse sickness virus is an orbivirus of the Reovirus family and as such infects the vascular endothelium and causes lesions associated with vascular fragility. There are 3 forms of febrile illness associated with AHS virus infection: a peracute pulmonary form (Dunkop), subacute cardiac form (Dikkop) and a milder form of disease (horse sickness fever). Most clinical cases are a mixture of the cardiac and pulmonary form, although this is usually only apparent on postmortem examination.[105] Outbreaks of AHS are seasonal in nature and correspond to peaks in the invertebrate host population. In general, outbreaks in South Africa begin in February, peak in March and April, and decline in frequency in May as the weather gets colder. Currently, the only licensed vaccine available in South Africa is a polyvalent-modified live virus vaccine (Onderstepoort Biological Products) that contains 7 of the 9 serotypes. Although the

World Organisation for Animal Health (OIE) Manual of Diagnostic Tests and Vaccines for Terrestrial Animals lists virus isolation from whole blood as the only diagnostic test for detecting the virus, there are commercial quantitative group-specific RT-PCR tests available that can provide a diagnosis in less than 48 hours (Guthrie AJ, Personal Communication 2014). This test is currently being validated for inclusion in the OIE manual. A similar quantitative RT-PCR test to distinguish the serotype of the AHSV isolate is also currently being used and validated in South Africa.

SUMMARY

Viral respiratory disease is an important cause of morbidity in horses; however, the reliance on virus isolation in cell culture and the often transient nature of virus shedding has limited the historical importance placed on individual viruses. The advent of molecular diagnostic techniques for many of these agents may allow veterinary researchers to more fully describe the prevalence of these viruses in outbreaks of respiratory disease in performance horses and better describe their role in the pathogenesis of equine respiratory disease.

REFERENCES

1. Bailey CJ, Rose RJ, Reid SW, et al. Wastage in the Australian thoroughbred racing industry: a survey of Sydney trainers. Aust Vet J 1997;75(1):64–6.
2. Sovinova O, Tumova B, Pouska F, et al. Isolation of a virus causing respiratory disease in horses. Acta Virol 1958;2:52–61.
3. Waddell GH, Teigland MB, Sigel MM. A new influenza virus associated with equine respiratory disease. J Am Vet Med Assoc 1963;143:587–90.
4. Daly JM, Lai AC, Binns MM, et al. Antigenic and genetic evolution of equine H3N8 influenza A viruses. J Gen Virol 1996;77(Pt 4):661–71.
5. Lai AC, Chambers TM, Holland RE Jr, et al. Diverged evolution of recent equine-2 influenza (H3N8) viruses in the Western Hemisphere. Arch Virol 2001;146(6): 1063–74.
6. Wood J, Smith K, Daly J, et al. Viral infections of the equine respiratory tract. In: McGorum B, Dixon P, Robinson N, et al, editors. Equine respiratory medicine and surgery. Philadelphia: Saunders Elsevier; 2007. p. 287–326.
7. Cullinane A, Newton JR. Equine influenza–a global perspective. Vet Microbiol 2013;167(1–2):205–14.
8. Mumford JA, Hannant D, Jessett DM. Experimental infection of ponies with equine influenza (H3N8) viruses by intranasal inoculation or exposure to aerosols. Equine Vet J 1990;22(2):93–8.
9. Willoughby R, Ecker G, McKee S, et al. The effects of equine rhinovirus, influenza virus and herpesvirus infection on tracheal clearance rate in horses. Can J Vet Res 1992;56(2):115–21.
10. Mumford JA, Rossdale PD. Virus and its relationship to the "poor performance" syndrome. Equine Vet J 1980;12(1):3–9.
11. Powell DG, Watkins KL, Li PH, et al. Outbreak of equine influenza among horses in Hong Kong during 1992. Vet Rec 1995;136(21):531–6.
12. Paillot R, Prowse L, Montesso F, et al. Duration of equine influenza virus shedding and infectivity in immunised horses after experimental infection with EIV A/eq2/Richmond/1/07. Vet Microbiol 2013;166(1–2):22–34.
13. Livesay GJ, O'Neill T, Hannant D, et al. The outbreak of equine influenza (H3N8) in the United Kingdom in 1989: diagnostic use of an antigen capture ELISA. Vet Rec 1993;133(21):515–9.

14. Kirkland PD, Davis RJ, Gu X, et al. Application of high-throughput systems for the rapid detection of DNA and RNA viruses during the Australian equine influenza outbreak. Aust Vet J 2011;89(Suppl 1):38–9.

15. Quinlivan M, Dempsey E, Ryan F, et al. Real-time reverse transcription PCR for detection and quantitative analysis of equine influenza virus. J Clin Microbiol 2005;43(10):5055–7.

16. Quinlivan M, Cullinane A, Nelly M, et al. Comparison of sensitivities of virus isolation, antigen detection, and nucleic acid amplification for detection of equine influenza virus. J Clin Microbiol 2004;42(2):759–63.

17. Edlund Toulemonde C, Daly J, Sindle T, et al. Efficacy of a recombinant equine influenza vaccine against challenge with an American lineage H3N8 influenza virus responsible for the 2003 outbreak in the United Kingdom. Vet Rec 2005; 156(12):367–71.

18. Slater J. Equine herpesviruses. In: Sellon DC, Long MT, editors. Equine infectious diseases. St Louis (MO): Elsevier; 2007. p. 134–53.

19. Kydd JH, Smith KC, Hannant D, et al. Distribution of equid herpesvirus-1 (EHV-1) in respiratory tract associated lymphoid tissue: implications for cellular immunity. Equine Vet J 1994;26(6):470–3.

20. Kydd JH, Smith KC, Hannant D, et al. Distribution of equid herpesvirus-1 (EHV-1) in the respiratory tract of ponies: implications for vaccination strategies. Equine Vet J 1994;26(6):466–9.

21. Burrows R, Goodridge D. Experimental studies on equine herpesvirus type-1 infections. J Reprod Fertil 1975;23:611–5.

22. Allen GP, Bryans JT. Molecular epizootiology, pathogenesis and prophylaxis of equine herpesvirus-1 infections. In: Pandey R, editor. Progress in veterinary microbiology and immunology, vol. 2. Basel (Switzerland): S. Karger; 1986. p. 78–144.

23. Matsumura T, Sugiura T, Imagawa H, et al. Epizootiological aspects of type 1 and type 4 equine herpesvirus infections among horse populations. J Vet Med Sci 1992;54:207–11.

24. Edington N, Bridges CG, Huckle A. Experimental reactivation of equid herpesvirus 1 (EHV 1) following the administration of corticosteroids. Equine Vet J 1985;17:369–72.

25. Browning GF, Bulach DM, Ficorilli N, et al. Latency of equine herpesvirus 4 (equine rhinopneumonitis virus). Vet Rec 1988;123:518–9.

26. Gilkerson J, Whalley JM, Drummer HE, et al. Epidemiology of EHV-1 and EHV-4 in the mare and foal populations on a Hunter Valley stud farm: are mares the source of EHV-1 for unweaned foals. Vet Microbiol 1999;68(1–2):27–34.

27. Gilkerson J, Whalley JM, Drummer HE, et al. Epidemiological studies of equine herpesvirus 1 (EHV-1) in Thoroughbred foals: a reveiw of studies conducted in the Hunter Valley of New South Wales between 1995 and 1997. Vet Microbiol 1999;68(1–2):15–25.

28. Foote CE, Gilkerson J, Whalley JM, et al. Seroprevalence of equine herpesvirus 1 in mares and foals on a large hunter Valley stud farm in years pre- and post-vaccination. Aust Vet J 2003;81(5):283–8.

29. Foote CE, Love DN, Gilkerson JR, et al. Detection of EHV-1 and EHV-4 DNA in unweaned Thoroughbred foals from vaccinated mares on a large stud farm. Equine Vet J 2004;36(4):341–5.

30. Gilkerson J, Jorm LR, Love DN, et al. Epidemiologic investigation of equid herpesvirus 4 (EHV-4) excretion assessed by nasal swabs taken from thoroughbred foals. Vet Microbiol 1994;39:275–83.

31. Heldens JG, Hannant D, Cullinane AA, et al. Clinical and virological evaluation of the efficacy of an inactivated EHV1 and EHV4 whole virus vaccine (Duvaxyn EHV1,4). Vaccination/challenge experiments in foals and pregnant mares. Vaccine 2001;19(30):4307–17.
32. Browning GF, Studdert MJ. Genomic heterogeneity of equine betaherpesviruses. J Gen Virol 1987;68(Pt 5):1441–7.
33. Hartley CA, Dynon KJ, Mekuria ZH, et al. Equine gammaherpesviruses: perfect parasites? Vet Microbiol 2013;167(1–2):86–92.
34. Allen GP, Murray MJ. In: Coetzer J, Tustin R, editors. Infectious diseases of livestock. Cape Town (South Africa): Oxford Press; 2004. p. 860–7.
35. Drummer HE, Reubel GH, Studdert MJ. Equine gammaherpesvirus 2 (EHV2) is latent in B lymphocytes. Arch Virol 1996;141(3–4):495–504.
36. Nordengrahn A, Merza M, Ros C, et al. Prevalence of equine herpesvirus types 2 and 5 in horse populations by using type-specific PCR assays. Vet Res 2002; 33(3):251–9.
37. Bell SA, Balasuriya UB, Nordhausen RW, et al. Isolation of equine herpesvirus-5 from blood mononuclear cells of a gelding. J Vet Diagn Invest 2006;18(5):472–5.
38. Dutta SK, Campbell DL. Pathogenicity of equine herpesvirus: in vivo persistence in equine tissue macrophages of herpesviuus type 2 detected in monolayer macrophage cell culture. Am J Vet Res 1978;39(9):1422–7.
39. Telford EA, Watson MS, Aird HC, et al. The DNA sequence of equine herpesvirus 2. J Mol Biol 1995;249(3):520–8.
40. Nordengrahn A, Rusvai M, Merza M, et al. Equine herpesvirus type 2 (EHV-2) as a predisposing factor for Rhodococcus equi pneumonia in foals: prevention of the bifactorial disease with EHV-2 immunostimulating complexes. Vet Microbiol 1996;51(1–2):55–68.
41. Purewal AS, Smallwood AV, Kaushal A, et al. Identification and control of the cis-acting elements of the immediate early gene of equid herpesvirus type 1. J Gen Virol 1992;73(Pt 3):513–9.
42. Welch HM, Bridges CG, Lyon AM, et al. Latent equid herpesviruses 1 and 4: detection and distinction using the polymerase chain reaction and co-cultivation from lymphoid tissues. J Gen Virol 1992;73(Pt 2):261–8.
43. Borchers K, Wolfinger U, Goltz M, et al. Distribution and relevance of equine herpesvirus type 2 (EHV-2) infections. Arch Virol 1997;142(5):917–28.
44. Murray MJ, Eichorn ES, Dubovi EJ, et al. Equine herpesvirus type 2: prevalence and seroepidemiology in foals. Equine Vet J 1996;28(6):432–6.
45. Bell SA, Balasuriya UB, Gardner IA, et al. Temporal detection of equine herpesvirus infections of a cohort of mares and their foals. Vet Microbiol 2006;116(4): 249–57.
46. Dunowska M, Wilks CR, Studdert MJ, et al. Equine respiratory viruses in foals in New Zealand. N Z Vet J 2002;50(4):140–7.
47. Blakeslee JR Jr, Olsen RG, McAllister ES, et al. Evidence of respiratory tract infection induced by equine herpesvirus, type 2, in the horse. Can J Microbiol 1975;21(12):1940–6.
48. Borchers K, Wolfinger U, Ludwig H, et al. Virological and molecular biological investigations into equine herpes virus type 2 (EHV-2) experimental infections. Virus Res 1998;55(1):101–6.
49. Dunowska M, Wilks CR, Studdert MJ, et al. Viruses associated with outbreaks of equine respiratory disease in New Zealand. N Z Vet J 2002;50(4):132–9.
50. Fu ZF, Robinson AJ, Horner GW, et al. Respiratory disease in foals and the epizootiology of equine herpesvirus type 2 infection. N Z Vet J 1986;34(9):152–5.

51. Collinson P, O'Rielly JL, Ficorilli N, et al. Isolation of equine herpesvirus type 2 (equine gammaherpesvirus 2) from foals with keratoconjunctivitis. J Am Vet Med Assoc 1994;205(2):329–31.

52. Dunowska M, Howe L, Hanlon D, et al. Kinetics of Equid herpesvirus type 2 infections in a group of Thoroughbred foals. Vet Microbiol 2011;152(1–2):176–80.

53. Studdert MJ. Comparative aspects of equine herpesviruses. Cornell Vet 1974; 64(1):94–122.

54. Galosi CM, de la Paz VC, Fernandez LC, et al. Isolation of equine herpesvirus-2 from the lung of an aborted fetus. J Vet Diagn Invest 2005;17(5):500–2.

55. Herder V, Barsnick R, Walliser U, et al. Equid herpesvirus 5-associated dermatitis in a horse–Resembling herpes-associated erythema multiforme. Vet Microbiol 2012;155(2–4):420–4.

56. Sledge DG, Miller DL, Styer EL, et al. Equine herpesvirus 2-associated granulomatous dermatitis in a horse. Vet Pathol 2006;43(4):548–52.

57. Vengust M, Baird JD, van Dreumel T, et al. Equid herpesvirus 2-associated oral and esophageal ulceration in a foal. J Vet Diagn Invest 2008;20(6):811–5.

58. Back H, Kendall A, Grandon R, et al. Equine Multinodular Pulmonary Fibrosis in association with asinine herpesvirus type 5 and equine herpesvirus type 5: a case report. Acta Vet Scand 2012;54(1):57.

59. Dunowska M, Hardcastle MR, Tonkin FB. Identification of the first New Zealand case of equine multinodular pulmonary fibrosis. N Z Vet J 2014;62(4):226–31.

60. Marenzoni ML, Passamonti F, Lepri E, et al. Quantification of Equid herpesvirus 5 DNA in clinical and necropsy specimens collected from a horse with equine multinodular pulmonary fibrosis. J Vet Diagn Invest 2011;23(4):802–6.

61. Niedermaier G, Poth T, Gehlen H. Clinical aspects of multinodular pulmonary fibrosis in two warmblood horses. Vet Rec 2010;166(14):426–30.

62. Soare T, Leeming G, Morgan R, et al. Equine multinodular pulmonary fibrosis in horses in the UK. Vet Rec 2011;169(12):313.

63. Williams KJ, Maes R, Del Piero F, et al. Equine multinodular pulmonary fibrosis: a newly recognized herpesvirus-associated fibrotic lung disease. Vet Pathol 2007; 44(6):849–62.

64. Wong DM, Belgrave RL, Williams KJ, et al. Multinodular pulmonary fibrosis in five horses. J Am Vet Med Assoc 2008;232(6):898–905.

65. Williams KJ, Robinson NE, Lim A, et al. Experimental induction of pulmonary fibrosis in horses with the gammaherpesvirus equine herpesvirus 5. PLoS One 2013;8(10):e77754.

66. Varga J, Fodor L, Rusvai M, et al. Prevention of Rhodococcus equi pneumonia of foals using two different inactivated vaccines. Vet Microbiol 1997;56(3–4): 205–12.

67. Kershaw O, von Oppen T, Glitz F, et al. Detection of equine herpesvirus type 2 (EHV-2) in horses with keratoconjunctivitis. Virus Res 2001;80(1–2):93–9.

68. Thein P, Bohm D. Etiology and clinical aspects of a viral keratoconjunctivitis in foals. Zentralbl Veterinarmed B 1976;23(5–6):507–19 [in German].

69. Schwarz B, Schwendenwein I, van den Hoven R. Successful outcome in a case of equine multinodular pulmonary fibrosis (EMPF) treated with valacyclovir. Equine Vet Educ 2013;25(8):389–92.

70. Black WD, Hartley CA, Ficorilli NP, et al. Sequence variation divides Equine rhinitis B virus into three distinct phylogenetic groups that correlate with serotype and acid stability. J Gen Virol 2005;86(Pt 8):2323–32.

71. Hartley CA, Ficorilli N, Dynon K, et al. Equine rhinitis A virus: structural proteins and immune response. J Gen Virol 2001;82(Pt 7):1725–8.

72. Horsington JJ, Gilkerson JR, Hartley CA. Identification of mixed equine rhinitis B virus infections leading to further insight on the relationship between genotype, serotype and acid stability phenotype. Virus Res 2011;155(2):506–13.
73. Li F, Browning GF, Studdert MJ, et al. Equine rhinovirus 1 is more closely related to foot-and-mouth disease virus than to other picornaviruses. Proc Natl Acad Sci U S A 1996;93(3):990–5.
74. Carman S, Rosendal S, Huber L, et al. Infectious agents in acute respiratory disease in horses in Ontario. J Vet Diagn Invest 1997;9(1):17–23.
75. Diaz-Mendez A, Viel L, Hewson J, et al. Surveillance of equine respiratory viruses in Ontario. Can J Vet Res 2010;74(4):271–8.
76. Diaz-Mendez A, Hewson J, Shewen P, et al. Characteristics of respiratory tract disease in horses inoculated with equine rhinitis A virus. Am J Vet Res 2014; 75(2):169–78.
77. Lynch SE, Gilkerson JR, Symes SJ, et al. Persistence and chronic urinary shedding of the aphthovirus equine rhinitis A virus. Comp Immunol Microbiol Infect Dis 2013;36(1):95–103.
78. Dynon K, Black WD, Ficorilli N, et al. Detection of viruses in nasal swab samples from horses with acute, febrile, respiratory disease using virus isolation, polymerase chain reaction and serology. Aust Vet J 2007;85(1–2):46–50.
79. McCollum WH, Timoney PJ. Studies on the seroprevalence and frequency of equine rhinovirus-I and -II infection in normal horse urine. Paper presented at: Cambridge(United Kingdom): Equine Infectious Diseases VI. July 7–11, 1991, 1992.
80. Quinlivan M, Maxwell G, Lyons P, et al. Real-time RT-PCR for the detection and quantitative analysis of equine rhinitis viruses. Equine Vet J 2010;42(2):98–104.
81. Plummer G. An equine respiratory virus with enterovirus properties. Nature 1962;195:519–20.
82. Black WD, Wilcox RS, Stevenson RA, et al. Prevalence of serum neutralising antibody to equine rhinitis A virus (ERAV), equine rhinitis B virus 1 (ERBV1) and ERBV2. Vet Microbiol 2007;119(1):65–71.
83. Dynon K, Varrasso A, Ficorilli N, et al. Identification of equine herpesvirus 3 (equine coital exanthema virus), equine gammaherpesviruses 2 and 5, equine adenoviruses 1 and 2, equine arteritis virus and equine rhinitis A virus by polymerase chain reaction. Aust Vet J 2001;79(10):695–702.
84. Bryans JT, Crowe ME, Doll ER, et al. Isolation of a filterable agent causing arteritis of horses and abortion by mares; its differentiation from the equine abortion (influenza) virus. Cornell Vet 1957;47(1):3–41.
85. Timoney PJ, McCollum WH. Equine viral arteritis. Vet Clin North Am Equine Pract 1993;9(2):295–309.
86. Balasuriya UB, Go YY, MacLachlan NJ. Equine arteritis virus. Vet Microbiol 2013; 167(1–2):93–122.
87. Balasuriya UB, MacLachlan NJ. Equine viral arteritis. In: Sellon DC, Long MT, editors. Equine infectious diseases. St Louis (MO): Elsevier; 2014. p. 169–81.
88. Broaddus CC, Balasuriya UB, White JL, et al. Evaluation of the safety of vaccinating mares against equine viral arteritis during mid or late gestation or during the immediate postpartum period. J Am Vet Med Assoc 2011;238(6):741–50.
89. Murray K, Rogers R, Selvey L, et al. A novel morbillivirus pneumonia of horses and its transmission to humans. Emerg Infect Dis 1995;1(1):31–3.
90. Murray K, Selleck P, Hooper P, et al. A morbillivirus that caused fatal disease in horses and humans. Science 1995;268(5207):94–7.
91. Playford EG, McCall B, Smith G, et al. Human Hendra virus encephalitis associated with equine outbreak, Australia, 2008. Emerg Infect Dis 2010;16(2):219–23.

92. Halpin K, Hyatt AD, Fogarty R, et al. Pteropid bats are confirmed as the reservoir hosts of henipaviruses: a comprehensive experimental study of virus transmission. Am J Trop Med Hyg 2011;85(5):946–51.

93. Halpin K, Young PL, Field HE, et al. Isolation of Hendra virus from pteropid bats: a natural reservoir of Hendra virus. J Gen Virol 2000;81(Pt 8):1927–32.

94. Williamson MM, Hooper PT, Selleck PW, et al. Experimental hendra virus infectionin pregnant guinea-pigs and fruit Bats (Pteropus poliocephalus). J Comp Pathol 2000;122(2–3):201–7.

95. Field H, de Jong C, Melville D, et al. Hendra virus infection dynamics in Australian fruit bats. PLoS One 2011;6(12):e28678.

96. Marsh GA, Haining J, Hancock TJ, et al. Experimental infection of horses with Hendra virus/Australia/horse/2008/Redlands. Emerg Infect Dis 2011;17(12):2232–8.

97. Bossart KN, Crameri G, Dimitrov AS, et al. Receptor binding, fusion inhibition, and induction of cross-reactive neutralizing antibodies by a soluble G glycoprotein of Hendra virus. J Virol 2005;79(11):6690–702.

98. Pallister J, Middleton D, Wang LF, et al. A recombinant Hendra virus G glycoprotein-based subunit vaccine protects ferrets from lethal Hendra virus challenge. Vaccine 2011;29(34):5623–30.

99. Middleton D, Pallister J, Klein R, et al. Hendra virus vaccine, a one health approach to protecting horse, human, and environmental health. Emerg Infect Dis 2014;20(3):372–9.

100. Howell PG. The 1960 epizootic of African Horsesickness in the Middle East and S. W. Asia. J S Afr Vet Med Assoc 1960;31:329–34.

101. Lubroth J. African horse sickness and the epizootic in Spain 1987. Equine Pract 1988;10(2):26–33.

102. Rodriguez M, Hooghuis H, Castano M. African horse sickness in Spain. Vet Microbiol 1992;33(1–4):129–42.

103. MacLachlan NJ, Guthrie AJ. Re-emergence of bluetongue, African horse sickness, and other orbivirus diseases. Vet Res 2010;41(6):35.

104. Sellers RF, Pedgley DE, Tucker MR. Possible spread of African horse sickness on the wind. J Hyg 1977;79:279–98.

105. Guthrie AJ. African horse sickness. In: Sellon DC, Long MT, editors. Equine infectious diseases. St Louis (MO): Elsevier; 2007. p. 164–71.

Update on Bacterial Pneumonia and Pleuropneumonia in the Adult Horse

Sarah M. Reuss, VMD[a],*, Steeve Giguère, DVM, PhD[b]

KEYWORDS

- Bronchopneumonia • Pleuropneumonia • Pneumonia • Tracheobronchial aspirate
- Thoracocentesis

KEY POINTS

- Adult horses most commonly acquire pneumonia when bacteria from the nasal or oropharynx reach the lower airways and overwhelm the pulmonary defense mechanisms.
- Although *Streptococcus equi* subsp *zooepidemicus* is the most common bacterium isolated from horses with pneumonia, mixed infections are possible and may include both aerobes and anaerobes.
- Knowledge of likely causative organisms can help with empirical treatment, but microbiologic culture and antimicrobial sensitivity testing is necessary in cases presenting with severe clinical signs or not responding to treatment.
- Thoracocentesis can be both diagnostic and therapeutic in horses with significant pleural effusion.
- The prognosis for survival and return to athletic function is good for horses with pneumonia that is recognized early and treated appropriately.

INTRODUCTION

Bacterial infections of the lower respiratory tract are common in adult horses. Infection involving both the bronchi and the lung parenchyma is bronchopneumonia. When the infection extends from the pulmonary parenchyma to the pleural space, pleuropneumonia occurs. The clinical signs shown by affected horses vary with the severity of the disease and may dictate the extent of the diagnostic evaluation as well as the

The authors have nothing to disclose.
[a] Department of Large Animal Clinical Sciences, University of Florida College of Veterinary Medicine, PO Box 100136, Gainesville, FL 32610, USA; [b] Department of Large Animal Medicine, 501 DW Brooks Drive, University of Georgia College of Veterinary Medicine, Athens, GA 30602, USA
* Corresponding author.
E-mail address: sreuss@ufl.edu

intensiveness of treatment. Early recognition of disease and implementation of appropriate therapy minimizes morbidity and mortality.

ETIOLOGY/PATHOGENESIS

Adult horses most commonly acquire bacterial pneumonia by aspiration of microorganisms that normally inhabit their nasopharynx or oral cavity.[1,2] β-Hemolytic streptococci, particularly S equi subspecies zooepidemicus, are by far the most common bacterial pathogens isolated from adult horses with bronchopneumonia.[3] Other bacteria isolated from horses with pneumonia are listed in **Table 1**. Synergy between aerobic, facultative aerobic, and anaerobic bacteria results in many mixed bacterial infections. Anaerobic bacteria are isolated from approximately one-third of adult horses with pleuropneumonia or pulmonary abscessation.[3,4] The importance of Mycoplasma spp in the development of equine bronchopneumonia and pleuropneumonia is controversial, with Mycoplasma felis and Mycoplasma equirhinis being the most common isolates.[5–9]

Opportunistic bacteria can colonize the lungs when the pulmonary defense mechanisms are compromised or are overwhelmed by large numbers of bacteria. Pulmonary defense mechanisms can be altered by numerous factors, including stress, viral infections, malnutrition, exposure to dust or noxious gases, immunosuppressive therapy, immunodeficiency disorders, and general anesthesia. Infections with influenza virus and equine herpesvirus 4 have been shown to significantly decrease mucociliary clearance for up to approximately 30 days after, potentially leaving horses predisposed to secondary bacterial infections.[10] Horses with a recent viral respiratory tract infection or exposure to other horses with viral infections have an increased risk of developing pleuropneumonia.[11,12] Long-distance transportation may result in a significant reduction in phagocytosis by peripheral blood neutrophils for approximately 36 h after transportation.[13] In general, moderate exercise enhances immune function, whereas strenuous exercise tends to be detrimental to immune function.[14–20] General anesthesia is also a risk factor, with 12.2% of 90 horses with pleuropneumonia having recently undergone anesthesia.[21]

Factors that increase bacterial contamination and therefore the risk for pneumonia include confinement with the head elevated, transportation, and high-intensity exercise.[22–24] Horses depend on periods of lowered head posture for normal mucociliary

Table 1
Possible causative organisms in cases of bronchopneumonia or pleuropneumonia

Nonenteric Gram-Negative Bacteria	Enteric Gram-Negative Bacteria	Gram-Positive Aerobes	Anaerobes
Pasteurella spp	Klebsiella spp	β-Hemolytic streptococci[a]	Bacteroides spp
Actinobacillus spp	Escherichia coli	Staphylococcus spp	Clostridium spp
Bordetella spp	Enterobacter spp	Rhodococcus equi[b]	Peptostreptococcus spp
Pseudomonas spp[c]	Salmonella enterica	Streptococcus pneumoniae[d]	Fusobacterium spp
			Prevotella spp

[a] Streptococcus equi subsp zooepidemicus most commonly.
[b] Rare in immunocompetent adults.
[c] Rarely a primary cause of pneumonia and more commonly due to sampling equipment contamination.
[d] Common pathogen of humans and has been correlated with disease in young Thoroughbred racehorses in the United Kingdom but rarely isolated from horses in the United States.[11,61]

clearance.[25] In one study, as early as 6 hours after initiating confinement and head elevation there was a significant increase in bacterial numbers and neutrophilic inflammation in the lower respiratory tract.[23] The duration with a raised head position seems to be more important than the stress of transport alone, as horses transported with their heads elevated for 12 hours had increased bacterial contamination and neutrophilic inflammation in tracheal aspirate fluid,[13] whereas those transported for 12 hours with their heads free had no significant cytologic or bacteriologic changes in bronchoalveolar lavage (BAL) fluid.[26] Regardless, long-distance transport within the week before the onset of clinical signs was the most significant risk factor for development of pleuropneumonia in one study, and in another, 24.4% of 90 horses with pleuropneumonia had recently been transported over long distances.[12,21] High-intensity exercise can also result in a 10-fold increase in aerobic bacterial counts and 100-fold increase in anaerobic bacterial counts in tracheal aspirate samples compared with preexercise values.[22]

Regardless of the exact mechanism predisposing to bacterial colonization, bacterial invasion induces infiltration with neutrophils and other inflammatory cells into the airways and pulmonary parenchyma resulting in various degrees of consolidation or focal abscesses. These lesions interfere with gas exchange and, if severe enough, the resulting ventilation-perfusion mismatch leads to hypoxemia and clinical signs of respiratory disease.

In animals with severe bronchopneumonia, inflammation extends to the pleural space. During the exudative stage, sterile fluid fills the pleural space in response to inflammation. If appropriate antimicrobial therapy is not initiated, the bacteria from the lung parenchyma invade the pleural fluid, resulting in septic exudate and the fibrinopurulent stage. Fibrin is deposited in continuous sheets covering both the visceral and parietal pleura resulting in loculation. In the organization stage, fibroblasts grow into the exudate from both pleural surfaces and produce an inelastic pleural peel that encases the lung, leaving it virtually functionless. Although bacterial extension is the most common cause of pleuropneumonia, other causes of pleural effusion include trauma, esophageal perforation, neoplasia, pericarditis, congestive heart failure, diaphragmatic hernia, hypoproteinemia, and chylothorax.

PATIENT DIAGNOSTIC EVALUATION

Presumptive diagnosis of pneumonia may be based on clinical signs and auscultation of the lungs. The goal of additional diagnostic evaluation is to rule out diseases of the upper respiratory tract and to determine the cause and severity of lung involvement.

Physical Examination

The clinical signs shown by a horse with bacterial pneumonia reflect the severity of the disease process. Horses with septic bronchitis and no or minimal involvement of the lung parenchyma may be normal at rest with signs only seen with exercise. As bronchopneumonia progresses, clinical signs may include fever, anorexia, bilateral nasal discharge, cough, weight loss, tachypnea, and respiratory distress. Nasal discharge is usually mucopurulent but may be hemorrhagic with pulmonary infarction and necrotizing pneumonia.[27] Halitosis and foul-smelling nasal discharge are frequently present with anaerobic infections, but their absence does not rule out infection with anaerobic bacteria.

Horses with acute pleuropneumonia often exhibit pleurodynia by grunting, evading pressure applied to the thorax, pawing, moving with a stiff forelimb gait, standing with abducted elbows, and being overall reluctant to move. As more fluid accumulates in the pleural space and the disease becomes chronic, pain is less evident. A plaque of sternal edema is a common nonspecific clinical finding in horses with pleuropneumonia.

Careful auscultation of the thorax with a rebreathing bag can define the presence and extent of lung involvement. Adventitious sounds may be heard over affected areas during inspiration or expiration and are more commonly located ventrally. Mild consolidation may result in increased bronchial sounds, whereas severe consolidation or pleural effusion may result in diminished or absent bronchovesicular sounds. Absence of lung sounds ventrally with excessively loud, radiating cardiac sounds is suggestive of pleural fluid. If pleural friction rubs are heard, they are present predominantly at the end of inspiration and the early part of expiration; however, they disappear as inflammation decreases or as pleural fluids accumulate.

Hematology and Biochemistry

Bacterial bronchopneumonia frequently results in a leukocytosis and absolute neutrophilia with or without a left shift; however, a normal leukogram does not rule out bacterial bronchopneumonia. Severely affected animals may have a neutropenia with a toxic left shift. Hyperfibrinogenemia and hyperglobulinemia might be seen with active and chronic inflammation, respectively, and an anemia of chronic inflammation may also develop.

Diagnostic Imaging

Radiographic abnormalities in horses with mild disease may range from normal to a mild bronchointerstitial pattern. In more severely affected animals, an alveolar pattern may be seen with air bronchograms and border effacement (**Fig. 1**). Abscesses may

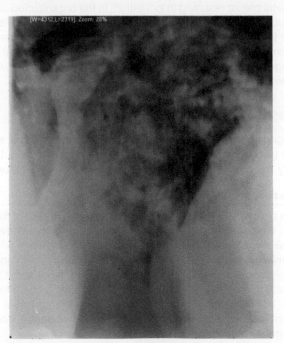

Fig. 1. Lateral thoracic radiograph of the caudoventral lung field from a 13-year-old Lusitano stallion. There is a unstructured interstitial to alveolar pattern, moderate to severe, with air bronchograms and border effacement of the cardiac silhouette.

be present as circular soft-tissue opacities, some of which may have a distinct horizontal line representing fluid gas interface. Pleural effusion appears as a horizontal line demarcating the fluid ventrally. When severe pleural effusion is present, pleural fluid should be drained before obtaining radiographs so as to not miss deep pulmonary lesions.

Thoracic ultrasonography is an effective tool to evaluate the periphery of the lung and the pleural space, but parenchymal lesions with overlying aerated lung are not be detected. Early sonographic lesions may include only irregularities of the pleural surface (often referred to as comet tails), which may progress to form focal areas of pulmonary consolidation and/or abscesses with loss of normal pulmonary architecture. Pleural fluid can be assessed for approximate volume and cellularity (**Fig. 2**). Fibrin strands may also be detected floating within the effusion progressing to loculation (**Fig. 3**). With anaerobic infection or bronchopleural fistulae, small, bright gas echoes may be seen (**Fig. 4**) but should not be confused with air leakage from thoracocentesis.[28]

Tracheobronchial Aspirate

A tracheobronchial aspirate (TBA) or transtracheal wash for cytologic examination and bacterial culture is one of the most helpful diagnostic procedures available when bronchopneumonia is suspected. Ideally, the sample should be collected before initiation of antimicrobial therapy or with at least 24 hours since last treatment. BAL is not useful as it is contaminated by the upper airway and is only representative of a localized area of lung. In one study of 22 horses diagnosed with pneumonia or pleuropneumonia, cytologic examination of BAL fluid showed abnormal results in only 10 horses despite attempts at selectively sampling the affected area, whereas all horses had evidence of septic inflammation based on cytologic examination of TBA.[29] TBA is preferably obtained by sterile percutaneous transtracheal aspiration to avoid contamination from the upper airway but can also be collected through the biopsy channel of a flexible endoscope with a sterile guarded aspiration catheter.[30,31] Airway fluid specimens should be submitted for cytology, gram staining, and aerobic and anaerobic bacterial culture. Fluid from horses with lower respiratory tract infections has increased numbers of degenerated neutrophils, as well as

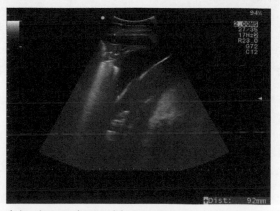

Fig. 2. Sonogram of the thorax obtained from a 12-year-old Tennessee Walking Mare with pleuropneumonia. The ventral lung tip is consolidated and is surrounded by anechoic pleural fluid of 9 cm depth between the chest wall and the diaphragm.

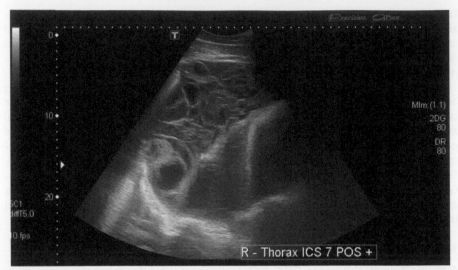

Fig. 3. Sonogram of the thorax obtained from a 6-year-old quarter horse gelding with pleuritis of 2 weeks' duration. There is severe fibrin deposition resulting in loculation of the pleural space.

intracellular and extracellular bacteria. Culture results should always be interpreted in the context of clinical signs and cytologic examination. If small numbers of bacteria are cultured in the absence of cytologic evidence of sepsis, it is unlikely that they are the cause of the respiratory problem. The presence of squamous epithelial cells

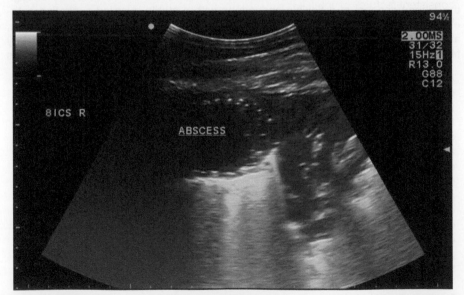

Fig. 4. Sonogram of the thorax from the same horse as in **Fig. 2** showing a pleural abscess. There are hyperechoic gas echoes within the abscess suggestive of anaerobic infection. Two species of *Prevotella* were obtained on culture.

indicates upper airway contamination, and occasional plant spores or fungal hyphae are more likely due to the horse's environment than due to true infection. Similarly, growth of various molds is common in TBA cultures, and the clinical signs and cytologic findings should be considered before initiating treatment with antifungal agents. In horses with pleural effusion, a TBA should always be obtained even if pleural fluid is available for bacterial culture. Culture of the pleural fluid showed negative results in 43% of 111 horses with pleuropneumonia, whereas tracheobronchial fluid yielded growth in all cases.[3] Only approximately 5% of cases had growth from the pleural fluid but not from TBA.[3]

Thoracocentesis

Thoracocentesis should be considered in horses with pleural effusion. The procedure can be of diagnostic value by allowing differentiation between septic pleural effusion and nonseptic effusion caused by other disease processes. It can also be of therapeutic value by allowing pulmonary reexpansion and a reduction in respiratory distress. Thoracocentesis is best performed using ultrasound guidance to determine the most appropriate site. A blunt teat cannula is typically used if a small volume of effusion is being sampled strictly for diagnostic purposes. Depending on the volume of effusion, a 16F, 24F, or 32F chest tube is used when pleural drainage is also indicated. Pleural fluid should be submitted for cytologic examination, gram staining, and aerobic and anaerobic bacterial culture.

Normal equine pleural fluid is clear to light yellow and odorless, with a protein concentration less than 2.5 g/dL and nucleated cell count less than 8000/μL.[32] Bacterial pleuropneumonia typically results in increases in the protein and nucleated cell count, as well as a visible cloudiness or color change. The increased cell count usually contains greater than 90% neutrophils, most of which exhibit degenerative changes. Bacteria may be cytologically visible. Low pleural fluid pH (<7.1), pleural fluid lactate level greater than blood lactate level, and glucose concentrations less than 40 mg/dL are consistent features of septic pleural effusion.[33,34] Fluid with a putrid odor indicates necrosis and suggests anaerobic infection.

PHARMACOLOGIC TREATMENT OPTIONS

Appropriate antimicrobial therapy is based on the severity of the disease, cost, route of administration, and results of culture and susceptibility testing of a TBA if available. Dosages for commonly used antimicrobial agents are presented in **Table 2**. It is reasonable to suspect S zooepidemicus as the likely causative microorganism in early cases of mild bronchopneumonia and to therefore treat accordingly with penicillin, ampicillin, or cephalosporins such as ceftiofur (**Table 3**). Ceftiofur offers the advantage of having a good spectrum of activity against S zooepidemicus in addition to many common enteric and nonenteric gram-negative pathogens that might contribute to a mixed infection (see **Table 3**). Ceftiofur is available as a sodium salt that requires daily intramuscular administration or as ceftiofur crystalline free acid. Two intramuscular doses of ceftiofur crystalline administered 4 days apart provide therapeutic concentrations of ceftiofur and desfuroylceftiofur-related metabolites in plasma and pulmonary epithelial lining fluid for approximately 10 days from the beginning of treatment.[35,36]

As horses with bronchopneumonia should generally be treated for a minimum of 10 days or until clinical signs resolve, oral options are often desired for patient and owner compliance. Trimethoprim-sulfonamide (TMS) combinations offer the advantage of oral administration, but TMS is generally not effective in vivo against S

Table 2
Antimicrobial agents commonly used to treat bacterial bronchopneumonia in adult horses

Antimicrobial[a]	Dose	Frequency (h)	Route
β-Lactams			
Benzyl penicillins			
Penicillin G (Na, K)	25,000 IU/kg	6	IV
Penicillin G (procaine)	25,000 IU/kg	12	IM
Aminobenzyl penicillins			
Ampicillin sodium	20 mg/kg	6–8	IV
Ampicillin trihydrate	20 mg/kg	12–24	IM
Cephalosporins			
Cefazolin	10–20 mg/kg	6	IV
Ceftiofur sodium	2.2–4.4 mg/kg	12–24	IM
Ceftiofur crystalline free acid	6.6 mg/kg	96[b]	IM
Cefotaxime	40	6	IV
Ceftriazone	25	12	IV or IM
Cefepime	2.2	8	IV or IM
Aminoglycosides			
Amikacin	10 mg/kg	24	IV or IM
Gentamicin	6.6 mg/kg	24	IV or IM
Fluoroquinolones			
Enrofloxacin[c]	5 mg/kg	24	IV
	7.5 mg/kg	24	PO
Tetracyclines			
Oxytetracycline[d]	6.6 mg/kg	12	IV[d]
Doxycycline	10 mg/kg	12	PO
Minocycline	4 mg/kg	12	PO
	2.2 mg/kg	12	IV
Others			
Chloramphenicol (palmitate or base)	50 mg/kg	6	PO
Metronidazole	25 mg/kg	12	PO
	35 mg/kg	12	Per rectum
Rifampin	5 mg/kg	12	PO
Trimethoprim-sulfonamide	30 mg/kg (combined)	12	PO

Abbreviations: IM, intramuscular; IV, intravenous; PO, by mouth.

  [a] Pharmacokinetics data are available for horses, but in most cases safety studies have not been performed in the equine species.

  [b] Two doses 4 days apart provide 10 days of coverage. If a longer treatment period is necessary, weekly (q 7 days) administration is sufficient after the initial 2 doses.

  [c] Should not be used in young growing horses because of the risk of arthropathy.

  [d] Dilute and give by slow IV infusion.

  From Giguère S. Bacterial pneumonia and pleuropneumonia in adult horses. In: Smith BP, editor. Large animal internal medicine. 5th edition. St Louis (MO): Elsevier; 2015. p. 477; with permission.

zooepidemicus, the most likely cause of bronchopneumonia. In a tissue chamber model of infection, despite in vitro susceptibility and high concentrations of TMS in the tissue chamber fluid, TMS was ineffective in eradicating *S equi* subspecies *zooepidemicus* in horses.[37,38]

Table 3
In vitro antimicrobial susceptibility of aerobic bacterial isolates that are commonly isolated from horses with bronchopneumonia or pleuropneumonia[a]

Microorganisms (n)	Antimicrobials[b]														
	GM	AMI	CHL	TMS	TE	RIF	P	AM	TIM	CFZ	CFT	XNL	CPE	ENR	CIP
Gram-positive bacteria															
Streptococcus zooepidemicus (192)	19	0	100	62	43	98	100	100	100	100	100	98	c	69	c
Staphylococcus aureus (43)	70	86	100	95	78	89	41	41	79	68	68	67[d]	68	79	81
Other staphylococci (48)	91	100	97	85	71	97	30	30	c	65	65	85[d]	65	94	97
Gram-negative bacteria															
Escherichia coli (127)	62	90	72	43	51	c	c	51	73	70	87	69	97	82	83
Klebsiella pneumoniae (52)	88	96	94	79	96	c	c	6	88	90	98	69	98	88	100
Enterobacter spp (32)	40	83	41	40	57	c	c	3	43	10	53	34	80	78	80
Pseudomonas aeruginosa (48)	70	97	c	c	c	c	c	c	94	c	15	6	91	65	97
Pasteurella spp (40)	94	94	100	91	100	c	c	100	100	94	100	95	100	100	100
Actinobacillus spp (31)	100	87	100	93	90	c	c	95	100	100	100	97	100	100	100

Abbreviations: AM, ampicillin; AMI, amikacin; CFT, cefotaxime; CFZ, cefazolin; CHL, chloramphenicol; CIP, ciprofloxacin; CPE, cefepime; ENR, enrofloxacin; GM, gentamicin; P, penicillin; RIF, rifampin; TE, tetracycline; TIM, ticarcillin-clavulanic acid (Timentin); TMS, trimethoprim-sulfonamide; XNL, ceftiofur.

[a] Data from the Clinical Microbiology Laboratory, University of Florida (2003–2005). Isolates were obtained from multiple equine clinical specimens including but not restricted to tracheobronchial aspirates and pleural fluid.

[b] Percentage of susceptible isolates (number of susceptible isolates/number of isolates tested × 100).

[c] Not tested or testing not warranted.

[d] In vivo, ceftiofur is rapidly metabolized to desfuroylceftiofur. Desfuroylceftiofur is as effective as ceftiofur against most bacterial pathogens, but most coagulase-positive *Staphylococcus* spp are resistant. Therefore, despite in vitro susceptibility, ceftiofur is not the ideal choice for the treatment staphylococcal infections.

From Giguère S. Bacterial pneumonia and pleuropneumonia in adult horses. In: Smith BP, editor. Large animal internal medicine. 5th edition. St Louis (MO): Elsevier; 2015. p. 478; with permission.

With more severe bronchopneumonia or pleuropneumonia, it becomes more important to base antimicrobial selection on results of culture and in vitro susceptibility testing. While awaiting those results, broad-spectrum antimicrobial therapy is initially required, as polymicrobial infections are common. In the early stages of treatment, parenteral antimicrobials are preferred to achieve higher plasma concentrations. A common initial empiric combination is gentamicin for gram-negative coverage and penicillin for gram-positive and anaerobic coverage. In adult horses, enrofloxacin can be used as a substitute to gentamicin with greater activity against Enterobacteriaceae, better penetration in phagocytic cells and tissues, and better activity in purulent material. However, enrofloxacin should never be used as stand-alone initial therapy in horses with bronchopneumonia because of its lack of activity against streptococci and anaerobes.

Treatment of anaerobes is frequently empiric because of difficulty in obtaining antimicrobial susceptibility testing of these fastidious organisms. Although most anaerobic isolates are susceptible to low concentrations of penicillin, *Bacteroides fragilis*, a frequently encountered anaerobe in horses with pleuropneumonia, is routinely resistant to penicillin. Other members of the *Bacteroides* family are known to produce β-lactamases and are potentially also resistant to penicillin. Metronidazole, however, has excellent in vitro activity *B fragilis* and other anaerobes and therefore should be added if anaerobic infection is suspected. Metronidazole should always be used in combination therapy, however, as it is not effective against aerobes. Chloramphenicol is active against most aerobes and anaerobes cultured from horses with pneumonia, but its use should be limited to severe refractory cases because of its human health concerns. Rifampin can also be added to combination therapies, as it is bactericidal, active against streptococci and some species of anaerobes, and penetrates well into abscesses.

Aerosolized antimicrobial agents may be a useful adjunct to systemic antimicrobial agents, particularly in horses with minimal involvement of the lung parenchyma. Aerosol administration can result in higher drug concentrations in the bronchial secretions and pulmonary epithelial fluid lining than systemically administered drugs.[39] Local delivery also minimizes systemic concentrations and their resulting toxicity; however, aerosol use of intravenous formulations can expose the airways to potentially irritating or toxic additives and inappropriate pH or osmolality ranges. The product formulation and type of nebulizer also affects drug delivery. In healthy horses, aerosolization of 20 mL of gentamicin sulfate solution diluted to 50 mg/mL resulted in bronchial lavage fluid concentrations approximately 12 times higher than concentrations achieved by a 6.6-mg/kg systemic dose while maintaining serum concentrations less than 1 µg/mL at all times.[40] Aerosol administration of gentamicin to healthy horses once daily for 7 consecutive days also did not result in pulmonary inflammation or drug accumulation in the respiratory tract.[41] The clinical utility of these findings is limited by the lack of efficacy of gentamicin against *S zooepidemicus*. In another study, nebulization of ceftiofur sodium (diluted to 50 mg/mL in sterile water) at a dose of 2.2 mg/kg was well tolerated and resulted in drug concentrations in pulmonary epithelial lining fluid more than the minimum inhibitory concentration of the drug required to inhibit the growth of 90% of *S zooepidemicus*, *Pasteurella* spp, and *Actinobacillus* spp for approximately 24 h after administration.[42] Additional studies are necessary to assess the efficacy of nebulized antimicrobial agents in horses with bacterial infections of the lower respiratory tract.

Many horses with pneumonia necessitate ancillary care. Nonsteroidal anti-inflammatory agents such as flunixin meglumine or phenylbutazone may also be used for their anti-inflammatory, analgesic, and antipyrexic effects. Additional analgesia with opioids may be necessary in horses with pleuropneumonia and severe pleurodynia. As patients are frequently receiving multiple potentially nephrotoxic agents, adequate hydration should be ensured using intravenous fluids if needed. Oxygen supplementation may be required in persistently severely hypoxemic horses, and distal limb cryotherapy may be beneficial to prevent laminitis in horses with signs of systemic inflammation or endotoxemia.

NONPHARMACOLOGIC TREATMENT OPTIONS
Pleural Drainage and Lavage

Although small amounts of pleural effusion may resolve with antimicrobial therapy alone, some horses necessitate drainage, including horses with fluid volumes resulting in respiratory distress or fluid with evidence of sepsis and/or a fetid odor. Early intervention is preferred, as fibrin deposition forms loculations that impair drainage. Although normal horses have an incomplete mediastinum, those perforations may become obstructed by fibrin, resulting in the inability to resolve bilateral pleural effusion by draining only one side of the thorax. Intermittent thoracocentesis may be performed in horses not rapidly reaccumulating fluid, whereas indwelling chest tubes with 1-way valves may be used with continued fluid production. These tubes may be maintained for several days. Potential complications include pneumothorax and local cellulitis at the site of entry into the chest.

Pleural lavage with warm, sterile isotonic fluids may be used in the subacute stages to dilute viscous pleural fluid for removal before loculations can occur or in later stages to break down fibrous adhesions and establish communication between loculae. Up to 5 L of fluid may be infused through the ventral drainage tube or through a specifically placed dorsal tube. Coughing and drainage of lavage fluid from the nose during infusion suggests the presence of a bronchopleural fistula, and lavage should be discontinued as it may result in spread of septic debris up the airways and into normal areas of the lungs.[43]

Intrapleural fibrinolytics such as streptokinase, urokinase, and recombinant tissue plasminogen activators (rtPA) have been investigated in human medicine for the treatment of loculated pleural effusion.[44] Although case series in people have shown that such therapy is fairly safe and may facilitate drainage, the few controlled trials performed have given conflicting results. In one study, intrapleural administration of streptokinase did not improve survival, the need for surgery, or the length of the hospital stay when compared with patients who had received a placebo.[45] In contrast, another study demonstrated a significant decrease in the need for surgical intervention and in the length of hospital stay with intrapleural streptokinase before drainage when compared with pleural drainage alone.[46] rtPA has largely replaced streptokinase in the treatment of people with pleural effusion, and although several case series have indicated a potential benefit for rtPA, large randomized placebo-controlled clinical trials are lacking.[44,47,48] Fibrinolytic drugs do not decrease the viscosity of purulent material, as that characteristic is mainly due to the DNA content. Therefore, intrapleural recombinant human deoxyribonuclease I (rhDNaseI) may be beneficial and has been used with apparent success in a single human patient who did not respond to fibrinolytic therapy.[49]

Intrapleural fibrinolytics have been used in horses with pleuropneumonia with isolated reports of the use of rtPA products. Alteplase (12 mg in 250 mL−2 L of 0.9% saline)[50] and tenecteplase (12–30 mg in 500 mL of 0.9% saline, alone or in combination with 25 mg of rhDNaseI)[51] resulted in a subjective decrease in the amount of fibrin seen sonographically in the thoracic cavity in treated horses. Additional studies evaluating the safety and efficacy of rtPA and rhDNaseI are required before the widespread use of these agents can be recommended in horses.

Thoracoscopy/Thoracotomy

Thoracoscopy is usually well tolerated in the standing sedated horse with local anesthesia.[52] It allows direct evaluation of the lungs and pleural cavity and may therefore be used to facilitate placement of thoracic drains into abscesses, transect pleural adhesions, or disrupt loculations.[53] Thoracoscopy can also be used to biopsy or aspirate specific lesions affecting the periphery of the lungs.

When medical therapy with antimicrobials and pleural drainage/lavage has failed, surgical intervention may be considered. Surgical intervention is most beneficial in chronic cases with large unilateral localized pockets of thick debris and improvement or resolution of disease in the opposite hemithorax. Surgical candidates should be systemically stable and have either a walled off lesion or complete mediastinum to avoid creation of a bilateral pneumothorax. Ultrasound imaging and thoracoscopy can be used to define the appropriate surgical site, and an open chest tube can be inserted into the targeted area before surgery to monitor for development of pneumothorax.[43]

Thoracotomy is typically performed with the horse standing and is done via an intercostal approach or rib resection. Although the intercostal approach preserves thoracic wall integrity and compliance, myectomy may be necessary to achieve adequate access and drainage. When the cavity is large and extensive debridement is necessary, thoracotomy with rib resection is the preferred procedure. Complications during thoracotomy may include bilateral pneumothorax and cardiac arrhythmias if the lesion is in close proximity to the heart. With either approach, the incision is left open, irrigated daily with a sterile isotonic fluid solution, and periodically manually debrided. Depending on the size of the incision, it may take a few weeks to 2 to 3 months for complete closure by second intention and a chronic draining fistula may remain. In a retrospective study of 16 horses that had a standing lateral thoracotomy for pleural disease, 14 horses (88%) survived to discharge and 46% of horses that survived returned to their previous level of athletic activity.[54]

COMPLICATIONS

In addition to the complications described previously for pleural drainage, other systemic complications include intravenous catheter-associated thrombophlebitis, antimicrobial-associated diarrhea, endotoxemia, coagulopathies, and laminitis. In a retrospective study of 153 horses with pleuropneumonia presented to a referral hospital, complications included pleural abscesses (21.6%), cranial thoracic masses (7.2%), bronchopleural fistulas (6.5%), pericarditis (2.6%), and laminitis (1.3%).[55] Cranial thoracic masses may form when the heart acts as a valve, trapping effusion in the cranial thorax. If these masses become large enough, they may result in sternal edema, jugular vein distension, pointing of the forelimbs, and caudal displacement of the heart. Most horses with cranial thoracic masses respond to conservative therapy with antimicrobial agents, although drainage may be performed if the mass interferes with cardiac funcion.[56] This procedure may be performed in the standing horse with the limb pulled forward or under short-term general anesthesia. Indwelling tubes are difficult to maintain in this region because of the triceps musculature, so repeated drainage and lavage may be necessary. A bronchopleural fistula develops when lung tissue necrosis results in a tract between the airways and pleural cavity. Most bronchopleural fistulas resolve in a period of weeks to months, with development of fibrin deposition or adhesions; however, partial pneumonectomy has been performed successfully to resolve a bronchopleural fistula and pulmonary abscess in 1 horse.[57]

EVALUATION OF OUTCOME

The prognosis for survival and return to athletic function depends on the severity of disease. In a retrospective study of 327 horses with either pneumonia or pleuropneumonia, the overall survival rate was 75%; however, only 38% of the 81 horses from which anaerobic bacteria were cultured survived.[3] The association between anaerobic bacteria and decreased survival was not seen in another study.[58] Pulmonary abscess also does not seem to affect survival, with 45 of 50 (90%) surviving and 36 of 50 (72%) returning to racing.[59] In cases of specifically pleuropneumonia, retrospective studies have shown survival rates ranging from 43.3% to 87.6%.[21,55,58] This range in rates is likely due to differences in referral populations as well as advances in medical and surgical therapies over the years saving horses that might have otherwise been euthanized. One retrospective study of 153 horses with pleuropneumonia showed a survival rate of 95.7% when horses electively euthanized were excluded.[55]

In addition to a good prognosis for survival, horses with mild to moderate bronchopneumonia also have a good prognosis for a return to previous athletic performance. After treatment of pulmonary abscesses, 23 of 25 (92%) of Standardbreds and 13 of 20 (52%) of Thoroughbreds raced, and their performance was not significantly different from that before the illness.[59] Horses recovering from uncomplicated pleuropneumonia also seem to have a fair return to athletic performance, although it has not been evaluated extensively. In one retrospective study, 43 of 70 (61%) horses that had recovered from pleuropneumonia returned to racing, and 24 of the 43 (56%) won at least 1 race.[60] The prognosis for return to performance did not seem to vary for horses that required an indwelling thoracic drain compared with those that did not.[60] In contrast, horses that developed complications such as pulmonary abscesses, cranial thoracic masses, or bronchopleural fistulas were significantly less likely to return to racing.[60]

REFERENCES

1. Bailey GD, Love DN. Oral associated bacterial infection in horses: studies on the normal anaerobic flora from the pharyngeal tonsillar surface and its association with lower respiratory tract and paraoral infections. Vet Microbiol 1991;26:367.
2. Hoquet F, Higgins R, Lessard P, et al. Comparison of the bacterial and fungal flora in the pharynx of normal horses and horses affected with pharyngitis. Can Vet J 1985;26:342.
3. Sweeney CR, Holcombe SJ, Barningham SC, et al. Aerobic and anaerobic bacterial isolates from horses with pneumonia or pleuropneumonia and antimicrobial susceptibility patterns of the aerobes. J Am Vet Med Assoc 1991;198:839.
4. Sweeney CR, Divers TJ, Benson CE. Anaerobic bacteria in 21 horses with pleuropneumonia. J Am Vet Med Assoc 1985;187:721.
5. Wood JL, Newton JR, Chanter N, et al. Inflammatory airway disease, nasal discharge and respiratory infections in young British racehorses. Equine Vet J 2005;37:236.
6. Christley RM, Hodgson DR, Rose RJ, et al. A case-control study of respiratory disease in Thoroughbred racehorses in Sydney, Australia. Equine Vet J 2001; 33:256.
7. Wood JL, Chanter N, Newton JR, et al. An outbreak of respiratory disease in horses associated with Mycoplasma felis infection. Vet Rec 1997;140:388.
8. Hoffman AM, Baird JD, Kloeze HJ, et al. Mycoplasma felis pleuritis in two show-jumper horses. Cornell Vet 1992;82:155.
9. Ogilvie TH, Rosendal S, Blackwell TE, et al. Mycoplasma felis as a cause of pleuritis in horses. J Am Vet Med Assoc 1983;182:1374.
10. Willoughby R, Ecker G, McKee S, et al. The effects of equine rhinovirus, influenza virus and herpesvirus infection on tracheal clearance rate in horses. Can J Vet Res 1992;56:115.

11. Wood JL, Newton JR, Chanter N, et al. Association between respiratory disease and bacterial and viral infections in British racehorses. J Clin Microbiol 2005;43:120.

12. Austin SM, Foreman JH, Hungerford LL. Case-control study of risk factors for development of pleuropneumonia in horses. J Am Vet Med Assoc 1995; 207:325.

13. Raidal SL, Bailey GD, Love DN. Effect of transportation on lower respiratory tract contamination and peripheral blood neutrophil function. Aust Vet J 1997; 75:433.

14. Horohov DW. Is exercise bad for the immune system? Equine Vet J 2003;35:113.

15. Raidal SL, Love DN, Bailey GD, et al. The effect of high intensity exercise on the functional capacity of equine pulmonary alveolar macrophages and BAL-derived lymphocytes. Res Vet Sci 2000;68:249.

16. Raidal SL, Love DN, Bailey GD, et al. Effect of single bouts of moderate and high intensity exercise and training on equine peripheral blood neutrophil function. Res Vet Sci 2000;68:141.

17. Raidal SL, Rose RJ, Love DN. Effects of training on resting peripheral blood and BAL-derived leucocyte function in horses. Equine Vet J 2001;33:238.

18. Folsom RW, Littlefield-Chabaud MA, French DD, et al. Exercise alters the immune response to equine influenza virus and increases susceptibility to infection. Equine Vet J 2001;33:664.

19. Horohov DW, Dimock A, Guirnalda P, et al. Effect of exercise on the immune response of young and old horses. Am J Vet Res 1999;60:643.

20. Nesse LL, Johansen GI, Blom AK. Effects of racing on lymphocyte proliferation in horses. Am J Vet Res 2002;63:528.

21. Raphel CF, Beech J. Pleuritis secondary to pneumonia or lung abscessation in 90 horses. J Am Vet Med Assoc 1982;181:808.

22. Raidal SL, Love DN, Bailey GD. Effect of a single bout of high intensity exercise on lower respiratory tract contamination in the horse. Aust Vet J 1997;75:293.

23. Raidal SL, Love DN, Bailey GD. Inflammation and increased numbers of bacteria in the lower respiratory tract of horses within 6 to 12 hours of confinement with the head elevated. Aust Vet J 1995;72:45.

24. Racklyeft DJ, Love DN. Influence of head posture on the respiratory tract of healthy horses. Aust Vet J 1990;67:402.

25. Raidal SL, Love DN, Bailey GD. Effects of posture and accumulated airway secretions on tracheal mucociliary transport in the horse. Aust Vet J 1996;73:45.

26. Traub-Dargatz JL, McKinnon AO, Bruyninckx WJ, et al. Effect of transportation stress on bronchoalveolar lavage fluid analysis in female horses. Am J Vet Res 1988;49:1026.

27. Carr EA, Carlson GP, Wilson WD, et al. Acute hemorrhagic pulmonary infarction and necrotizing pneumonia in horses: 21 cases (1967–1993). J Am Vet Med Assoc 1997;210:1774.

28. Reimer JM, Reef VB, Spencer PA. Ultrasonography as a diagnostic aid in horses with anaerobic bacterial pleuropneumonia and/or pulmonary abscessation: 27 cases (1984–1986). J Am Vet Med Assoc 1989;194:278.

29. Rossier Y, Sweeney CR, Ziemer EL. Bronchoalveolar lavage fluid cytologic findings in horses with pneumonia or pleuropneumonia. J Am Vet Med Assoc 1991;198:1001.

30. Darien BJ, Brown CM, Walker RD, et al. A tracheoscopic technique for obtaining uncontaminated lower airway secretions for bacterial culture in the horse. Equine Vet J 1990;22:170.

31. Christley RM, Hodgson DR, Rose RJ, et al. Comparison of bacteriology and cytology of tracheal fluid samples collected by percutaneous transtracheal aspiration or via an endoscope using a plugged, guarded catheter. Equine Vet J 1999;31:197.
32. Wagner AE, Bennett DG. Analysis of equine thoracic fluid. Vet Clin Pathol 1982;11:13.
33. Brumbaugh GW, Benson PA. Partial pressures of oxygen and carbon dioxide, pH, and concentrations of bicarbonate, lactate, and glucose in pleural fluid from horses. Am J Vet Res 1990;51:1032.
34. Schott HC, Mansmann RA. Thoracic drainage in horses. Compend Contin Educ Vet 1990;12:251.
35. Credille RC, Giguere S, Berghaus LJ, et al. Plasma and pulmonary disposition of ceftiofur and its metabolites after intramuscular administration of ceftiofur crystalline free acid in weanling foals. J Vet Pharmacol Ther 2012;35:259.
36. Giguere S, Sturgill TL, Berghaus LJ, et al. Effects of two methods of administration on the pharmacokinetics of ceftiofur crystalline free acid in horses. J Vet Pharmacol Ther 2011;34:193.
37. Ensink JM, Smit JA, van Duijkeren E. Clinical efficacy of trimethoprim/sulfadiazine and procaine penicillin G in a *Streptococcus equi* subsp. *zooepidemicus* infection model in ponies. J Vet Pharmacol Ther 2003;26:247.
38. Ensink JM, Bosch G, van Duijkeren E. Clinical efficacy of prophylactic administration of trimethoprim/sulfadiazine in a *Streptococcus equi* subsp. *zooepidemicus* infection model in ponies. J Vet Pharmacol Ther 2005;28:45.
39. Baldwin DR, Honeybourne D, Wise R. Pulmonary disposition of antimicrobial agents: in vivo observations and clinical relevance. Antimicrob Agents Chemother 1992;36:1176.
40. McKenzie HC III, Murray MJ. Concentrations of gentamicin in serum and bronchial lavage fluid after intravenous and aerosol administration of gentamicin to horses. Am J Vet Res 2000;61:1185.
41. McKenzie HC III, Murray MJ. Concentrations of gentamicin in serum and bronchial lavage fluid after once-daily aerosol administration to horses for seven days. Am J Vet Res 2004;65:173.
42. Fultz L, Giguere S, Berghaus LJ, et al. Pulmonary pharmacokinetics of desfuroyl-ceftiofur acetamide after nebulisation or intramuscular administration of ceftiofur sodium to weanling foals. Equine Vet J 2014. http://dx.doi.org/10.1111/evj.12316.
43. Chaffin MK, Carter GK, Byars TD. Equine bacterial pleuropneumonia. Part III. Treatment, sequelae, and prognosis. Compend Contin Educ Vet 1994;15:1585.
44. Singh G, Pitoyo CW, Nasir AU, et al. Update on the role of intrapleural fibrinolytic therapy in the management of complicated parapneumonic effusions and empyema. Acta Med Indones 2012;44:258.
45. Maskell NA, Davies CW, Nunn AJ, et al. U.K. Controlled trial of intrapleural streptokinase for pleural infection. N Engl J Med 2005;352:865.
46. Misthos P, Sepsas E, Konstantinou M, et al. Early use of intrapleural fibrinolytics in the management of postpneumonic empyema. A prospective study. Eur J Cardiothorac Surg 2005;28:599.
47. Gervais DA, Levis DA, Hahn PF, et al. Adjunctive intrapleural tissue plasminogen activator administered via chest tubes placed with imaging guidance: effectiveness and risk for hemorrhage. Radiology 2008;246:956.
48. Thommi G, Nair CK, Aronow WS, et al. Efficacy and safety of intrapleural instillation of alteplase in the management of complicated pleural effusion or empyema. Am J Ther 2007;14:341.
49. Simpson G, Roomes D, Reeves B. Successful treatment of empyema thoracis with human recombinant deoxyribonuclease. Thorax 2003;58:365.

50. Hilton H, Pusterla N. Intrapleural fibrinolytic therapy in the management of septic pleuropneumonia in a horse. Vet Rec 2009;164:558.
51. Rendle DI, Armstrong SK, Hughes KJ. Combination fibrinolytic therapy in the treatment of chronic septic pleuropneumonia in a Thoroughbred gelding. Aust Vet J 2012;90:358.
52. Peroni JF, Horner NT, Robinson NE, et al. Equine thoracoscopy: normal anatomy and surgical technique. Equine Vet J 2001;33:231.
53. Vachon AM, Fischer AT. Thoracoscopy in the horse: diagnostic and therapeutic indications in 28 cases. Equine Vet J 1998;30:467.
54. Hilton H, Aleman M, Madigan J, et al. Standing lateral thoracotomy in horses: indications, complications, and outcomes. Vet Surg 2010;39:847.
55. Byars TD, Becht JL. Pleuropneumonia. Vet Clin North Am Equine Pract 1991;7:63.
56. Byars TD, Dainis CM, Seltzer KL, et al. Cranial thoracic masses in the horse: a sequel to pleuropneumonia. Equine Vet J 1991;23:22.
57. Sanchez LC, Murphy DJ, Bryant JE, et al. Use of diagnostic thoracoscopy and partial pneumonectomy for the treatment of a pulmonary abscess and broncho-pleural fistula in a thoroughbred filly. Equine Vet Educ 2002;4:375.
58. Collins MB, Hodgson DR, Hutchins DR. Pleural effusion associated with acute and chronic pleuropneumonia and pleuritis secondary to thoracic wounds in horses: 43 cases (1982–1992). J Am Vet Med Assoc 1994;205:1753.
59. Ainsworth DM, Erb HN, Eicker SW, et al. Effects of pulmonary abscesses on racing performance of horses treated at referral veterinary medical teaching hospitals: 45 cases (1985–1997). J Am Vet Med Assoc 2000;216:1282.
60. Seltzer KL, Byars TD. Prognosis for return to racing after recovery from infectious pleuropneumonia in thoroughbred racehorses: 70 cases (1984–1989). J Am Vet Med Assoc 1996;208:1300.
61. Blunden AS, Hannant D, Livesay G, et al. Susceptibility of ponies to infection with *Streptococcus pneumoniae* (capsular type 3). Equine Vet J 1994;26:22.

Update on Bacterial Pneumonia in the Foal and Weanling

Sarah M. Reuss, VMD[a],*, Noah D. Cohen, VMD, MPH, PhD[b]

KEYWORDS

- Equine • Foal • Weanling • Pneumonia • Sepsis • Aspiration • *Rhodococcus equi*

KEY POINTS

- Bacterial pneumonia is a common cause of morbidity and mortality in foals of all ages.
- The most likely causal agents of bacterial pneumonia vary with the age of the foal, and knowledge of likely agents and their antimicrobial-resistance profiles is important for treatment selection.
- Macrolide antibiotics remain the treatment of choice for *Rhodococcus equi* infections, but resistance is emerging and effective alternatives are exiguous.

INTRODUCTION

Bacterial pneumonia is a common problem in foals of all ages. The causal agents of that pneumonia, however, vary with the age of the foal. Neonatal foals are more likely to have pneumonia as a component of systemic sepsis, whereas older foals and weanlings can have primary pneumonia. Knowledge of the likely agents is especially important when selecting empirical antimicrobials while awaiting microbial culture results. With appropriate treatment, prognosis for survival and athletic performance is good.

ETIOLOGY

Neonates

Neonatal foals may acquire pneumonia as a primary condition, but are more likely to develop bacterial pneumonia secondary to sepsis, the major cause of morbidity and mortality in the neonatal foal. Infection may occur in utero because of ascending

---

The authors have nothing to disclose.
[a] Department of Large Animal Clinical Sciences, University of Florida College of Veterinary Medicine, PO Box 100136, Gainesville, FL 32610, USA; [b] Department of Large Animal Clinical Sciences, Texas A&M University College of Veterinary Medicine, 4475 TAMU, College Station, TX 77845, USA
* Corresponding author.
E-mail address: sreuss@ufl.edu

infection of the fetal membranes or aspiration of contaminated fetal fluids. It also can occur at the time of parturition or during the postnatal period, whereby the respiratory tract, gastrointestinal tract, and umbilicus are all possible portals of pathogen entry. Microbial invasion of the bloodstream may result in systemic inflammatory response syndrome, causing the classical signs of sepsis, including fever, depression, anorexia, dehydration, tachycardia, and tachypnea. Signs of disease may remain generalized or may become localized. Localization may result either indirectly from septic shock-induced organ failure (eg, hemodynamic renal failure) or from infection localizing at sites, such as the lungs, gastrointestinal tract, umbilical remnants, synovial structures, bones, or meninges. Acute lung injury or acute respiratory distress syndrome may develop as part of the systemic inflammatory response to sepsis. In one study of 423 bacteremic foals, 79 (19%) were diagnosed with pneumonia. In that population, the presence of diarrhea was negatively associated with the presence of pneumonia; this may reflect the incidence of infections in that hospital population, routes of infection, or different localization patterns.[1] Other studies have reported the prevalence of pneumonia in septic foals as 28%[2] to 50%.[3] The most common bacterial organisms associated with pulmonary disease in neonates are identical to those that cause systemic sepsis. *Escherichia coli* has consistently been the most common etiologic organism isolated from the blood of septic foals.[1,4] The relative reported incidence of other bacteria varies with time and geographic location, but common organisms include *Klebsiella* spp, *Actinobacillus* spp, *Salmonella* spp, and other gram-negative aerobes. Mixed infections with gram-positive bacteria, such as *Enterococcus* spp, *Streptococcus* spp, and *Staphylococcus* spp also occur.[2,4,5]

Neonates may acquire primary bacterial pneumonia secondary to aspiration. Milk aspiration is generally related to a poor suckle reflex, weakness, or dysphagia associated with prematurity or neonatal maladjustment syndrome. Other causes of aspiration may include congenital diseases, such as cleft palate, subepiglottic cysts, megaesophagus, esophageal compression due to vascular anomalies, hyperkalemic periodic paralysis, or other causes of pharyngeal dysfunction.[6,7] Improper bottle feeding or incorrect placement or use of a nasoesophageal or nasogastric feeding tube may also result in aspiration pneumonia.

Meconium may also be aspirated in utero or at the time of parturition. Neonates with meconium aspiration syndrome have respiratory compromise because of a combination of mechanical airway obstruction, chemical pneumonitis, alveolar edema, and displacement of surfactant, which results in reduced lung compliance and small airway obstruction, leading to ventilation/perfusion mismatching.[8] Although meconium is sterile, secondary bacterial infection often can result as a complication of meconium aspiration.

Suckling and Weaning Foals

Pneumonia is the most common cause of morbidity and mortality in foals aged 1 to 6 months[9] and is usually acquired via inhalation. The most common bacterial cause of primary foal pneumonia is *Streptococcus equi* subsp *zooepidemicus*, which may be isolated alone or as part of a mixed infection. *S zooepidemicus* is a normal inhabitant of the upper respiratory tract, but viral infections (eg, equine herpes virus 1 or 4, equine influenza, or equine arteritis virus) may damage the mucous membranes, allowing for establishment of disease. Stressors such as high ambient temperature, weaning, and transport also have been implicated. Although isolates of *S zooepidemicus* from pneumonic foals and horses tend to be clonal (ie, the same) within individuals,[10] they are highly variable among individuals. Evidence of clones of *S zooepidemicus* causing epizootics has been described.[11]

Rhodococcus equi is a common cause of pneumonia in foals between 3 weeks and 6 months of age at endemic farms. *R equi* pneumonia is often insidious with vague clinical signs that can progress to acute respiratory distress or sudden death. Affected foals often have extrapulmonary lesions in addition to suppurative bronchopneumonia with abscessation.[12] Although clinical signs are generally not seen until 30 days of age, evidence supports foals becoming infected shortly after birth. Experimental infection is more successful in foals less than 1 week of age,[13] and epidemiologic data also are consistent with early exposure.[14] The occurrence of disease in exposed foals is due to a combination of agent, environment, and foal factors.

Agent

R equi isolates found in pneumonic foals carry an 80-kbp to 95-kbp virulence-associated plasmid (Vap). The expression of VapA is necessary, but not sufficient alone, to cause disease in foals and results in the classification of that isolate as virulent. Other plasmid-encoded genes also influence virulence,[15] and these factors may interact with chromosomal genes to influence virulence (ie, survival within macrophages). A wide array of virulent isolates occurs in nature,[16] not only within the same farm but even within the same foal.[17] Thus, it appears that specific clones do not cause infection at farms or in foals, and that any isolate bearing the Vap may cause disease in a susceptible foal. Organisms without this plasmid do not replicate in macrophages and fail to cause disease in foals. These avirulent isolates are abundant in the environment and in equine feces. Unfortunately, transfer of the virulence plasmid from virulent to avirulent isolates is possible and in one study occurred among field strains at a frequency of 0.15%,[18] making eradication of virulent *R equi* from the environment virtually impossible.

Environment

Foals are thought to acquire *R equi* by inhalation. Although evidence has shown that the concentration of virulent bacteria in maternal feces or the soil is not associated with increased odds of development of pneumonia,[19,20] there is evidence that the presence of bacteria in the air is associated. The concentration of virulent *R equi* in air samples collected over the first 2 weeks of life has been shown to be higher in the stalls or pens of foals that went on to develop *R equi* pneumonia versus in those of foals that did not develop pneumonia.[21,22] Increases in airborne concentration are seen in stalls versus paddocks,[23,24] although there are conflicting results likely because of differences in individual farm management and methods for and conditions of sampling. The month during which the highest concentrations are found has varied among studies and is also likely due to management factors and geographic differences (eg, northern vs southern hemispheres). Other factors linked to increased incidence of *R equi* pneumonia in foals include increased density of mares and foals.[25,26] Dusty conditions are also putatively associated with increased incidence of pneumonia.[27]

Foal

Affected foals also likely have ineffective immune responses. Considerable evidence exists that adaptive immune responses are important for controlling *R equi* infection.[28,29] Innate immunity also seems to play a critical role. Neutrophil concentrations of foals that subsequently developed pneumonia were lower at 2 and 4 weeks of age compared with age-matched unaffected control foals.[30] Neutrophils have also been demonstrated to be critical for protection of mice against infection with *R equi*.[31]

Recent work has identified a genetic locus associated with *R equi* pneumonia, including a region on chromosome 26 that encodes a protein associated with neutrophil function. Foals with a single nucleotide polymorphism in this region were 3-fold to 4-fold more likely to have clinical *R equi* pneumonia than their herd mates with either subclinical pneumonia or no pneumonia (ie, lacking clinical or ultrasonographic signs of pneumonia).[32]

PATIENT DIAGNOSTIC EVALUATION
Physical Examination

The clinical evaluation of all animals should include thorough auscultation of the thorax. A rebreathing examination can be performed in animals not in respiratory distress to accentuate any abnormalities. It is important to note, however, that foals with significant pulmonary disease may have unremarkable thoracic auscultation.

Hematology and Biochemistry

Determining the white blood cell concentration with its differential cell count, plasma fibrinogen, and plasma chemistry with globulin determination can be helpful in assessing the timing and severity of disease, and for monitoring response to therapy. Systemic disease and chemistry abnormalities such as azotemia may also influence the antimicrobials selected for treatment.

Respiratory Function Monitoring

Hypoxemia is a common problem in many septic neonatal foals because of hypoventilation, ventilation perfusion mismatch, diffusion impairment, and shunting. The presence of severe bacterial pneumonia in these foals may worsen the hypoxemia as well as potentially lead to respiratory failure. Pulse oximetry is a noninvasive technique that can be used to monitor oxygen saturation of the blood with the goal to maintain a SaO_2 greater than 92%. Arterial blood gas measurement (ABG), however, provides a more complete assessment of the function of the respiratory system. ABG samples can be obtained from the dorsal metatarsal or brachial artery in most neonates. The goal for foals greater than 1 day of age is generally to maintain the PaO_2 between 80 mm Hg and 120 mm Hg, using supplemental oxygen if needed. The amount of struggling and position of the foal during sampling must be taken into account.

Diagnostic Imaging

Thoracic radiographs can be used to define the distribution and severity of pneumonia. Length of recumbency before imaging in neonates must be taken into account, however, because it can be difficult to differentiate pneumonia from atelectasis. Neonatal pneumonia secondary to sepsis is often diffuse, whereas pneumonia secondary to aspiration is generally ventrally distributed (**Figs. 1** and **2**). Foals with *R equi* pneumonia may have a variety of radiographic abnormalities (**Fig. 3**). A scoring system using severity of the interstitial or alveolar pattern, tracheobronchial lymphadenopathy, pleural effusion, number of nodules and cavitary lesions, and number of affected quadrants has been published with nonsurviving foals having higher median scores than survivors.[33] The severity of the alveolar pattern and number of cavitary lesions were the only 2 factors found to be associated with decreased survival.[33] Thoracic ultrasound is easily performed in both referral hospitals and the field. Ultrasonography is most useful for determining pathologic abnormalities in the periphery of the lung or pleural space and will fail to identify axial lesions in foals that lack peripheral (abaxial) lesions.

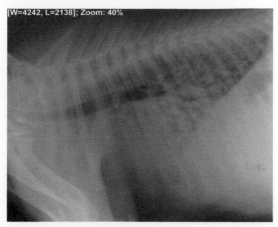

Fig. 1. Lateral radiograph of the thorax of an 8-day-old foal. There is a severe, diffuse interstitial to alveolar pulmonary pattern. Heavy growth of *Klebsiella pneumonia* subsp *pneumoniae* was identified on aerobic culture of the blood as well as postmortem culture of the lung.

Organism Identification

Blood culture should be obtained in all neonates with systemic signs of sepsis. In older foals, transtracheal aspirates are necessary for cytology and culture to identify the causal organism or organisms. Cytologic analysis is used to confirm the presence of intracellular bacteria as well as provide preliminary identification of gram-positive, gram-negative, or mixed infections. For *R equi*, mixed infection does not appear to influence prognosis.[34] Culture allows for a definitive diagnosis and sensitivity testing. Polymerase chain reaction can also be performed for the detection of VapA-positive *R equi*.[35]

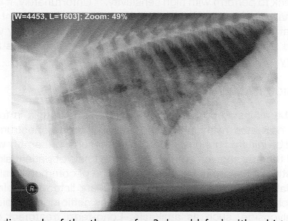

Fig. 2. Lateral radiograph of the thorax of a 3-day-old foal with a history of meconium staining of the fetal membranes as well as signs of neonatal maladjustment syndrome. A multinodular interstitial pattern coalescing to an alveolar pattern in the caudal ventral lung fields is seen consistent with aspiration pneumonia. A nasoesophageal feeding tube is present within the esophagus, and an intravenous catheter is seen within the cranial great vessels with the tip in the region of the right atrium.

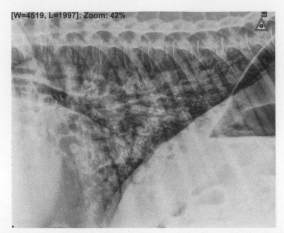

Fig. 3. Lateral radiograph of the thorax of a 3-month-old foal with a history of lethargy and fever. There is a moderate unstructured interstitial pattern throughout the lung lobes that coalesces to multifocal regions of an alveolar pattern ventrally. There are multifocal, round, well-defined soft tissue opacities up to 14 mm in diameter consistent with abscesses. *R equi* was identified by microbiologic culture of the transtracheal aspirate.

Screening

Various screening programs for the detection of *R equi* pneumonia have been implemented because of the insidious nature of the disease, resulting in affected foals not being recognized until pneumonia is severe. These screenings include physical examination, white blood cell concentration, fibrinogen measurement, serum amyloid A concentration, and thoracic imaging. Serologic testing,[36] serum amyloid A concentrations,[37] and fibrinogen concentrations[38,39] have not been shown to be as accurate as screening tests. White blood cell concentrations as a means of screening have produced conflicting results.[38,39] Thoracic ultrasonography is specific for lung lesions and relatively quick to perform with high sensitivity.[40] Unfortunately, it lacks specificity and results in many foals being unnecessarily treated. Development of a screening test program that retains the sensitivity of thoracic ultrasonography while improving specificity would be of considerable benefit to equine practitioners and the equine breeding industry.

PHARMACOLOGIC TREATMENT OPTIONS

Antibiotics are the mainstay of therapy for bacterial pneumonia in foals of all ages. When treating neonates with presumed sepsis, broad-spectrum antimicrobial coverage should be initiated pending blood culture results, preferably with bactericidal drugs. Empirical therapy should be selected on the basis of patient signalment, cytologic characteristics of the organism, and knowledge of common local isolates. Common antimicrobials and suggested doses for foals are listed in **Table 1**. A common initial treatment plan is a β-lactam antibiotic, such as ceftiofur or ampicillin, combined with an aminoglycoside, such as amikacin. Long-term treatment can be altered depending on the identification and sensitivity patterns of the pathogens isolated from the transtracheal aspirate or blood culture. A minimum course of 4 weeks is recommended for foals with localized sepsis such as pneumonia.

Treatment in older foals and weanlings often may be more targeted given the preponderance of *Streptococcus* or *Rhodococcus* as the causative organism. Although

Table 1
Antimicrobial agents commonly used to treat bacterial bronchopneumonia in foals

Antimicrobial	Dose	Notes
Amikacin sulfate	21–25 mg/kg IV or IM q24h	Potentially nephrotoxic
Amoxicillin sodium	20–40 mg/kg IV q6–12h	
Ampicillin sodium	25 mg/kg IV q6h	
Azithromycin	10 mg/kg PO q24–48h	May cause hyperthermia. Not recommended for use in foals >4 mo due to risk of enterocolitis
Cefapirin	20 mg/kg IM q8h, 20–30 mg/kg IV q6h	
Cefazolin	20 mg/kg IV or IM q6–8h	
Cefepime	11 mg/kg IV q8h	
Cefotaxime sodium	25–40 mg/kg IV q6h or 40 mg/kg loading then 6.66 mg/kg/h constant rate infusion (CRI) IV	
Cefpodoxime	10 mg/kg PO q6–12h	
Cefquinome	1–4.5 mg/kg IV or IM q6–12h	4th generation cephalosporin
Ceftazidime	40 mg/kg IV q6–8h	3rd generation cephalosporin, good blood brain barrier penetration
Ceftiofur sodium	5–10 mg/kg IV or IM q12h or 1.2–2.2 mg/kg loading dose, then 2.8–12.5 µg/kg/min CRI	
Ceftiofur free crystalline acid	6.6 mg/kg SQ q72h	
Ceftriaxone	25–50 mg/kg IV or IM q12h	
Chloramphenicol (palmitate or base)	50 mg/kg PO q6–12h	
Chloramphenicol sodium succinate	25–50 mg/kg IV q6–12h	
Clarithromycin	7.5 mg/kg PO q12h	May cause hyperthermia. Not recommended for use in foals >4 mo due to risk of enterocolitis
Doxycycline	10–20 mg/kg PO q12h	
Erythromycin	25 mg/kg PO q6–8h	May cause hyperthermia. Not recommended for use in foals >4 mo due to risk of enterocolitis
Florfenicol	20 mg/kg IM q48h	Risk of colitis in older foals and adults
Gentamicin sulfate	11–15 mg/kg IV or IM q36h until 2 wk of age, then 6.6 mg/kg IV or IM q24h	
Imipenem-cilastatin	10–15 mg/kg IV or IM q8–12h	
Metronidazole	15–20 mg/kg PO q6–8h 25 mg/kg PO q12h	
Minocycline	4 mg/kg PO q12h	

(continued on next page)

Table 1 (continued)		
Antimicrobial	Dose	Notes
Oxytetracycline hydrochloride	5–10 mg/kg IV q12–24h	Dilute and give slowly
Penicillin G potassium	22,000–40,000 IU/kg IV q6h	Give slowly
Penicillin G procaine	22,000 IU/kg IM q12–24h	
Rifampin	5–10 mg/kg PO q12h	Do not use alone
Ticarcillin-clavulanic acid	50 mg/kg IV q6h	
Trimethoprim-sulfonamide	30 mg/kg PO q12h	
Vancomycin	4.5–7.5 mg/kg IV q8h	Dilute and give over 1 h. Reserve only for use with bacteria resistant to all other drugs

many antimicrobials show in vitro efficacy against R equi, many are ineffective in vivo primarily because of low intracellular concentrations failing to reach intracellular R equi. For example, despite in vitro susceptibility to gentamicin, in one study, all 17 R equi–infected foals treated with penicillin and gentamicin died.[41] The combination of a macrolide antimicrobial with rifampin became the standard treatment in the 1980s, resulting in increased foal survival. Erythromycin was originally used but has been replaced primarily by either clarithromycin or azithromycin. Based on a retrospective evaluation as well as pharmacokinetic and pharmacodynamics considerations, the combination of clarithromycin plus rifampin appears superior to azithromycin or erythromycin combined with rifampin.[42] The combination of macrolides and rifampin has been shown to be synergistic in vitro and in vivo, and the combination of macrolides with rifampin is thought to reduce the resistance to either drug given alone.[43] The mutant prevention concentration (MPC) is the drug concentration that prevents the selective enrichment of resistant mutants. One study looking at the MPC for 10 antimicrobials found that the MPC and MPC/minimum inhibitory concentration ratio for erythromycin, clarithromycin, or azithromycin in combination were significantly lower than that of each drug tested individually.[44]

Despite these findings and decades of positive clinical experience, recent evidence indicates that the combination of rifampin with macrolides may be undesirable. The concentration of tulathromycin in plasma and bronchoalveolar lavage fluid was reduced by coadministration of rifampin in foals.[45] The bioavailability and pulmonary distribution of clarithromycin were evaluated before and after comedication with rifampin in 9 healthy foals. After rifampin, the relative bioavailability of clarithromycin decreased by more than 90%, resulting in plasma levels below the minimal inhibitory concentration for R equi[46]; this appears to occur largely as a result of inhibition of intestinal absorption.[47] Despite these results, the concentrations of clarithromycin in BAL fluid cells and pulmonary epithelial lining fluid, although reduced by rifampin, are still well above the minimal inhibitory concentration for macrolide-susceptible strains.[46] A recent small-scale clinical trial at a breeding farm in Germany revealed that azithromycin or azithromycin plus rifampin was significantly more effective than placebo among foals with mild pneumonia and thoracic lesions attributed to R equi, but there was no significant difference between the success of the macrolide plus rifampin relative to the macrolide alone.[48] Although these results suggest that monotherapy is equally as effective, the sample size of the study was quite small. Moreover, the foals in this study had subclinical or mild pneumonia: about 67% of placebo-treated foals recovered. Nevertheless, this study did not demonstrate reduced efficacy of the combination of a macrolide with rifampin. Further work is needed to determine the necessity for combining macrolides with rifampin; however, such work is unlikely to be conducted because the necessary clinical trial would have to be large in scale and costs. At this time, the authors recommend a combination of a macrolide with rifampin for treatment of R equi pneumonia on the basis of synergistic effects in vivo in mice, effects on MPCs in vitro, and the evidence of the absence of negative effects from a clinical trial (albeit an underpowered study).

There have been investigations into the use of other macrolide antibiotics. Tulathromycin has no in vitro activity against R equi with a MIC_{90} greater than 64 μg/mL.[49] In a clinical trial, foals treated with tulathromycin had larger pulmonary abscesses at 1 week and significantly longer duration of treatment versus those treated with azithromycin plus rifampin, suggesting that tulathromycin is not effective in the treatment of R equi pneumonia.[50] Tilmicosin also appears poorly active in vitro against isolates of R equi with a MIC_{90} of 64 μg/mL.[49] Gamithromycin at a dose of 6 mg/kg intramuscularly results in phagocytic cell concentrations above the MIC_{90} for macrolide-susceptible R equi isolates (as well as S zooepidemicus) for approximately 7 days[51] but has not been evaluated clinically. Telithromycin is a ketolide antibiotic having a spectrum of activity similar to newer generation macrolides, while overcoming current bacterial mechanisms of resistance to macrolides. Following an intragastric dose of 15 mg/kg, therapeutic drug levels were reached for treatment of macrolide-susceptible R equi isolates. Although the MIC_{50} for telithromycin for macrolide-resistant R equi isolates was lower than for clarithromycin, azithromycin, and erythromycin, telithromycin still would not be expected to be active against most macrolide-resistant isolates.[52] Further study is needed to look at the safety and efficacy of these other macrolide and ketolide antimicrobials in foals.

There is recent evidence that foals with small pulmonary lesions (total abscess scores between 1 and 10 cm) attributed to R equi infections do not necessitate treatment at some farms. Treatment of foals with antimicrobials (azithromycin or azithromycin combined with rifampin) on one farm in Germany did not speed resolution of disease compared with a placebo.[53] Therefore, the recent American College of Veterinary Internal Medicine consensus statement on R equi calls for the establishment of better criteria to determine the necessity for treatment of subclinically affected foals,[54] especially with increasing recognition of and attention to the development of macrolide-resistant R equi.

NONPHARMACOLOGIC TREATMENT OPTIONS

Supplemental oxygen is indicated in any neonate with a level of Pao_2 less than 60 mm Hg or a level of SaO_2 less than 90%. Supplemental oxygen is most commonly performed with intranasal oxygen insufflation. It is difficult to predict the resulting fraction of inspired oxygen as it varies with cannula placement and patency as well as tidal and minute volume. Most foals necessitate between 2 and 15 L/min to maintain a level of Pao_2 within an appropriate range. Complications include nasal mucosal irritation and drying, which can be mitigated by preconditioning with a water-filled humidifier. Oxygen toxicity can also occur, so serial ABGs should be used to monitor response. Foals with hypercapnia in addition to hypoxemia may benefit from mechanical ventilation. The benefits of mechanical ventilation are to improve V/Q matching, increase ventilation, decrease intrapulmonary shunting, and decrease the work of breathing. Survival rates of up to 80% have been reported in foals being ventilated for neonatal maladjustment syndrome and botulism.[55] Unfortunately, foals with pneumonia do not often respond as favorably.

TREATMENT RESISTANCE/COMPLICATIONS

Antimicrobial susceptibility patterns for the various bacteria reported to cause systemic sepsis and therefore pneumonia in the neonatal foal are location-specific and time period–specific and are reported elsewhere. It is worth noting that overall antimicrobial sensitivity is low and gram-positive organisms have unpredictable sensitivity patterns.[1,4,5] Between the years of 1982 and 2007, there was no significant development of bacterial resistance to commonly used antimicrobials in one population.[1] Treatment may be associated with complications such as antimicrobial-associated diarrhea or catheter-associated thrombophlebitis. Specific antimicrobials have some associated risk. Aminoglycosides and tetracyclines may cause nephrotoxicity, especially with repeated dosing in hypovolemic or systemically ill patients. Enrofloxacin should not be used in neonates because of its effect on cartilage.[56]

The emergence of macrolide-resistant R equi is of concern, especially with the widespread use of early detection and treatment programs. Rifampin-resistant isolates were first reported[57] and were found to be caused by a single base mutation in the rpoB cluster I region.[58] Next, clinical cases with resistance to both erythromycin and rifampin were reported.[59] Then, in a study from 9 laboratories between 1997 and 2008, 24 R equi isolates classified as resistant to macrolide antimicrobials or rifampin were reported with an apparent increase in frequency after 2002. Although 2 isolates were resistant to rifampin only, 22 of 24 (92%) were resistant to azithromycin, clarithromycin, erythromycin, and rifampin.[60] In that same study, the overall presence of resistant isolates was 4% (12/328) for the R equi samples submitted to laboratories in Florida and Texas. Clinically, one farm in central Kentucky that has participated in an ultrasonographic screening program since 2001 began seeing macrolide-resistant R equi isolates in 2008 and found 24% (6/25) of pretreatment R equi isolates in 2011 were resistant to macrolides and rifampin. Posttreatment with clarithromycin and rifampin, 62% (8/13) of isolates were resistant to macrolides and rifampin.[61] These resistant agents seem to be associated with a worse prognosis than macrolide-susceptible organisms.[60] Moreover, evidence exists that they may be more genetically similar to each other than susceptible isolates,[61] suggesting that these strains might be more likely to become endemic than macrolide-susceptible isolates. In addition to treatment failure, administration of macrolide antibiotics also carries potential risk. Potentially life-threatening diarrhea can be seen in either the treated foal or its dam. Hyperthermia has also been reported in foals receiving treatment with macrolides.[62] Recent evidence suggests that this effect may be due to drug-induced anhidrosis.[63]

PREVENTION

Prevention of neonatal pneumonia relies on management practices such as appropriate vaccination of pregnant mares, verification of transfer of passive immunity, and minimizing the risk of inhalation of pathogenic bacteria. As the foal matures, appropriate deworming and vaccination will decrease the risk of parasitic and viral pneumonias impacting the development of bacterial pneumonia. Currently, there are no effective, licensed vaccines for use in foals for bacterial pneumonia, although there have been multiple attempts to develop a vaccine for the prevention of R equi pneumonia.[64] Although chemoprophylaxis with azithromycin has been shown to be effective,[65] it is not recommended because of concerns regarding development of antimicrobial resistance.[61] Gallium maltolate has also been evaluated for chemoprophylaxis against R equi pneumonia in foals but did not decrease the incidence of pneumonia.[66] Transfusion of hyperimmune plasma has been shown to decrease occurrence of pneumonia[67] but is expensive, labor-intensive to administer, incompletely effective, and carries some risk for foals from handling and transfusion, possibly including serum hepatitis.[68] Although use of a commercially available parapoxvirus ovis immunomodulator failed to protect foals against R equi pneumonia,[69] the concept of host-directed treatment or prevention remains a worthy field for investigation. Whether vaccines will be warranted or feasible for S zooepidemicus (enzootic or endogenous types) remains to be determined. Alternative preventive strategies merit consideration for both S zooepidemicus and S equi subsp equi.

EVALUATION OF OUTCOME

Survival rates of foals with sepsis have increased from 25% reported in the early 1980s[70] to 70% currently.[2,3] Multiple factors have been associated with survival of septic foals in retrospective studies, but pneumonia as a specific feature of sepsis has not been shown to affect survival. Thoroughbred foals surviving sepsis do not differ from their siblings with regard to percentage of starters, percentage of winners, or number of starts, but they do have significantly fewer wins and total earnings.[1] Odds of athletic performance have been negatively associated with factors such as septic arthritis,[71] but pneumonia as a form of localized sepsis has not been specifically evaluated as a predictor of performance.

Survival proportions have also increased over the years for R equi pneumonia. Survival proportions were as low as 20% before the implementation of macrolide treatment,[72] but are now consistently at least 60% even in referral hospitals where the more severe cases are likely to be prevalent.[42,73] The odds of survival in foals infected with macrolide-resistant R equi isolates, however, are approximately 7-fold less than in foals infected with susceptible isolates.[60] The impact of R equi on athletic performance has also been assessed. Foals that recover from R equi pneumonia are somewhat less likely to race as adults (54% vs 65% of their birth cohort), but their racing performance is not different.[73]

SUMMARY

Bacterial pneumonia remains an important cause of morbidity and mortality in foals of all ages. Early recognition and institution of appropriate treatment should result in a good prognosis for survival and athletic function.

REFERENCES

1. Sanchez LC, Giguère S, Lester GD. Factors associated with survival of neonatal foals with bacteremia and racing performance of surviving Thoroughbreds: 423 cases (1982-2007). J Am Vet Med Assoc 2008;233:1446–52.
2. Stewart AJ, Hinchcliff KW, Saville WJ, et al. Actinobacillus sp bacteremia in foals: clinical signs and prognosis. J Vet Intern Med 2002;16:464–71.
3. Freeman L, Paradis MR. Evaluating the effectiveness of equine neonatal care. Vet Med 1992;87:921–6.
4. Marsh PS, Palmer JE. Bacterial isolates from blood and their susceptibility patterns in critically ill foals: 543 cases (1991-1998). J Am Vet Med Assoc 2001; 218:1608–10.

5. Russell CM, Axon JE, Blishen A, et al. Blood culture isolates and antimicrobial sensitivities from 427 critically ill neonatal foals. Aust Vet J 2008;86:266–71.

6. Holcombe SJ, Hurcombe SD, Barr BS, et al. Dysphagia associated with presumed pharyngeal dysfunction in 16 neonatal foals. Equine Vet J 2012;44:105–8.

7. Traub-Dargatz JL, Ingram JT, Stashak TS, et al. Respiratory stridor associated with polymyopathy suspected to be hyperkalemic periodic paralysis in four quarter horse foals. J Am Vet Med Assoc 1992;201:85–9.

8. Wilkins PA. Lower respiratory problems of the neonate. Vet Clin North Am Equine Pract 2003;19:19–33.

9. Cohen ND. Causes of and farm management factors associated with disease and death in foals. J Am Vet Med Assoc 1994;204:1644–51.

10. Anzai T, Walker JA, Blair MB, et al. Comparison of the phenotypes of Streptococcus zooepidemicus isolated from tonsils of healthy horses and specimens obtained from foals and donkeys with pneumonia. Am J Vet Res 2000;61:162–6.

11. Velineni S, Despitter D, Perchec AM, et al. Characterization of a mucoid clone of Streptococcus zooepidemicus from an epizootic of equine respiratory disease in New Caledonia. Vet J 2014;200:82–7.

12. Reuss SM, Chaffin MK, Cohen ND. Extrapulmonary disorders associated with Rhodococcus equi infection in foals: 150 cases (1987-2007). J Am Vet Med Assoc 2009;235:855–63.

13. Sanz M, Loynachan A, Sun L, et al. The effect of bacterial dose and foal age at challenge on Rhodococcus equi infection. Vet Microbiol 2013;167:623–31.

14. Horowitz ML, Cohen ND, Takai S, et al. Application of Sartwell's model (logarithmic-normal distribution of incubation periods) to age at onset and age at death of foals with Rhodococcus equi pneumonia as evidence of perinatal infection. J Vet Intern Med 2001;15:171–5.

15. Wang X, Coulson GB, Miranda-Casoluengo AA, et al. IcgA is a virulence factor of Rhodococcus equi that modulates intracellular growth. Infect Immun 2014;82(5): 1793–800.

16. Cohen ND, Smith KE, Ficht TA, et al. Epidemiologic study of results of pulsed-field gel electrophoresis of isolates of Rhodococcus equi obtained from horses and horse farms. Am J Vet Res 2003;64:153–61.

17. Bolton TI, Kuskie K, Halbert N, et al. Detection of strain variation in isolates of Rhodococcus equi from an affected foal using repetitive sequence-based polymerase chain reaction. J Vet Diagn Invest 2010;22(4):611–5.

18. Stoughton W, Poole T, Kuskie K, et al. Transfer of the virulence-associated protein a-bearing plasmid between field strains of virulent and virulent Rhodococcus equi. J Vet Intern Med 2013;27:1555–62.

19. Grimm MB, Cohen ND, Slovis NM, et al. Evaluation of fecal samples from mares as a source of Rhodococcus equi for their foals by use of quantitative bacteriologic culture and colony immunoblot analyses. Am J Vet Res 2007; 68:63–71.

20. Muscatello G, Anderson GA, Gilkerson JR, et al. Associations between the ecology of virulent Rhodococcus equi and the epidemiology of R equi pneumonia on Australian Thoroughbred farms. Appl Environ Microbiol 2006;72:6152–60.

21. Cohen ND, Chaffin MK, Kuskie KR, et al. Association of perinatal exposure to airborne Rhodococcus equi with risk of pneumonia caused by R equi in foals. Am J Vet Res 2013;74:102–9.

22. Kuskie KR, Smith JL, Sinha S, et al. Associations between the exposure to airborne virulent Rhodococcus equi and the incidence of R equi pneumonia among individual foals. J Equine Vet Sci 2011;31:463–9.

23. Cohen ND, Kuskie KR, Smith JL, et al. Association of airborne concentration of virulent Rhodococcus equi with location (stall versus paddock) and month (January through June) on 30 horse breeding farms in central Kentucky. Am J Vet Res 2012;73:1603–9.

24. Muscatello G, Gerbaud S, Kennedy C, et al. Comparison of concentrations of Rhodococcus equi and virulent R. equi in air of stables and paddocks on horse breeding farms in a temperate climate. Equine Vet J 2006;38:263–5.

25. Chaffin MK, Cohen ND, Martens RJ. Evaluation of equine breeding farm characteristics as risk factors for development of Rhodococcus equi pneumonia in foals. J Am Vet Med Assoc 2003;222:467–75.

26. Cohen ND, Carter CN, Scott HM, et al. Association of soil concentrations of Rhodococcus equi and incidence of pneumonia attributable to Rhodococcus equi in foals on farms in central Kentucky. Am J Vet Res 2008;69:385–95.

27. Giguère S, Prescott JF. Clinical manifestations, diagnosis, treatment, and prevention of Rhodococcus equi infections in foals. Vet Microbiol 1997;56:313–34.

28. Giguère S, Cohen ND, Chaffin MK, et al. Rhodococcus equi: clinical manifestations, virulence, and immunity. J Vet Intern Med 2011;25(6):1221–30.

29. Dawson TR, Horohov DW, Meijer WG, et al. Current understanding of the equine immune response to Rhodococcus equi. An immunological review of R. equi pneumonia. Vet Immunol Immunopathol 2010;135:1–11.

30. Chaffin MK, Cohen ND, Martens RJ, et al. Hematologic and immunophenotypic factors associated with development of Rhodococcus equi pneumonia of foals at equine breeding farms with endemic infection. Vet Immunol Immunopathol 2004;100:33–48.

31. Martens RJ, Cohen ND, Jones SL, et al. Protective role of neutrophils in mice experimentally infected with Rhodococcus equi. Infect Immun 2005;73(10):7040–2.

32. McQueen CM, Doan R, Dindot SV, et al. Identification of genomic loci associated with Rhodococcus equi susceptibility in foals. PLoS One 2014;9(6):e98710. http://dx.doi.org/10.1371/journal.pone.0098710.

33. Giguère S, Roberts GD. Association between radiologic pattern and outcome in foals with pneumonia caused by Rhodococcus equi. Vet Radiol Ultrasound 2012; 53:601–4.

34. Giguère S, Jordan LM, Glass K, et al. Relationship of mixed bacterial infection to prognosis in foals with pneumonia caused by Rhodococcus equi. J Vet Intern Med 2012;26(6):1443–8.

35. Halbert ND, Reitzel RA, Martens RJ, et al. Evaluation of a multiplex polymerase chain reaction assay for simultaneous detection of Rhodococcus equi and the vapA gene. Am J Vet Res 2005;66:1380–5.

36. Martens RJ, Cohen ND, Chaffin MK, et al. Evaluation of 5 serologic assays to detect Rhodococcus equi pneumonia in foals. J Am Vet Med Assoc 2002;221: 825–33.

37. Cohen ND, Chaffin MK, Vandenplas M, et al. Study of serum amyloid A concentrations as a means of achieving early diagnosis of Rhodococcus equi pneumonia in foals. Equine Vet J 2005;37:212–6.

38. Chaffin MK, Cohen ND, Blodgett GP, et al. Evaluation of hematologic screening methods for predicting subsequent onset of clinically apparent Rhodococcus equi pneumonia in foals. Proc Am Assoc Equine Pract 2013;59:267.

39. Giguère S, Hernandez J, Gaskin JM, et al. Evaluation of WBC concentration, plasma fibrinogen concentration, and an agar gel immunodiffusion test for early identification of foals with Rhodococcus equi pneumonia. J Am Vet Med Assoc 2003;222:775–81.

40. Slovis NM, McCracken JL, Mundy G. How to use thoracic ultrasound to screen foals for Rhodococcus equi at affected farms, in Proceedings. Am Assoc Equine Pract 2005;51:274–8.
41. Sweeney CR, Sweeney RW, Divers TJ. Rhodococcus equi pneumonia in 48 foals: response to antimicrobial therapy. Vet Microbiol 1987;14:329–36.
42. Giguère S, Jacks S, Roberts GD, et al. Retrospective comparison of azithromycin, clarithromycin, and erythromycin for the treatment of foals with Rhodococcus equi pneumonia. J Vet Intern Med 2004;18:568–73.
43. Giguère S, Lee EA, Guldbech KM, et al. In vitro synergy, pharmacodynamics, and postantibiotic effect of 11 antimicrobial agents against Rhodococcus equi. Vet Microbiol 2012;160:207–13.
44. Berghaus LJ, Giguère S, Guldbech K. Mutant prevention concentration and mutant selection window for 10 antimicrobial agents against Rhodococcus equi. Vet Microbiol 2013;166:670–5.
45. Venner M, Peters J, Höhensteiger N, et al. Concentration of the macrolide antibiotic tulathromycin in broncho-alveolar cells is influenced by comedication of rifampicin in foals. Naunyn Schmiedebergs Arch Pharmacol 2010;381(2): 161–9.
46. Peters J, Block W, Oswald S, et al. Oral absorption of clarithromycin is nearly abolished by chronic comedication of rifampicin in foals. Drug Metab Dispos 2011;39:1643–9.
47. Peters J, Eggers K, Oswald S, et al. Clarithromycin is absorbed by an intestinal uptake mechanism that is sensitive to major inhibition by rifampicin: results of a short-term drug interaction study in foals. Drug Metab Dispos 2012;40:522–8.
48. Venner M, Credner N, Lammer M, et al. Comparison of Tulathromycin, azithromycin and azithromycin-rifampin for the treatment of mild pneumonia associated with Rhodococcus equi. Vet Rec 2013;173(16):397.
49. Carlson K, Kuskie K, Chaffin MK, et al. Antimicrobial activity of Tulathromycin and 14 other antimicrobials against virulent Rhodococcus equi in vitro. Vet Ther 2010; 11:1–9.
50. Venner M, Kerth R, Klug E. Evaluation of Tulathromycin in the treatment of pulmonary abscesses in foals. Vet J 2007;174:418–21.
51. Berghaus LJ, Giguère S, Sturgill TL, et al. Plasma pharmacokinetics, pulmonary distribution, and in vitro activity of gamithromycin in foals. J Vet Pharmacol Ther 2012;35:59–66.
52. Javsicas LH, Giguère S, Womble AY. Disposition of oral telithromycin in foals and in vitro activity of the drug against macrolide-susceptible and macrolide-resistant Rhodococcus equi isolates. J Vet Pharmacol Therap 2010;33:383–8.
53. Venner M, Rodiger A, Laemmer M, et al. Failure of antimicrobial therapy to accelerate spontaneous healing of subclinical pulmonary abscesses on a farm with endemic infections caused by Rhodococcus equi. Vet J 2012;192:293–8.
54. Giguère S, Cohen ND, Chaffin MK, et al. Diagnosis, treatment, control, and prevention of infections caused by Rhodococcus equi in foals. J Vet Intern Med 2011;25:1209–20.
55. Wilkins PA, Palmer JE. Mechanical ventilation in foals with botulism: 9 cases (1989-2002). J Vet Intern Med 2003;17:708–12.
56. Vivrette SL, Bostian A, Bermingham E. Quinolone-induced arthropathy in neonatal foals. In: Proceedings of the 47th Annual Convention of the American Association of Equine Practitioners. San Diego (CA): Wiley; 2001. p. 376–77.
57. Takai S, Takeda K, Nakano Y, et al. Emergence of rifampin-resistant Rhodococcus equi in an infected foal. J Clin Microbiol 1997;35:1904–8.

58. Fines M, Pronost S, Maillard K, et al. Characterization of mutations in the rpoB gene associated with rifampin resistance in Rhodococcus equi isolated from foals. J Clin Microbiol 2001;39:2784–7.

59. Kenney DG, Robbins SC, Prescott JF, et al. Development of reactive arthritis and resistance to erythromycin and rifampin in a foal during treatment for Rhodococcus equi pneumonia. Equine Vet J 1994;26:246–8.

60. Giguère S, Lee E, Williams E, et al. Determination of the prevalence of antimicrobial resistance to macrolide antimicrobials or rifampin in Rhodococcus equi isolates and treatment outcome in foals infected with antimicrobial-resistant isolates of R equi. J Am Vet Med Assoc 2010;237:74–81.

61. Burton AJ, Giguère S, Sturgill TL, et al. Macrolide- and rifampin-resistant Rhodococcus equi on a horse breeding farm, Kentucky, USA. Emerg Infect Dis 2013;19: 282–5.

62. Stratton-Phelps M, Wilson WD, Gardner IA. Risk of adverse effects in pneumonic foals treated with erythromycin versus other antibiotics: 143 cases (1986-1996). J Am Vet Med Assoc 2000;217:68–73.

63. Stieler AS, Sanchez LC, Mallicote MF, et al. Macrolide-induced hyperthermia in foals: role of impaired sweat responses [Abstract]. J Vet Intern Med 2014;28:1109.

64. Giles C, Vanniasinkam T, Ndi S, et al. Rhodococcus equi (Prescottella equi) vaccines; the future of vaccine development. Equine Vet J 2014. http://dx.doi.org/10.1111/evj.12310.

65. Chaffin MK, Cohen ND, Martens RJ. Chemoprophylactic effects of azithromycin against Rhodococcus equi pneumonia among foals at endemic equine breeding farms. J Am Vet Med Assoc 2008;232:1035–47.

66. Chaffin MK, Cohen ND, Martens RJ, et al. Evaluation of the efficacy of gallium maltolate for chemoprophylaxis against pneumonia caused by Rhodococcus equi infection in foals. Am J Vet Res 2001;72:945–57.

67. Madigan JE, Hietala S, Muller N. Protection against naturally acquired Rhodococcus equi pneumonia in foals by administration of hyperimmune plasma. J Reprod Fertil Suppl 1991;44:571–8.

68. Aleman M, Nieto JE, Carr EA, et al. Serum hepatitis associated with commercial plasma transfusion in horses. J Vet Intern Med 2005;19(1):120–2.

69. Sturgill TL, Giguère S, Franklin RP, et al. Effects of inactivated parapoxvirus ovis on the cumulative incidence of pneumonia and cytokine secretion in foals on a farm with endemic infections caused by Rhodococcus equi. Vet Immunol Immunopathol 2011;140(3–4):237–43.

70. Koterba AM, Brewer BD, Tarplee FA. Clinical and clinicopathological characteristics of the septicaemic neonatal foal: review of 38 cases. Equine Vet J 1984;16: 376–82.

71. Smith LJ, Marr CM, Payne RJ, et al. What is the likelihood that Thoroughbred foals treated for septic arthritis will race? Equine Vet J 2004;36:452–6.

72. Eilssalde GS, Renshaw HW, Walberg JA. Corynebacterium equi: an interhost review with emphasis on the foal. Comp Immunol Microbiol Infect Dis 1980;3: 433–45.

73. Ainsworth DM, Eicker SW, Yeager AE, et al. Associations between physical examination, laboratory, and radiographic findings and outcome and subsequent racing performance of foals with Rhodococcus equi infection: 115 cases (1984-1992). J Am Vet Med Assoc 1998;213:510–1.

Update on Interstitial Pneumonia

Pamela A. Wilkins, DVM, MS, PhD*, Kara M. Lascola, DVM, MS

KEYWORDS

- Equine • Respiratory • Pulmonary fibrosis • Inflammation • Toxin

KEY POINTS

- Interstitial pneumonia represents a group of acute and chronic inflammatory respiratory diseases that have the potential to cause marked alveolar damage and impairment of gas exchange within the lung in horses of all ages.
- Equine multinodular pulmonary fibrosis and acute lung injury/acute respiratory distress are recognized as specific categories of interstitial pneumonia.
- Treatment of interstitial pneumonia is often unrewarding. Therapy should include suppression of inflammation, maintenance of tissue oxygen delivery, and appropriate treatment of any underlying diseases.

The term interstitial pneumonia defines several diseases that can be acute, such as in acute lung injury (ALI)/ acute respiratory distress syndrome (ARDS), and become chronic, or be chronic and progress to pulmonary fibrosis. The course of most interstitial pneumonias is insidious with both acute and chronic forms ultimately characterized by alveolar structural derangements that lead to loss of functional gas exchange units and altered mechanical properties of the lung, characterizing these pneumonias as restrictive lung problems. Although interstitial pneumonia is an uncommon cause of acute or chronic disorders of the lower respiratory tract of horses, because of its severity, recognition and diagnosis are desirable as early as possible in its clinical course.[1–8]

GENERAL CLINICAL SIGNS

Horses affected with interstitial pneumonia frequently have cough, weight loss, nasal discharge, exercise intolerance, severe dyspnea, cyanosis, and a restrictive breathing pattern. Fever is variable and dependent on the causative agent and the chronicity of disease. A so-called heave line is frequently present; nostril flare and an anxious expression are usual. The history can be acute or chronic, and horses and foals

Department of Veterinary Clinical Medicine, University of Illinois College of Veterinary Medicine, 1008 West Hazelwood Drive, Urbana, IL 61801, USA
* Corresponding author.
E-mail address: pawilkin@illinois.edu

Vet Clin Equine 31 (2015) 137–157
http://dx.doi.org/10.1016/j.cveq.2014.11.006
0749-0739/15/$ – see front matter © 2015 Elsevier Inc. All rights reserved.

may be evaluated several times and treated for a variety of conditions before a diagnosis related to interstitial pneumonia is made. Affected foals are frequently depressed and anorectic, whereas adults may be bright and alert with a variable appetite. More than one foal at a farm may be affected. The disease may progress despite treatment, with progressive respiratory compromise, although some patients may also slowly improve with time and treatment.

PATHOPHYSIOLOGY

Interstitial pneumonia progresses through 4 phases. During the first phase, the initial insult causes parenchymal injury and alveolitis. This stage is followed by a proliferative phase characterized by cellular and parenchymal alterations in the tissues of the lung. Chronic cases progress to the development of interstitial fibrosis, and the final stage results in end-stage irreparable fibrosis of the lung.

The structural changes that occur in the lung reduce the number of functional alveoli, adversely affecting ventilation by altering ventilation-perfusion relationships, reducing surface area available for gas exchange, and increasing diffusion barrier thickness. Reduced lung compliance is associated with the loss of distensible alveoli, the presence of pulmonary edema, and fibrosis. Total and vital lung capacities are decreased in association with the loss of functional gas exchange units and reduced lung compliance. The work of breathing is increased, resulting in exercise intolerance and difficulty in breathing. Pulmonary hypertension and cor pulmonale may be complications of interstitial pneumonia, fibrosis, and hypoxemia/hypoxia. Although the origin of pulmonary hypertension is unclear, hypoxic vasoconstriction and generation of vasoactive compounds (such as endothelin-1) that alter pulmonary vascular resistance acutely and vessel anatomy chronically may play a role.

DIAGNOSTIC TESTING

In older horses, the primary differential diagnosis of heaves may be excluded by the leukocytosis and hyperfibrinogenemia that commonly occur in horses with interstitial pneumonia and fibrosis but do not generally occur in horses with heaves. However, these clinical abnormalities are common in horses with bacterial bronchopneumonia, which is another early differential diagnosis.

Thoracic imaging, both radiography and ultrasonography, are helpful and important in the establishment of a definitive diagnosis. Computed tomography (CT) is possible in neonatal foals because of their smaller size (**Fig. 1**).[9,10] Typically, thoracic radiographs reveal extensive interstitial and bronchointerstitial pulmonary patterns.[11] Nodular infiltrates may be present, either large or miliary, but are always diffusely distributed (**Fig. 2**).

Bacterial and fungal culture and viral isolation of transtracheal or bronchoalveolar lavage (BAL) aspirates often yield no significant growth of known or common pathogens. Cytologic evaluation of tracheal or BAL fluid (BALF) generally shows increased numbers of neutrophils and macrophages (**Fig. 3**). If *Pneumocystis carinii* is involved, BALF may reveal trophozoites or intracystic bodies with special stains, such as toluidine blue or methenamine silver.[12] Using polymerase chain reaction (PCR), equine herpes virus (EHV)-5 has been found in BALF from horses with equine multinodular pulmonary fibrosis (EMPF).[13]

Histologic examination of a transthoracic lung tissue biopsy specimen is the definitive antemortem diagnostic test for chronic interstitial pneumonia and fibrosis and for EMPF and may also be beneficial in fungal lung diseases. Care must be taken to ensure that the tissue biopsy is obtained from a representative area; ultrasonography

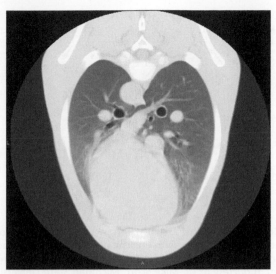

Fig. 1. Transverse thoracic CT image of a healthy 10-day-old foal. The foal is sedated, positioned in sternal recumbency, and breathing spontaneously (room air). Note the mild increase in attenuation of the ventral lungs caused by positional atelectasis.

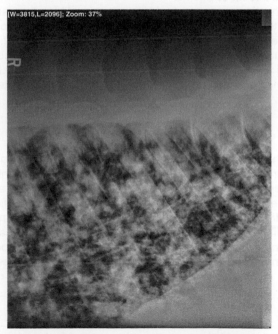

Fig. 2. Standing lateral radiographic appearance of caudal dorsal lung field of a horse affected by equine multinodular pulmonary fibrosis (EMPF). Note increased interstitial pattern and nodular alveolar pattern. (*Courtesy of* Dr. Sarah Reuss, University of Florida.)

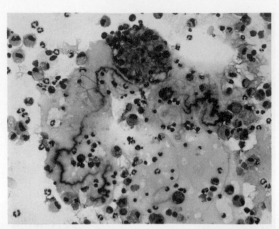

Fig. 3. Typical findings for cytocentrifuged BALF from a 12-year-old thoroughbred gelding with EMPF. Note the prominent mucus with Curschmann spirals, a multinucleated giant cell, and an increase in neutrophils. No viral inclusions or bacteria were present (Wright-Giemsa stain, 50× objective). (*Courtesy of* Dr. Mike Scott, Michigan State University.)

guidance is useful and should be used. Complications from this technique that are clinically important, such as hemorrhage or respiratory duress, are uncommon but can occur.[14,15] Biopsy can both confirm the clinical diagnosis and define the causative agent in some cases. Immunohistochemical and PCR evaluation of lung tissue may identify suspected infectious agents.

Additional diagnostic procedures could include arterial blood gas analysis, abdominocentesis, and thoracocentesis as attempts to rule out metastatic neoplastic disease. Serologic testing for antibody to fungi and chicken serum, if hypersensitivity pneumonitis is suspected, has been useful in some cases.[16,17] A complete cardiac evaluation should also be conducted, because pulmonary hypertension and cor pulmonale are common sequelae and, if present, are generally associated with a poorer prognosis.[13]

CAUSE

Multiple agents have been implicated in the genesis of interstitial pneumonia in animals, but fewer than 20 have been confirmed in horses (**Box 1**). Chief among these are infectious agents and ingested toxins. Frequently the causative agent cannot be identified because of the insidious nature of the process, and the final diagnosis is idiopathic interstitial pneumonia. The lung responds in a stereotypic manner to injury, and a limited ability to identify infectious, toxic, and immunologic causes frequently hinders the current ability to make an accurate identification of a specific cause. All efforts should be made to identify a causative agent early in the course of the disease, but practitioners need to be aware that treatment is frequently nonspecific and supportive.

Infectious Agents

Infectious causes of interstitial pneumonia in horses and foals include viral, bacterial, parasitic, protozoal, and fungal agents. Typically the pneumonia is acute and severe, characterized by severe damage to the lung parenchyma (alveolar region).

Box 1
Causes of interstitial pneumonia in horses

Acute

Infections (viral, bacterial, fungal, parasitic)

Inhaled chemicals

    Oxygen (high Fio_2, >50%)

    Smoke

Ingested toxins (or precursors)

    Perilla mint

    Crofton weed

    Crotalaria spp

    Senecio spp

Adverse drug reactions

Hypersensitivity

Endogenous metabolic or toxic conditions

    ALI/ARDS

    Endotoxemia

    Systemic inflammatory response syndrome

    Disseminated intravascular coagulation

Idiopathic or cryptogenic

Chronic

Infections (Viral, bacterial, fungal, parasitic)

    EMPF

Inhaled inorganic dust (pneumoconiosis)

    Silicosis

Hypersensitivity

Ingested toxins (or precursors)

    Perilla mint

    Crofton weed

    Crotalaria spp

    Senecio spp

Collagen/vascular disorders

Idiopathic or cryptogenic

Abbreviation: Fio_2, fraction of inspired oxygen (21% room air).

Viral diseases

Viral agents are frequently implicated or suspected but rarely identified by the usual serologic, histopathologic, and virus isolation methods. The advent of more sensitive and specific techniques, such as in situ PCR and monoclonal antibody immunohistochemistry (IHC), has resolved some of the diagnostic challenges. Equine viral arteritis

(EVA) and herpes viral infections (EHV-1 and EHV-4) have been implicated in in utero viral infections leading to lung disease.[18] Although involvement of adenovirus in the pathogenesis of pneumonia has also been reported in a thoroughbred foal, fatal adenoviral pneumonia is primarily associated with severe combined immunodeficiency (SCID) in Arabian foals.[19,20] In addition, influenza A virus has been isolated from a 7-day-old foal with bronchointerstitial pneumonia and reports from the Australian influenza outbreak include many affected foals.[20]

Influenza

Although sporadic infection in foals has been described, there are few published reports of widespread outbreaks in foals less than 6 months of age, the most recent being in Australia in 2007.[21–23] A lower incidence of disease in young foals is most likely a result of the presence of maternally derived antibodies in vaccinated or previously exposed mares. The Australian outbreak was unique in that it was an unvaccinated naive population; horse of all ages were severely affected, with many not surviving.[23] Influenza-specific serum antibody concentration is a highly accurate correlate to protection against infection and disease, and animals with high concentrations of homologous antibody are almost always protected against experimental challenge.[24,25] Immunization of horses against influenza has reduced the frequency of disease outbreaks and the frequency and severity of clinical signs when epizootic disease occurs among vaccinated animals.[26–28]

Outbreaks of equine influenza generally occur when unvaccinated or susceptible horses are housed in close contact with one another (eg, horse shows, racetracks, sale barns). Virus transmission occurs through direct contact with infected animals or via droplet or airborne transmission.[29] A usual clinical presentation of equine influenza consists of fever, anorexia, lethargy, nasal discharge, and cough with fever the first symptom recognized, generally between 48 to 96 hours after infection. Nasal discharge is serous in the first few days but may become mucopurulent 3 to 4 days postinfection. Coughing, typically dry and hacking, may still be present 3 weeks postinfection, long after other clinical signs have resolved.

Equine herpes viruses

The most important EHVs associated with respiratory disease in horses are the alpha-herpes viruses EHV-1 and EHV-4. EHV-1 commonly infects horses, donkeys, and mules and occasionally infects zebras and other species; EHV-4 is restricted to horses.[30] Gamma-herpes viruses EHV-2 and EHV-5 can be associated with respiratory disease, although their pathogenicity is reportedly low.[31] EHV-5 has been implicated in the pathogenesis of EMPF. Infections caused by EHV-1 and EHV-4 are particularly common in young performance horses and result in latent infection within the first weeks or months of life.[32] Viral reactivation can then result in clinical disease and viral shedding later in life.[30]

Both EHV-1 and EHV-4 cause respiratory signs, but signs are more severe for EHV-1, as is the likelihood of viremia. Clinical respiratory disease in susceptible horses has an incubation period of 1 to 3 days. Signs include fever, usually biphasic, with a first peak at 24 to 48 hours associated with upper respiratory tract infection and a second peak at 4 to 8 days associated with viremia. Depression and anorexia are often mild. Nasal discharge becomes mucopurulent by day 5 to 7. Neonatal foals infected with EHV-1 either in utero or shortly after birth show weakness, lethargy, and profound respiratory distress caused by interstitial pneumonia shortly after birth or infection.[33,34] Prognosis is poor for survival. Although EHV-1 respiratory disease is uncommon in horses more than 2 years of age because of prior infection and development of immunity, the occasional horse, generally less than 3 years of age, can be affected by a severe pulmonary vasculotropic form and die peracutely.[35]

Equine arteritis virus

Neonatal foals infected with equine arteritis virus (EAV) show severe respiratory signs and high mortality. In foals with congenital infection that survive for any length of time, or that acquire the virus following birth, fever and leukopenia with thrombocytopenia are present. Interstitial pneumonia, lymphocytic arteritis or periarteritis, renal tubular necrosis, and fibrinoid necrosis of the tunic media are seen on pathologic examination.[36] Old, debilitated, or immunosuppressed horse can be similarly predisposed to severe EVA.[37]

Hendra virus

Hendra virus (HeV) is able to cause natural disease in humans and horses and therefore has zoonotic potential, posing a serious public health and occupational safety risk for workers in the equine industry and equine veterinarians.[38] HeV has only been identified in Australia and the natural reservoir is the native Australian fruit bat. The first outbreak occurred 1994; the virus then disappeared for almost 10 years with subsequent years providing at least 1 case per year, the most recent being in 2014.[38,39] HeV infection in horses is characterized by an acute, febrile respiratory illness with variable facial swelling, ataxia, head pressing, and recumbency. Frothy nasal discharge and tachycardia are considered to be indicators of imminent death. The course of disease in infected horses is short, with animals dying within 36 hours after onset of clinical signs. Experimentally the incubation period is 6 to 12 days.[40] Histologically, HeV infection is associated with interstitial pneumonia with proteinaceous alveolar edema and hemorrhage. The presence of syncytial giant cells in the endothelium of pulmonary blood vessels is the most informative histologic finding.[41] There is no known effective antiviral medication. A vaccine has been developed and recently introduced.[42]

Bacterial/protozoal/parasitic/fungal diseases

Bacterial agents have been isolated from the lung in some horses with bronchointerstitial pneumonia of either unknown cause or caused by viral pneumonia. The usual distribution of bacterial bronchopneumonia in the horse is caudoventral, whereas the distribution in interstitial pneumonia is diffuse. In the latter cases the bacteria are most likely opportunistic pathogens and do not represent the primary causative agents, although infection by these opportunistic organisms may require treatment. An exception is *Rhodococcus equi* pneumonia of older foals. *R equi* has been cultured from foals with severe, acute bronchointerstitial pneumonia, probably ALI/ARDS, with a diffuse pulmonary distribution.[4,5,43]

Interstitial pneumonia associated with *P carinii* has been described in the foal, and *Mycoplasma* species have been isolated from the respiratory tract of adult horses.[12,44,45] *P carinii* pneumonia is thought to occur primarily in immunocompromised foals as a complication of some other serious disease, such as infectious pneumonia or SCID. It is characterized by plasmacytic lymphocytic interstitial pneumonia with flooding of alveoli with foamy acidophilic material, which can easily progress to pyogranulomatous bronchopneumonia.[12,46] *Mycoplasma* isolates tend to be considered innocent bystanders in the horse.

Parasitic pneumonia, an uncommon cause of chronic bronchointerstitial pneumonia, usually occurs in young foals secondary to migration of *Parascaris equorum* larvae through the pulmonary parenchyma.[47]

Fungal infections in horses are also uncommon, although geographic prevalence is highly variable. Fungi are ubiquitous, and their constant aerosol exposure to respiratory tissue is inevitable. Upper respiratory and pulmonary disease caused by fungi is frequently acquired by the inhalation route, with the sporular diameter small enough to allow penetration into the distal airways and alveoli. Important predisposing factors for fungal pneumonia include (1) qualitative and especially quantitative granulocyte abnormalities, and (2) the presence of devitalized tissue. Primary pathogenic fungi such as *Blastomyces dermatitidis*, *Histoplasma capsulatum*, *Coccidioides immitis*, *Cryptococcus neoformans*, and *Conidiobolus coronatus* usually infect immunologically normal horses, whereas a separate group of fungal pathogens tend to infect only equine patients with abnormal host defenses. Opportunistic fungi including *Aspergillus* species, *Candida* species, *Fusarium* species, and *Emmonsia crescens* have caused fungal disease in horses that are immunocompromised or neutropenic; have neoplasia, colitis, enteritis, or bacterial pneumonia; or have been treated with corticosteroids.[48-51] Pulmonary fungal infections with granulomas, diffuse pneumonia, or pleuropneumonia have clinical signs similar to those of bacterial infection with fever; cough; nasal discharge; tachypnea; respiratory distress; hemoptysis; and, if chronic, weight loss. The radiographic appearance of fungal pneumonia varies and may manifest as any infiltrative pattern; the most common initial finding is a patchy bronchopneumonia with a peripheral distribution. Treatment of *Aspergillus* species pneumonia is unrewarding in most cases, because diagnosis is often made late in the course of disease in a horse with severe underlying preexisting disease. Successful therapy has been reported for fungal pneumonia with other causes.[52-56]

Toxins

Ingested chemicals

Ingested chemicals rank second only to infectious agents as potential causes of interstitial pneumonia in horses. Ingestion of pyrrolizidine alkaloids from a variety of plants (mostly genera *Crotalaria*, *Trichodesma*, and *Senecio*) can cause interstitial pneumonia in horses.[57] Toxicity is associated with production of a toxic metabolite that is activated in the liver and then circulates to the lung. The toxic alkylating agents damage capillary endothelial cells, although the amount of alkaloid required to damage the lung is generally less than that required for hepatotoxicity.

Crofton weed (*Eupatorium adenophorum*), a poisonous plant found primarily in Australia, California, and Hawaii, can result in interstitial pneumonia in horses if the flowering plant is ingested.[58] The nature of the toxin is not known.

Perilla ketone, derived from the plant *Perilla fructans*, experimentally produces acute respiratory distress within a week of ingestion in ponies.[59] The lesions include diffuse alveolitis and type II pneumocyte proliferation with sparing of the bronchioles. Toxicity depends on additional metabolism of the 3-substituted furan by the mixed function oxidase system, which occurs directly in the lung of the horse.

Inhaled chemicals

Direct pulmonary injury by inhaled chemicals is an uncommon cause of interstitial pneumonia in horses. In people, this type of pneumonia is primarily related to occupational exposure.

Smoke inhalation

Smoke inhalation causes acute, diffuse interstitial pneumonia in horses, frequently followed within a few days by opportunistic bacterial pneumonia.[60] Insult to the respiratory system by smoke inhalation depends on the fuels that are burned, the completeness of combustion, and the generated heat intensity. In general, lesions are initiated by 3 mechanisms.

The first is direct thermal injury, which is often limited to the upper respiratory tract by laryngeal reflexes and efficient heat exchange within the nasal passages.[61] Second, toxic chemicals in the smoke can cause damage, both directly and indirectly, through inflammatory mediators. Carbon monoxide intoxication is commonly associated with human injuries from smoke and is a product of incomplete combustion.[62] In addition, with combustion there is consumption of oxygen, and the resulting low partial arterial oxygen pressure (Pao_2) can lead to pulmonary vasoconstriction as well as generalized hypoxia.

Three phases of pulmonary dysfunction have been described in the horse.[63,64] The first stage is acute pulmonary insufficiency caused by several mechanisms. Carbon monoxide may be present in sufficiently high concentration to cause toxicity within a short time after exposure. Carbon monoxide combines with hemoglobin to form carboxyhemoglobin. Hemoglobin has a 200 to 250 times greater affinity for carbon monoxide compared with its affinity for oxygen.[62] High levels of circulating carboxyhemoglobin result in a shift of the oxyhemoglobin dissociation curve to the left, thereby decreasing oxygen release at the tissue level and leading to tissue hypoxia.

Other processes occurring during this acute phase include progressive edema and necrosis in the upper respiratory tract, leading to airway obstruction, bronchoconstriction in the lower respiratory tract caused by the irritating effects of noxious products, and altered pulmonary blood flow.[65] These insults produce the second stage: formation of pulmonary edema, lower airway obstruction, and pulmonary parenchymal lesions. Within 48 to 72 hours after exposure, pulmonary macrophage-derived cytokines attract neutrophils to the area of insult. Neutrophils release additional cytokines, proteolytic enzymes, and oxygen-derived free radicals. Expression of the inflammatory cascade in excess of balance by antiinflammatory processes causes microvascular damage, leading to increased extravascular lung water. Local insult also results in the release of tissue factor, initiating the coagulation cascade to produce fibrin. Debris from the inflammatory cascade, along with fibrin and material directly deposited from smoke inhalation, create pseudomembranous casts, which may obstruct the small airways. Widespread unidirectional plugging of the small airways may significantly increase airway pressure, causing barotrauma and additional alveolar damage.[65] The last stage, bronchopneumonia, occurs as a result of an impaired host immune system, both locally and systemically. This phase may occur up to 1 to 2 weeks after the initial injury.

Horses exposed to fire with smoke have a variety of clinical signs depending on the duration and type of exposure and the length of time from the insult. Acutely, within the first 6 hours, signs of carbon monoxide toxicity and shock may occur. The patient shows signs of severe hypoxemia and may be depressed, disoriented, irritable, ataxic, or even moribund and comatose. As edema and necrosis progress in the upper respiratory tract, dyspnea and stridor may develop. Auscultation of the thorax may reveal decreased air movement, crackles, or wheezes, but these may not become apparent for 12 to 24 hours. If edema of the airways is sufficiently severe, airflow may be severely restricted. Edema fluid may be visible at the nostrils and, later, may be replaced by inflammatory exudate. Signs of infection may be difficult to differentiate from signs associated with the primary insult. All that may be noticed is a fever and a worsening of respiratory signs after initial improvement.

Diagnosis is typically based on history of exposure to fire and smoke, such as a barn fire, and physical examination. A normal initial examination does not rule out exposure because the onset of clinical signs may be delayed for several days. Within a short time after exposure, carboxyhemoglobin concentration in venous blood can be measured. A level of more than 10% is consistent with carbon monoxide toxicity.[62]

Oxygen

Oxygen toxicity can theoretically produce interstitial pneumonia and alveolar type II cell proliferation. This problem is more likely to be seen in neonatal foals mechanically ventilated with increased levels of oxygen (fraction of inspired oxygen [Fio_2] >50%) for several days, although this may be a form of ventilator-associated lung injury caused by mechanical stretch of the airspaces. Damage is thought to be caused by production of reactive oxygen metabolites, which attack a lung already injured by barotrauma resulting from ventilator-driven increases in airway pressure.[66]

Other chemicals

Agrichemicals or herbicides, such as paraquat, may cause acute interstitial pneumonia in horses and should be considered in horses with a history of possible exposure.[67]

Silicosis is a specific chronic granulomatous pneumonia of horses associated with inhalation of silicon dioxide crystals.[11,68] This syndrome has been described in horses originating from the Carmel Valley region of California. The inhaled particles are ingested by alveolar macrophages and result in lysis of the macrophage, chronic alveolitis, and fibrosis. Multiple granulomas are present, and submicrometer intracytoplasmic crystalline particles can be identified in macrophages. A concurrent osteoporosislike syndrome may be seen in affected horses.

Hypersensitivity Reactions

In the most specific sense, hypersensitivity pneumonitis refers to pulmonary disease caused by inhalation of organic antigens. Lymphocytic, plasmacytic bronchitis and bronchiolitis, combined with lymphocytic interstitial pneumonia, characterize the disease in horse lung. Granuloma formation and fibrosis can be observed. Chicken dust and fungi have been implicated as causes of severe, chronic bronchointerstitial pneumonia, but the syndrome is rare.[16,17]

Endogenous Metabolic and Toxic Conditions

Various conditions cause acute pulmonary injury with inflammatory edema or severe alveolar wall damage and serofibrinous exudation similar to that described for acute interstitial pneumonia. Acute uremia, shock, burns, and trauma can produce an acute pulmonary injury termed ALI or ARDS, depending on severity.[69] Although endotoxin does not directly injure the lung, endotoxemia in the horse initiates inflammatory and metabolic cascades, potentially mediated via Toll-like receptor-9 and pulmonary intravascular macrophages (PIMs), which can lead to pulmonary injury.[70] Activation of these pathways produces vasoactive and chemoattractant molecules that increase vascular permeability, activate complement, produce proinflammatory cytokines, and release neutrophil enzymes that can adversely affect the lungs of horses.[70] Horses as a species are sensitive to the negative effects of endotoxemia, and their lungs are particularly sensitive, perhaps because of the presence of PIMs, which further amplify the inflammatory cascade.[70]

EQUINE MULTINODULAR PULMONARY FIBROSIS

A novel gamma-EHV, EHV type 5 (EHV-5), has been found to be associated with a nodular form of interstitial pneumonia of horses characterized by pulmonary interstitial fibrosis, suggesting that these unusual cases may have an underlying infectious cause.[71–74] This disease has been termed EMPF by the investigators describing the pathology and clinical presentation of the disease.[13,71] Like people with idiopathic pulmonary fibrosis, which is also thought to be associated with gamma-herpesvirus infection.[72,75] EMPF seems to be a disease of the middle-aged to older individual, although the diagnosis has been made in horses as young as 2 years.[76,77] Abnormal physical examination findings of horses with EMPF include variable hyperthermia, weight loss, tachypnea, and tachycardia. Thoracic auscultation is usually abnormal with wheezes and crackles commonly reported both with and without rebreathing examination. Affected horses have generally been treated for heaves or infectious bronchopneumonia with little to no improvement and progression of clinical signs before receiving a diagnosis of EMPF.

Commonly reported clinical pathology findings in EMPF include hyperfibrinogenemia, leukocytosis, neutrophilia, monocytosis, anemia, and hypoxemia, particularly in cases that have had diagnosis delayed.[72,78,79] In evaluating these cases clinically, recurrent airway obstruction (RAO) (or summer pasture associated obstructive pulmonary disease [SPAOPD]) needs to be effectively ruled out. The clinician should determine whether reversible bronchospasm is contributing to the observed clinical signs of tachypnea, dyspnea, and in some cases significant arterial hypoxemia. In horses with RAO or SPAOPD, bronchodilator administration significantly improves the horse's breathing effort and pattern within 20 to 30 minutes of administration, whereas horses with EMPF show little improvement. Eosinophilic intranuclear inclusion bodies, although rare, may be found in macrophages in BALF if carefully examined.

Typical radiographs reveal multiple discreet to coalescing nodular densities overlying a diffuse interstitial pattern (see **Fig. 2**). Ultrasonographic examination reveals bilateral, diffuse roughening of the pleural surface and, as the disease progresses, the existence of multiple superficial discrete nodules of varying size (**Fig. 4**). Histologic appearance is diagnostic of this disease. EHV-5 has been identified in both BALF and lung biopsy samples from affected patients by both PCR assay and IHC.[13,71,78]

Based on current limited experience, the diagnosis of EMPF is associated with a fair to poor prognosis. Of the treated cases reported in the literature, about 50% have responded to therapy as shown by an improvement in demeanor, weight gain, and radiographic changes, or have self-cured.[72,78,79] Anecdotally, the cure rate might be a bit higher. It also seems that the response is improved in horses diagnosed early in the clinical course.

ACUTE LUNG INJURY/ACUTE RESPIRATORY DISTRESS SYNDROME

ALI and the more severe ARDS represent complex clinical syndromes of overwhelming pulmonary inflammation. These clinical syndromes involve the acute onset of pulmonary disease in response to a variety of pulmonary (direct) or extrapulmonary (indirect) inflammatory stimuli. In humans, the highest incidence of ALI/ARDS is found in septic patients.[80] ARDS is most widely defined by the presence of bilateral pulmonary infiltrates, noncardiogenic pulmonary edema, and severe hypoxemia as defined by a Pao_2/F_io_2 ratio of less than 200 mm Hg. ALI, considered by many to be a precursor to ARDS, is distinguished by a Pao_2/F_io_2 ratio of less than 300 mm Hg.[81]

ALI and ARDS have been described in several veterinary species, including adult and juvenile horses, and a veterinary-specific consensus definition for these syndromes (veterinary ALI [VetALI]/veterinary ARDS [VetARDS]) has been developed (**Box 2**).[69] A specific subcategory of VetALI/VetARDS was created to define these conditions in neonatal foals, equine neonatal ARDS (EqNARDS), and equine neonatal ALI (EqNALI), to account for the relative hypoxemia of normal neonatal foals compared with adults during the first week of life (**Table 1**).[69] EqNARDS/EqNALI are

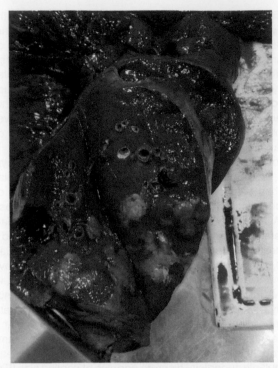

Fig. 4. Cut section of lung from a horse with EMPF. Note large areas of fibrosis within the parenchyma. (*Courtesy of* Dr. Sarah Reuss, University of Florida.)

distinguished from neonatal equine respiratory distress syndrome, which represents a distinct clinical syndrome resulting from a primary surfactant deficiency in foals less than 24 hours of age.[69] Identified direct and indirect risk factors in veterinary species are similar to those in humans and include sepsis, systemic inflammatory response syndrome, local or systemic infection or inflammation, severe trauma, smoke inhalation, near-drowning, multiple transfusions, and exposure to certain drugs or toxins.

The best documentation of VetALI and VetARDS is for older foals (1–12 months of age), with the earliest reports referring to these syndromes as proliferative interstitial lung disease or acute bronchointerstitial pneumonia.[3–5,43,82] Affected foals typically present with sudden and severe respiratory distress. Various initial bacterial or viral insults, such as *R equi*, have been reported in the history of foals presenting with VetALI and VetARDS and concurrent primary pulmonary disease is possible.[4,5,43] Foals may also present without any known previous respiratory or systemic disease.[5,43,82] Documentation of probable ALI/ARDS in adult horses is limited but includes isolated reports of near-drowning, smoke inhalation injury, and experimental endotoxin exposure.[83,84] In neonatal foals, perinatal viral infection or progression of bacterial sepsis or any form of pulmonary disease to EqNALI or EqNARDS are significant risks.[22,36,85–88]

The pathogenesis of ALI/ARDS has been extensively reviewed and represents an imbalance between proinflammatory and antiinflammatory processes within the lung.[89–92] Direct (intrapulmonary) or indirect (extrapulmonary) insults trigger upregulation of local humoral and cellular-mediated inflammation. Early lung injury occurs within minutes to hours of the insult and is characterized by increased alveolar-capillary permeability edema (a hallmark of ALI/ARDS), infiltration and activation of

Box 2
Diagnostic criteria for VetALI and VetARDS

At least 1 of each of the first 4 criteria must be met; criterion 5 is optional but recommended

1. Acute onset (<72 hours) of tachypnea and labored breathing at rest

2. Known risk factors

3. Evidence of noncardiogenic pulmonary edema (no clinical or diagnostic evidence of left heart failure) based on one of the following:

    a. Bilateral/diffuse infiltrates on thoracic radiographs (more than 1 quadrant/lobe)

    b. Bilateral dependent density gradient on CT (neonatal foals)

4. Hypoxemia without PEEP (mechanical ventilation) and known Fio_2

    a. Pao_2/Fio_2 ratio

        i. Less than or equal to 300 for VetALI

        ii. Less than or equal to 200 for VetARDS

    b. Increased alveolar-arterial oxygen gradient

5. Evidence of diffuse pulmonary inflammation

    a. Transtracheal wash/BAL sample neutrophilia

    b. Transtracheal wash/BAL biomarkers of inflammation

Abbreviation: PEEP, positive end-expiratory pressure.
Adapted from Wilkins PA, Otto CM, Dunkel B, et al. Acute lung injury (ALI) and acute respiratory distress syndromes (ARDS) in veterinary medicine: consensus definitions. J Vet Emerg Crit Care 2007;17(4):333–9.

inflammatory cells, atelectasis, and pulmonary hypertension.[89–92] This is represented clinically by dyspnea, profound hypoxemia secondary to V/Q mismatch, and reduced lung compliance.[89–92]

Pulmonary edema develops in response to damage to both the pulmonary microvascular endothelium and the alveolar epithelium. Endothelial activation and injury after insult involves altered vasomotor tone as well as destruction and obstruction of the vascular bed. Loss of alveolar epithelial integrity not only disrupts the fluid transport

Table 1
EqNALI/EqNARDS age-dependent diagnostic criteria

Postnatal Age	Normal Pao_2 (mm Hg)[a]	Normal Pao_2/Fio_2 (mm Hg)	EqNALI Pao_2/Fio_2 (mm Hg)	EqNARDS Pao_2/Fio_2 (mm Hg)
60 min	60.9 ± 2.7	>300	<175	<115
12 h	73.5 ± 3.0	>350	<200	<140
24 h	67.6 ± 4.4	>350	<200	<140
48 h	74.9 ± 3.3	>350	<200	<140
4 d	81.2 ± 3.1	>400	<250	<160
7 d	90.0 ± 3.1	>430	<280	<190

[a] Breathing room air, in lateral recumbency, and sample obtained from lateral metatarsal artery.
Adapted from Wilkins PA, Otto CM, Dunkel B, et al. Acute lung injury (ALI) and acute respiratory distress syndromes (ARDS) in veterinary medicine: consensus definitions. J Vet Emerg Crit Care 2007;17(4):333–9.

mechanisms of the alveoli but may also impair normal surfactant production. The combination of endothelial dysfunction, internal and external vascular occlusion, and increased vascular tone contributes to pulmonary hypertension, which is a characteristic of ALI/ARDS.[93] Neutrophil migration, activation, and sequestration within the alveoli and microvasculature along with upregulation of vasoactive (eg, endothelin [ET]-1), proinflammatory (eg, tumor necrosis factor-alpha, interleukin [IL]-1, IL-8), and procoagulant (eg, tissue factor) mediators are noted early and are central to the pathogenesis of ALI/ARDS.[89–92] Progression of ALI/ARDS may include resolution of edema and inflammation and restoration of the alveolar epithelial membrane or may involve maladaptive fibroproliferative repair.[89]

The clinical presentation of VetALI/VetARDS is best described in older foals.[5,43,82] Acute respiratory distress characterized by tachypnea and increased respiratory effort, nasal flare, and occasionally paradoxic breathing is the most consistent finding. Cyanosis may also be observed. Reduced to absent peripheral bronchovesicular sounds along with bronchial sounds over the central airways or adventitial lung sounds of crackles and wheezes over the dorsal lung field have both been described on thoracic auscultation. Other findings on physical examination are nonspecific and may include pyrexia, tachycardia, injected mucous membranes, depression, or other signs of concurrent systemic disease. Additional diagnostics should be directed toward confirming the diagnosis of VetALI/VetARDS or EqNALI/EqNARDS and identifying the underlying cause or concurrent disease. The specific diagnostic criteria for VetALI/VetARDS in horses are similar to those in humans, with an added recommendation for evidence of diffuse pulmonary inflammation and accounting for age-related differences in gas exchange (see **Box 2**, **Table 1**).[69] Serial measurement of Pao_2 is not only useful for confirming a diagnosis of VetALI or VetARDS but also for monitoring the patient's response to therapy. Radiographic findings may include a diffuse bronchointerstitial pattern or a multifocal to diffuse coalescing alveolar pattern with air bronchograms.[5,43,82] Descriptions of CT images of the lungs of neonatal foals with EqALI/EqARDS are limited, but may show a diffuse, bilateral, patchy to coalescing alveolar pattern with air bronchograms most pronounced in the ventral lungs but extending into the caudodorsal lungs (**Fig. 5**). Thoracic ultrasonography may be useful for

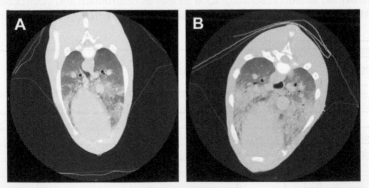

Fig. 5. Transverse thoracic CT images of neonatal foals with mild (A) and severe (B) ALI. Both foals were sedated, positioned in sternal recumbency, and breathing spontaneously. (A) Seven-day-old foal with a Pao_2/Fio_2 of 260 mm Hg on room air. Note the patchy-to-coalescing alveolar pattern that is most pronounced in the ventral lungs. (B) Four-day-old foal with a Pao_2/Fio_2 of 214 mm Hg on room air. A diffuse, coalescing alveolar pattern with air bronchograms is noted throughout the right and left lung fields.

identification of concurrent bacterial pneumonia, to rule out cardiac disease, or in patients for whom radiography is not an option. Described findings on ultrasonography include multiple coalescing comet-tail artifacts in the caudodorsal lung field.[82] In addition to providing evidence of pulmonary inflammation, culture of transtracheal wash is useful when underlying bacterial pneumonia is suspected.

Mortality is reported to be between 30% and 40% in older foals with VetALI/ VetARDS.[5,43,82] In neonatal foals, the prognosis may be worse because other comorbidities, such as sepsis, are common. However, reports on long-term follow-up and athletic performance in horses recovering from VetALI/VetARDS are lacking.

TREATMENT

Treatment of these cases is often unrewarding, especially in neonatal foals with ALI/ARDS. Therapeutic goals are treatment of any underlying or secondary infection, suppression of inflammation, maintenance of tissue oxygen delivery within appropriate limits, relief of any associated bronchoconstriction, and prevention or treatment of complications (**Tables 2** and **3**). Environmental control, with appropriate temperature and humidity control and good ventilation, is beneficial.

Parenteral corticosteroid therapy is the mainstay of treatment, with early and aggressive therapy providing the best long-term outcome, particularly in foals. In one report of 23 foals affected with acute bronchointerstitial pneumonia, 9 of 10 treated with corticosteroids survived, but none of those not receiving steroid treatment lived, with a second report later showing similar findings in 15 cases.[5,43]

Horses with EMPF have reportedly responded to treatment with antiviral and corticosteroid therapy.[75,78,79] The course of therapy is generally prolonged (6–12 weeks); clinical and radiographic improvement has been noted in a few cases to date.

Broad-spectrum antimicrobial treatment should be instituted initially, particularly in foals, as described for treatment of infectious bronchopneumonia. The choice of antimicrobial agent and duration of therapy should be dictated by the culture and sensitivity results from the transtracheal aspirate (TTA) and by the patient's clinical course.

Table 2
Agents used to treat equine herpes viral infections (EHV-1 and EHV-5) and EMPF and ALI/ARDS in horses

Agent	Dose (mg/kg)	Frequency (h)	Route
Antiviral Agents Used to Treat Equine Herpes Viral Infections (EHV-1 and EHV-5)			
Acyclovir	20	8	PO
	10[a]	12	IV
Valacyclovir	40	8	PO
	27 (loading dose)	8	PO
	18 (maintenance dose)		
Corticosteroids used in the Treatment of EMPF and ALI/ARDS			
Methylprednisolone sodium succinate	1	12–24	IM or IV (slowly)
Hydrocortisone sodium succinate	1	12	IM or IV
Dexamethasone	0.01–0.02	12–24	IM or IV
Prednisolone	1	12–24	PO

Abbreviations: EMPF, equine multinodular pulmonary fibrosis; IM, intramuscular; IV, intravenous; PO, by mouth.
[a] Dilute in 1 L of isotonic crystalloid and give slowly over 1 hour.

Table 3 Other medications used in the treatment of interstitial pneumonia in horses[a]				
Class	Drug	Dose	Frequency (h)	Route
Bronchodilators	Clenbuterol	0.8 µg/kg	12	PO
	Albuterol	450 µg	8–12	MDI
	Albuterol plus ipratropium[b]	550 µg albuterol 100 µg ipratropium	8–12	MDI
	Ipratropium	90 µg	8–12	MDI
	Furosemide	250 mg	8–12	Nebulized
Inhaled steroids	Fluticasone	2000 µg	12–24	MDI
Inhaled antimicrobials	Ceftiofur sodium	500 mg	12	Nebulized
	Gentamicin	250 mg	12	Nebulized

Abbreviation: MDI, metered dose inhaler.
  [a] In some cases these drugs have been studied for efficacy in horses, but in most cases pharmacokinetics/pharmacodynamics (PK/PD) and safety studies have not been performed in the equine species. Antimicrobial dosages are extrapolated from human use. There currently are no data supporting dosages of nebulized antimicrobials in adult horses.
  [b] Combivent.

There is potential benefit in antimicrobial nebulization in the airway for cases with either primary or secondary bacterial infection.[94,95]

Foals, in particular, and adults with severe respiratory distress may benefit from nasal insufflation of humidified oxygen, with flow rates of 10 L/min for foals and 15 L/min in adults.[96,97] If necessary, as determined by persistent hypoxemia with intranasal insufflation at the rates given, a second nasal cannula can be placed in the opposite nostril to increase the Fio_2. Care must be taken to avoid obstruction of the nasal passages. Alternatively, intratracheal or transtracheal insufflation can be considered to further increase Fio_2 and improve oxygenation.[98] If available, mechanical ventilation can be lifesaving in severely affected neonates.[99,100]

Systemic bronchodilator therapy may or may not be indicated in these cases. If used, bronchodilators may worsen ventilation-perfusion inequalities. Therefore bronchodilator therapy should be accompanied by supplemental oxygen, and the effects should be monitored with serial blood gas measurements and discontinued if hypoxemia worsens. Nebulized or aerosolized bronchodilator therapy may be more judicious, and beneficial effects are evident in some foals with respiratory distress. Aminophylline and theophylline should not be used, owing to their narrow therapeutic range.[101] Furosemide, inhaled or parenteral, may be appropriate for its bronchodilator effect and its effect on reducing pulmonary artery pressure, particularly if cor pulmonale develops.[102]

PROGNOSIS

The prognosis for horses with interstitial pneumonia is uniformly poor to guarded. Affected foals, treated early and aggressively with corticosteroid and antimicrobial therapy, have the best outlook for life. The disease is usually progressive in adults and eventually results in the demise of the horse, although some horses recover sufficiently to return to previous performance levels. A fair number of adult horses, with continuous intense management, live for a period of time but are severely compromised, which limits their usefulness. Exceptions to the poor prognosis may be seen in cases of older foals with ALI/ARDS, P carinii pneumonia in foals if they are treated early and aggressively, cases of smoke inhalation that survive the burn injuries, and possibly also in cases of idiopathic interstitial pneumonia or EMPF in adult horses that are treated early with corticosteroids and antiviral drugs. A trial of treatment of peracute interstitial disease for 48 to 96 hours is warranted, with a goal of signs of improvement in that time but not disease resolution. Patients with chronic interstitial pneumonia should be treated for a minimum of 4 to 6 weeks, if practical, before the possibility of recovery is discarded.

REFERENCES

1. Wilkins PA. Interstitial pneumonia. In: Robinson E, editor. Current veterinary therapy. 5 edition. Philadelphia: WB Saunders; 2003. p. 425–8.
2. Bruce EH. Interstitial pneumonia in horses. Compend Cont Educ (Pract Vet) 1995;17:1145–55.
3. Buergelt CD, Hines SA, Cantor G, et al. A retrospective study of proliferative interstitial lung disease of horses in Florida. Vet Pathol 1986;23(6):750–6.
4. Prescott JF, Wilcock BP, Carman PS, et al. Sporadic, severe bronchointerstitial pneumonia of foals. Can Vet J 1991;32(7):421–5.
5. Lakritz J, Wilson W, Berry CR, et al. Bronchointerstitial pneumonia and respiratory distress in young horses: clinical, clinicopathologic, radiographic, and pathological findings in 23 cases. (1984-1989). J Vet Intern Med 1993;7(5): 277–88.
6. Derksen FJ, Slocombe RF, Brown CM, et al. Chronic restrictive pulmonary disease in a horse. J Am Vet Med Assoc 1982;180(8):887–9.
7. Donaldson MT, Beech J, Ennulat D, et al. Interstitial pneumonia and pulmonary fibrosis in a horse. Equine Vet J 1998;30(2):173–5.
8. Wilkins PA, Del Piero F, Williams KJ. Interstitial pneumonia. In: Smith BP, editor. Respiratory diseases. Large animal internal medicine. 5th edition. Philadelphia: Elsevier Inc; 2014. p. 510–2.
9. Lascola KM, O'Brien RT, Wilkins PA, et al. Qualitative and quantitative interpretation of computed tomography of the lungs in healthy neonatal foals. Am J Vet Res 2013;74(9):1239–46.
10. Schliewert EC, Lascola KM, O'Brien RT, et al. Comparison of radiographic and computed tomography images of the lung in healthy neonatal foals. Am J Vet Res 2015 Jan;76(1):42–52.
11. Berry CR, O'Brien TR, Madigan JE, et al. Thoracic radiographic features of silicosis in 19 horses. J Vet Intern Med 1991;5(4):248–56.
12. Ainsworth DM, Weldon AD, Beck KA, et al. Recognition of *Pneumocystis carinii* in foals with respiratory distress. Equine Vet J 1993;25(2):103–8.
13. Wong DM, Belgrave R, Williams KJ, et al. Equine multinodular pulmonary fibrosis in five horses. J Am Vet Med Assoc 2008;232(6):898–905.
14. Raphel CF, Gunson DE. Percutaneous lung biopsy in the horse. Cornell Vet 1981;71(4):439–48.
15. Savage CJ, Traub-Dargatz JL, Mumford EL. Survey of the large animal diplomates of the American College of Veterinary Internal Medicine regarding percutaneous lung biopsy in the horse. J Vet Intern Med 1998;12(6):456–64.
16. Mansmann RA, Osburn BI, Wheat JD, et al. Chicken hypersensitivity pneumonitis in horses. J Am Vet Med Assoc 1975;166(7):673–7.
17. Asmundsson T, Gunnarsson E, Johannesson T. "Haysickness" in Icelandic horses: precipitin tests and other studies. Equine Vet J 1983;15(3):229–32.
18. Vaala WE, Hamir AN, Dubovi EJ, et al. Fatal congenital acquired infection with equine arteritis virus in a neonatal thoroughbred. Equine Vet J 1992;24(2):155–8.

19. Webb RF, Knight PR, Walker KH. Involvement of adenovirus in pneumonia in a thoroughbred foal. Aust Vet J 1981;57(3):142–3.
20. Thompson DB, Spradborw PB, Studdert M. Isolation of an adenovirus from an Arab foal with a combined immunodeficiency disease. Aust Vet J 1976;52(10):435–7.
21. Smith BP. Influenza in foals. J Am Vet Med Assoc 1979;174(3):289–90.
22. Peek SF, Landolt G, Karasin AI, et al. Acute respiratory distress syndrome and fatal interstitial pneumonia associated with equine influenza in a neonatal foal. J Vet Intern Med 2004;18(1):132–4.
23. Begg AP, Reece RL, Hum S, et al. Pathological changes in horses dying with equine influenza in Australia, 2007. Aust Vet J 2011;89(Suppl 1):19–22.
24. Mumford JA, Wood JM, Folkers C, et al. Protection against experimental infection with influenza virus A/equine/Miami/63 (H3N8) provided by inactivated whole virus vaccines containing homologous virus. Epidemiol Infect 1988; 100(3):501–10.
25. Mumford JA, Wood JM, Scott AM, et al. Studies with inactivated equine influenza vaccine. 2. Protection against experimental infection with influenza virus A/equine/Newmarket/79 (H3N8). J Hyg 1983;90(3):385–95.
26. Nyaga PN, Wiggins AD, Priester WA. Epidemiology of equine influenza, risk by age, breed and sex. Comp Immunol Microbiol Infect Dis 1980;3(1–2):67–73.
27. Newton JR, Verheyen K, Wood JL, et al. Equine influenza in the United Kingdom in 1998. Vet Rec 1999;145(16):449–52.
28. Wood J, Mumford J. Epidemiology of equine influenza. Vet Rec 1992;130(6):126.
29. Bridges CB, Kuehnert MJ, Hall CB. Transmission of influenza: implications for control in health care settings. Clin Infect Dis 2003;37(8):1094–101.
30. Allen GP, Kydd JH, Slater JD, et al. Equid herpesvirus 1 and equid herpesvirus 4 infections. In: Coetzer JA, Tustin RC, editors. Infectious diseases of livestock. Newmarket (United Kingdom): Oxford University Press; 2004. p. 829.
31. Allen GP, Murray MJ. Equid herpesvirus 2 and equid herpesvirus 5 infections. In: Coetzer JA, Tustin RC, editors. Infectious diseases of livestock. Newmarket (United Kingdom): Oxford University Press; 2004. p. 860.
32. Foote CE, Love DN, Gilkerson JR, et al. Detection of EHV-1 and EHV-4 DNA in unweaned thoroughbred foals from vaccinated mares on a large stud farm. Equine Vet J 2004;36(5):341–5.
33. Perkins G, Ainsworth DM, Erb HN, et al. Clinical, haematological and biochemical findings in foals with neonatal equine herpesvirus-1 infection compared with septic and premature foals. Equine Vet J 1999;31(5):422–6.
34. Murray MJ, del Piero F, Jeffrey SC, et al. Neonatal equine herpesvirus type 1 infection on a thoroughbred breeding farm. J Vet Intern Med 1998;12(1):36–41.
35. Del Piero F, Wilkins PA, Timoney PJ, et al. Fatal nonneurological EHV-1 infection in a yearling filly. Vet Pathol 2000;37(6):672–6.
36. Del Piero F, Wilkins PA, Lopez JW, et al. Equine viral arteritis in newborn foals: clinical, pathological, serological, microbiological and immunohistochemical observations. Equine Vet J 1997;29(3):178–85.
37. MacLachlan NJ, Balasuriya UB. Equine viral arteritis. Adv Exp Med Biol 2006; 581:429–33.
38. Murray K, Selleck P, Hooper P, et al. A morbillivirus that caused fatal disease in horses and humans. Science 1995;268(5207):94–7.
39. Ball M, Dewberry T, Freeman P, et al. Clinical review of Hendra virus infection in 11 horses in New South Wales, Australia. Aust Vet J 2014;92(6):213–8.
40. Rogers RJ, Douglas IC, Baldock FC, et al. Investigation of a second focus of equine morbillivirus infection in coastal Queensland. Aust Vet J 1996;74(3):243–4.

41. Westbury HA. Hendra virus disease in horses. Rev Sci Tech 2000;19(1):151–9.
42. Middleton D, Pallister J, Klein R, et al. Hendra virus vaccine, a one health approach to protecting horse, human, and environmental health. Emerg Infect Dis 2014;20(3):372–9.
43. Dunkel B, Dolente B, Boston RC. Acute lung injury/acute respiratory distress syndrome in 15 foals. Equine Vet J 2005;37(5):435–40.
44. Ammar A, Kirchhoff H, Heitmann J, et al. Demonstration and differentiation of mycoplasmas in bronchial secretions including serological study of horses with acute and chronic respiratory tract diseases. Berl Munch Tierarztl Wochenschr 1980;93(23):457–62 [in German].
45. Wood JL, Chanter N, Newton JR, et al. An outbreak of respiratory disease in horses associated with *Mycoplasma felis* infection. Vet Rec 1997;140(15): 388–91.
46. Ewing PJ, Cowell RL, Tyler RD, et al. *Pneumocystis carinii* pneumonia in foals. J Am Vet Med Assoc 1994;204(6):929–33.
47. Srihakim S, Swerczek TW. Pathologic changes and pathogenesis of *Parascaris equorum* infection in parasite-free pony foals. Am J Vet Res 1978;39(7): 1155–60.
48. Sweeney CR, Habecker PL. Pulmonary aspergillosis in horses: 29 cases (1974–1997). J Am Vet Med Assoc 1999;214(6):808–11.
49. Tunev SS, Ehrhart EJ, Jensen HE, et al. Necrotizing mycotic vasculitis with cerebral infarction caused by *Aspergillus niger* in a horse with acute typhlocolitis. Vet Pathol 1999;36(4):347–51.
50. Pusterla N, Pesavento PA, Leutenegger CM, et al. Disseminated pulmonary adiaspiromycosis caused by *Emmonsia crescens* in a horse. Equine Vet J 2002;34(7):749–52.
51. Reilly LK, Palmer JE. Systemic candidiasis in four foals. J Am Vet Med Assoc 1994;205(3):464–6.
52. Pusterla N, Holmberg TA, Lorenzo-Figueras M, et al. *Acremonium strictum* pulmonary infection in a horse. Vet Clin Pathol 2005;43(4):413–6.
53. Cornick JL. Diagnosis and treatment of pulmonary histoplasmosis in a horse. Cornell Vet 1990;80(1):97–103.
54. Begg M, Hughes KJ, Kessell A, et al. Successful treatment of cryptococcal pneumonia in a pony mare. Aust Vet J 2004;82(11):686–92.
55. Higgins JC, Leith GS, Pappagianis D, et al. Successful treatment of *Coccidioides immitis* pneumonia with fluconazole in two horses. J Vet Intern Med 2005;19(11):482–3.
56. Nappert G, Van Dyck T, Papich M, et al. Successful treatment of a fever associated with consistent pulmonary isolation of *Scopulariopsis* sp in a mare. Equine Vet J 1996;28(5):421–4.
57. Nobre D, Dagli ML, Haraguchi M. *Crotalaria juncea* intoxication in horses. Vet Hum Toxicol 1994;36(5):445–8.
58. O'Sullivan BM. Investigations into Crofton weed (*Eupatorium adenophorum*) toxicity in horses. Aust Vet J 1985;62(1):30–2.
59. Schmidbauer SM, Venner M, von Samson-Himmelstjerna G, et al. Compensated overexpression of procollagens alpha 1(I) and alpha 1(III) following perilla mint ketone-induced acute pulmonary damage in horses. J Comp Pathol 2004; 131(2–3):186–98.
60. Marsh PS. Fire and smoke inhalation in horses. Vet Clin Equine 2007;23(1):19–30.
61. Toon MH, Maybauer MO, Greenwood JE, et al. Management of acute smoke inhalation injury. Crit Care Resusc 2010;12(1):53–61.

62. Ernst A, Zibrak JD. Carbon monoxide poisoning. N Engl J Med 1998;339(13):1603–8.
63. Geor RJ, Ames TR. Smoke inhalation injury in horses. Compend Cont Educ (Pract Vet) 1991;13:1162–9.
64. Kirkland KD, Goetz TE, Foreman JH, et al. Smoke inhalation injury in a pony. Vet Emerg Crit Care 1992;3:83–9.
65. Murakami K, Tabor DL. Pathophysiological basis of smoke inhalation injury. News Physiol Sci 2003;18:125–9.
66. Bast A, Weseler AR, Haenen GR, et al. Oxidative stress and antioxidants in interstitial lung disease. Curr Opin Pulm Med 2010;16(5):516–20.
67. Takahashi T, Takahashi Y, Nio M. Remodeling of the alveolar structure in the paraquat lung of humans: a morphometric study. Hum Pathol 1994;25(7):702–8.
68. Schwartz LW, Knight HD, Whittig LD, et al. Silicate pneumoconiosis and pulmonary fibrosis in horses from the Monterey-Carmel peninsula. Chest 1981;80(1 Suppl):82–5.
69. Wilkins PA, Otto CM, Dunkel B, et al. Acute lung injury (ALI) and acute respiratory distress syndromes (ARDS) in veterinary medicine: consensus definitions [Special commentary]. J Vet Emerg Crit Care 2007;17(4):333–9.
70. Aharonson-Raz K, Singh B. Pulmonary intravascular macrophages and endotoxin-induced pulmonary pathophysiology in horses. Can J Vet Res 2010;74(1):45–9.
71. Williams KJ, Maes R, Del Piero F, et al. Equine multinodular pulmonary fibrosis: a newly recognised herpesvirus-associated fibrotic lung disease. Vet Pathol 2007; 44(6):849–62.
72. Doran P, Egan JJ. Herpesviruses: a cofactor in the pathogenesis of idiopathic pulmonary fibrosis? Am J Physiol Lung Cell Mol Physiol 2005;289(5): L709–710.
73. Williams KJ, Robinson NE, Lim A, et al. Experimental induction of pulmonary fibrosis in horses with the gammaherpesvirus equine herpesvirus 5. PLoS One 2013;8(10):e77754.
74. Williams KJ. Gammaherpesviruses and pulmonary fibrosis: evidence from humans, horses, and rodents. Vet Pathol 2014;51(2):372–84.
75. Nalysnyk L, Cid-Ruzafa J, Rotella P, et al. Incidence and prevalence of idiopathic pulmonary fibrosis: review of the literature. Eur Respir Rev 2012; 21(126):355–61.
76. Kubiski SV, Rech RR, Camus MS, et al. Pathology in practice. J Am Vet Med Assoc 2009;235:381–3.
77. Marenzoni ML, Coppola G, Maranesi M, et al. Age-dependent prevalence of equid herpesvirus 5 infection. Vet Res Commun 2010;34(8):703–8.
78. Wilkins PA. Equine multinodular pulmonary fibrosis: diagnosis and treatment. Eq Vet Educ 2013;25(8):393–7.
79. Wong DM, Maxwell LK, Wilkins PA. Use of antiviral medications against equine herpes virus associated disorders. Eq Vet Educ 2010;22(5):244–52.
80. Perl M, Lomas-Neira J, Venet F, et al. Pathogenesis of indirect (secondary) acute lung injury. Expert Rev Respir Med 2011;5(1):115–26.
81. Bernard GR, Artigas A, Brigham KL, et al. The American-European consensus conference on ARDS. Definitions, mechanisms, relevant outcomes and clinical trial coordination. Am J Respir Crit Care Med 1994;149(3 part 1):818–24.
82. Dunkel B. Acute lung injury and acute respiratory distress syndrome in foals. Clin Tech Equine Pract 2006;5:127–33.
83. Sembrat R, Di Stazio J, Reese J, et al. Acute pulmonary failure in the conscious pony with Escherichia coli septicemia. Am J Vet Res 1978;39(7):1147–54.

84. Kemper T, Spier S, Barratt-Boyes SM, et al. Treatment of smoke inhalation in five horses. J Am Vet Med 1993;202(1):91–4.
85. Frymus T, Kita J, Woyciechowska S, et al. Foetal and neonatal foal losses on equine herpesvirus 1 infected farms before and after EHV-1 vaccination was introduced. Pol Arch Med Wewn 1986;26(3–4):7–14.
86. Gilkerson JR, Whalley JM, Drummer HE, et al. Epidemiology of EHV-1 and EHV-4 in the mare and foal populations on a Hunter Valley stud farm: are mares the source of EHV-1 for unweaned foals? Vet Microbiol 1999;68(1–2):27–34.
87. Wilkins PA. Lower respiratory problems of the neonate. Vet Clin North Am Equine Pract 2003;19(1):19–33.
88. Hoffman AM, Viel L, Prescott J, et al. Association of microbiologic flora with clinical, endoscopic, and pulmonary cytologic findings in foals with distal respiratory tract infection. Am J Vet Res 1993;54(10):1615–22.
89. Ware LB. Pathophysiology of acute lung injury and the acute respiratory distress syndrome. Sem Respiratory Crit Care Med 2006;27(4):337–46.
90. Bhatia M, Moochhala S. Role of inflammatory mediators in the pathophysiology of acute respiratory distress syndrome. J Pathol 2004;202(2):145–56.
91. Wheeler AP, Bernard GR. Acute lung injury and the acute respiratory distress syndrome: a clinical review. Lancet 2007;369(9572):1553–65.
92. Cehovic GA, Hatton KW, Fahy BG. Adult respiratory distress syndrome. Int Anesthesiol Clin 2009;47(1):83–95.
93. Price LC, McAuley DF, Marino PS, et al. Pathophysiology of pulmonary hypertension in acute lung injury. Am J Physiol Lung Cell Mol Physiol 2012;302(9):L803–15.
94. Quon BS, Goss CH, Ramsey BW. Inhaled antibiotics for lower airway infections. Ann Am Thorac Soc 2014;11(3):425–34.
95. Fultz L, Giguère S, Berghaus LJ, et al. Pulmonary pharmacokinetics of desfuroylceftiofur acetamide after nebulisation or intramuscular administration of ceftiofur sodium to weanling foals. Equine Vet J 2014. http://dx.doi.org/10.1111/evj.12316.
96. Wong DM, Alcott CJ, Wang C, et al. Physiologic effects of nasopharyngeal administration of supplemental oxygen at various flow rates in healthy neonatal foals. Am J Vet Res 2010;71(9):1081–8.
97. Wilson DV, Schott HC 2nd, Robinson NE, et al. Response to nasopharyngeal oxygen administration in horses with lung disease. Equine Vet J 2006;38(3):219–23.
98. Hoffman AM, Viel L. A percutaneous transtracheal catheter system for improved oxygenation in foals with respiratory distress. Equine Vet J 1992;24(3):239–41.
99. Palmer JE. Ventilatory support of the neonatal foal. Vet Clin North Am Equine Pract 1994;10(1):167–85.
100. Palmer JE. Ventilatory support of the critically ill foal. Vet Clin North Am Equine Pract 2005;21(2):457–86.
101. McKiernan BC, Koritz GD, Scott JS, et al. Plasma theophylline concentration and lung function in ponies with recurrent obstructive lung disease. Equine Vet J 1990;22(3):194–7.
102. Prandota J. Furosemide: progress in understanding its diuretic, anti-inflammatory, and bronchodilating mechanism of action, and use in the treatment of respiratory tract diseases. Am J Ther 2002;9(4):317–28.

Update on Noninfectious Inflammatory Diseases of the Lower Airway

Melissa R. Mazan, DVM

KEYWORDS

- Inflammatory airway disease • Recurrent airway obstruction • Bronchodilator
- Environmental remediation • Airway inflammation • Corticosteroid • Lung function

KEY POINTS

- Inflammatory airway disease and recurrent airway obstruction are 2 nonseptic diseases with a shared cause of exposure to particulate matter and are likely 2 ends of a spectrum of disease.
- Diagnosis and differentiation of the 2 conditions can be made based on clinical signs, lung function testing, and cytologic analysis of bronchoalveolar fluid.
- Treatment consists of environmental modification and pharmacologic treatment, with each equally important.
- Corticosteroids, either systemic or inhaled, along with environmental remediation, are the cornerstone of successful treatment with bronchodilators indicated for short-term, rescue therapy.

Both inflammatory airway disease (IAD) and recurrent airway obstruction (RAO, better known as heaves) are inflammatory but *not* septic diseases of the equine respiratory system. The causes of both IAD and RAO share similarities, both being diseases of domestication and exposure to particulate matter, whereas it is at present unclear if it is the pathogenesis itself or the severity of pathogenesis that differs. The distinction between the 2 diseases becomes more apparent when history, clinical signs, and response to treatment are considered. Although they are considered separate diseases, there are recent data[1] to support the idea offered by Viel[2] decades ago that a spectrum of disease exists, with low-grade IAD on one end and RAO on the other end. This review begins with a discussion of what is known about the cause and pathogenesis of IAD and RAO and then considers the clinical signs; diagnostic approach, including sampling of respiratory fluids, lung function testing, and imaging; and concludes with a discussion of treatment options, including environmental modifications and pharmacologic treatments.

Disclosures: None.
Large Animal Department of Clinical Sciences, Cummings School of Veterinary Medicine at Tufts University, 200 Westborough Road, North Grafton, MA 01536, USA
E-mail address: Melissa.mazan@tufts.edu

Vet Clin Equine 31 (2015) 159–185
http://dx.doi.org/10.1016/j.cveq.2014.11.008
0749-0739/15/$ – see front matter © 2015 Elsevier Inc. All rights reserved.

CAUSE OF INFLAMMATORY AIRWAY DISEASE

The exact cause of IAD is as yet unknown. It is probable that there is no one cause of this pervasive disease; rather, many different causes likely contribute to the constellation of signs that is recognized as IAD. The most commonly invoked contributors remain high levels of particulates in the environment, viral disease, air pollution, genetic predisposition, and bacterial infection. Although IAD is often referred to as allergic airway disease, this entity, defined as an immunoglobulin E (IgE)–mediated airway inflammatory condition, has not been shown to exist in horses.[3] This finding does not, however, imply that the immune system is uninvolved in the cause and pathogenesis of IAD.

Environment has long been associated with airway inflammation in horses. More than a decade ago, Sweeney and colleagues[4] noted that racehorses with clinical signs of IAD lived in poorly ventilated stables and speculated that organic dusts and molds were to blame. There is more than just an association of environment with airway inflammation: previously unaffected horses were shown in multiple studies to develop bronchoalveolar lavage (BAL) neutrophilia when introduced to a stable environment.[5] There is a plethora of substances found in bedding and feed that may be responsible for this response. The 2 components of the barn environment that have been best studied are particulate matter and endotoxin. The role of ammonia in inducing airway inflammation is being increasingly scrutinized as well. Airborne particulate matter in the stable environment is largely organic, including plant debris, mold spores primarily from hay, β-glucans, live and dead microbes, proteases, and animal dander to name a few. Inorganic particulates are of less importance, but still contribute, with silicates from dusty arenas or oil fly ash from diesel machinery being used inside large barns.[6]

It has long been recognized that the stable environment frequently presents an unacceptably high level of airborne particulates. Even the best of hay contains mold spores, such as *Aspergillosus fumigatus*, *Faenia rectivirgula*, and *Thermoactinomyces vulgaris*.[7] The role these molds play in disease cause is more clearly understood in RAO (see later discussion), but there is increasing evidence that exposure to hay and its accompanying organic particulates is important in the cause of IAD as well. When unaffected horses are exposed to endotoxin, they develop airway neutrophilia,[8] and the unsurprising finding that endotoxin concentrations are higher in stables than at pasture[9] goes far in explaining hay-eating as a risk factor for increased tracheal mucus in pleasure horses.[10] Not only is stabling a risk factor, but the horse's position in the stable may also affect development of IAD: being in a stall near high levels of activity, such as near the trainer's office, near entrances to the stable, or where fans are being used to improve ventilation are all risk factors.[5] Recent studies have found that levels of particulates and endotoxin at the horse's immediate breathing zone can be significantly and importantly greater than in the surrounding barn environs, and that the worst offender in increasing exposure to airborne particulates is the hay net.[11]

Previous exposure to respiratory viral disease is often invoked, especially by trainers, as a predisposing factor in the development of IAD. Recent infection with a respiratory virus is the most common trigger for exacerbation of the similar disease, asthma, in humans, so it is logical to make the connection to IAD. There are no clear data to support this idea, but indirect evidence is building. Recently, a large study looking for evidence of herpesvirus in horses with a clinical diagnosis of IAD or poor performance, but specifically excluding horses with signs of acute infectious disease, found that the affected group was more likely to have a positive tracheal wash (polymerase chain reaction [PCR]) for herpesvirus, with EHV-2 being most prevalent.[12] Long-lasting airway neutrophilia (21 days) was seen with experimental induction of EHV-2, but clinical signs concordant with IAD were not seen.[13] A recent study in the author's laboratory has shown that horses with hyperresponsive airways have a correspondingly higher titer to equine rhinitis A virus (unpublished data, Mazan MR, 2014). The role of bacterial infection in IAD remains a point of contention. A strong relationship between inflammation of the lower respiratory tract and the presence of Streptococcal species has been noted.[14] It is debatable whether there is a causal relationship or whether poor clearance secondary to airway inflammation allows a transient population of bacteria to accumulate.

As with viral disease, it is tempting to speculate on the role of air pollution (as opposed to the particulates due to hay in the breathing zone in the immediate barn environment) in the development of IAD. Horses sample the ambient air on a continual basis, and the air that they sample is seldom conditioned or filtered. Clinically normal horses experimentally exposed to ozone did have a significant increase in total iron levels in the pulmonary lining fluid as well as an increase in the glutathione redox ratio, indicating that there was a corrective response to the exposure[15]; however, there is little else in the literature to refute or support this finding.

There are multiple other possible contributors to the development of airway inflammation in horses, including cold air and pulmonary hemorrhage, but again, there are few data to either refute or support these causes.[16]

PATHOGENESIS OF INFLAMMATORY AIRWAY DISEASE

Although there is a strong argument that IAD is indeed caused by environmental exposures, little is still known about the actual pathogenesis of IAD.

The role of cytokine production in the pathogenesis of IAD is increasingly well-studied. Interestingly, healthy horses seem to down-regulate inflammatory cytokine production in the lung as they age, whereas horses with airway inflammation do the opposite.[17] Exactly which cytokines are up-regulated, and whether this up-regulation invokes a Th-1 or Th-2 pathway, remains a matter of debate.[18–20]

However, the presence of elevated numbers of mast cells in bronchoalveolar lavage fluid (BALF) of horses with poor performance and the association of BAL mastocytosis with airway hyperresponsiveness are suggestive of a degree of allergic response.[21] When regarding recent studies looking at gene expression profiles in BALF in horses with IAD, it is important to note whether the horses were diagnosed as having IAD on the basis of a generalized increase in inflammatory cells, or if the study group was parsed more thoroughly into horses with increased mast cells or horses with increased neutrophils. One study looking at horses with a generalized increase in inflammatory cells found an up-regulation of interleukin (IL)-1β, IL-23, and tumor necrosis factor (TNF)-α, but no evidence of a polarized cytokine response.[19] On the other hand, when horses are stratified into mast cell versus neutrophil groups, mRNA for IL-4 correlated with mast cells but not neutrophils; whereas for all groups, similar to the previous study, TNF-α and IL-1β were increased.[18,22] It is most likely that multiple factors contribute to the development of IAD in individual horses; a critical level of risk factors or exposure is probably necessary for the disease to manifest itself.

HISTOPATHOLOGY OF INFLAMMATORY AIRWAY DISEASE

Much of what is known about the histopathology of IAD must be gleaned from older studies of horses diagnosed with chronic obstructive pulmonary disease (COPD), but in retrospect, more closely fit the definition of a younger, athletic horse with IAD. Bronchiolar biopsies of athletic young horses with lower airway inflammation have shown inflammatory mucosal cellular infiltrates and luminal exudates, bronchiolar hyperplasia, and goblet cell metaplasia.[23] It is interesting to note that 80% of supposedly normal horses had minimal evidence of peribronchiolitis—raising the question, of course, of what constitutes normal. An extensive study of young racehorses with a primary diagnosis of exercise induced pulmonary hemorrhage (EIPH) found plentiful evidence of multifocal, small airway–centered disease, including increased mucosal and peribronchiolar connective tissue, mononuclear bronchiolar cuffing, and epithelial hyperplasia.[24] Other studies of young thoroughbred horses in training found increased collagen, and evidence of epithelial injury, which correlated with an interstitial pattern on radiographs.[25] Nevertheless, another study of young horses with "mild COPD" revealed decreased Clara cell function and goblet cell metaplasia within the bronchioles without signs of inflammation typical of RAO.[26] These data in sum certainly suggest that the histopathologic lesion of IAD is not only local bronchiolar inflammation, but also remodeling and thickening of the bronchioles themselves, which lends itself to at least low-grade airway obstruction. Viel's suggestion, many years ago, that IAD and RAO were simply on a continuum, is supported by these data[2] as well as by recent data that horses with early signs of IAD were more likely to develop RAO in later years.[1]

RECURRENT AIRWAY OBSTRUCTION CAUSE

In concert with IAD, RAO/heaves has a clear environmental cause. Although exposure to moldy hay and endotoxin[27] or a combination of fungal spores, lipopolysaccharide, and silicates[28] all caused airway neutrophilia in control horses, clinical disease and clearly evident pulmonary dysfunction only developed in horses with a history of RAO. Unlike IAD, there is an emerging genetic basis to RAO, which may explain the difference in clinical signs on exposure to airborne particulates, especially molds from hay.[29,30] The exact mode of inheritance is incompletely understood and likely to be complex[30]; however, our understanding is increasing with the knowledge that chromosomal regions have been identified in affected warmblood horses,[31] including the IL-4 receptor gene in some families, supporting a Th-2-mediated pathway.[32] Recently, connections have been made between RAO and susceptibility to parasitic disease and development of allergic skin diseases.[30] The condition, known as Summer Pasture Associated Recurrent Airway Obstruction, or the rather ungainly acronym, SPARAO, shares many of the features of RAO, but is seen in horses in more southern climates when they are turned out in spring and summer. Recent work in this area has shown that although a clear causal relationship has not yet been established, clinical exacerbations of SPARAO, which echo those of RAO, are associated with hot humid weather and high environmental contamination with fungal spores and grass pollens.[33]

RECURRENT AIRWAY OBSTRUCTION PATHOGENESIS

The pathogenesis of RAO is far more clearly understood than that of IAD; nonetheless, much remains to be learned. It has long been clear that horses with RAO develop a profound neutrophilia in the epithelial lining fluid in response to certain stimuli, especially moldy hay,[34] but although clinically there appears to be a hypersensitivity component to RAO, and there are many similarities to asthma in humans, there is no clear evidence for a type I hypersensitivity. There is mixed evidence for and against the role of IgE in RAO, with studies showing both increased levels of mold-specific IgE in serum of RAO versus controls,[34] and, conversely, no difference between the 2 groups.[35,36] On a functional level, although only 15% of serum samples from horses with RAO reacted positively in a reaginic assay to determine type I hypersensitivity, none of the serum samples from control horses did so.[37] As with IAD, there has been an ongoing effort to establish a Th-1 versus Th-2 type pathogenesis for RAO based on cytokine expression, but the results are similarly unclear: studies that show increased expression of IL-4 and IL-5 and decreased expression of IFN-γ seem to support an allergic mechanism, whereas other studies show either increased expression of IFN-γ, or a mixed response.[38] It is likely that differences in exposure and time and type of sampling combine to contribute to these inconsistent findings. It may also be that there are multiple types of RAO just as there are suspected to be types of IAD.

There is, however, evidence that a late or delayed-type hypersensitivity may be a more important mechanism in RAO, with involvement of CD4$^+$ T cells.[39,40] Macrophages likely play an important role with production of the chemoattractant cytokine IL-8, which recruits neutrophils to the lung.[41 43] Recently, both PI3K and MAP kinase pathways were shown to be important in signals in recruiting neutrophils to the airways.[44] In addition to this increased signaling, dysregulation of apoptosis retards the removal of neutrophils from the airspaces.[45-47] Other important inflammatory mediators and cytokines have been identified, including IL-1β, TLR4, TNF-α, transforming growth factor–β1[48] as well as matrix metalloproteases,[49] tryptase from mast cells that are elevated in the epithelium of horses with RAO,[50] and adenosine.[51] Horses, along with calves, sheep, goats, cats, and pigs (but not dogs, laboratory animals, and humans), rely on pulmonary intravascular macrophages (PIMs) to clear blood-borne bacteria and other particulates and to increase the horse's sensitivity to endotoxin.[52] There is new information that these PIMs may mediate the response in horses to inhaled endotoxin, because depletion of PIMs in horses with RAO resulted in attenuated clinical scores, reduced the migration of neutrophils to the alveolar space, and decreased the expression of IL-8 and TLR4 mRNA in the BAL fluid.[53] The end result of these combined insults is an inflammatory infiltrate around the airways,[26] profound airway remodeling with goblet cell and epithelial hyperplasia,[23] variable airway smooth muscle hypertrophy or hyperplasia, and alveolar fibrosis. Interestingly, although exposure to a dusty environment causes increases in BAL neutrophils in control horses as well as affected horses, in one study, only horses with RAO had an increase in tracheal mucus with such exposure, implicating mucus plugging as an important cause of lung dysfunction in heaves.[23] Clara cell secretory protein is decreased in horses with RAO, likely because it is consumed in the attempt to counter inflammation.[54] The role of airway innervation in the pathogenesis of heaves has also been explored. It appears that dysfunction of the inhibitory nonadrenergic, noncholinergic system may be the most important neurogenic factor in RAO.[55] However, multiple other possibilities exist, including a decreased density of β-2 adrenergic receptors in the lower airways of horses with RAO[56] and increased excitatory NANC pathways.[57]

There has been considerable interest in the role of oxidative stress in the pathogenesis of RAO. Several studies have shown increases in oxidative stress,[58-60] reactive oxygen (ROS), and nitrogen species (RNS).[57] Although work has not yet been done in vivo, both pentoxifylline and endothelin antagonists decreased ROS and RNS in vitro in equine pulmonary tissues, suggesting future therapeutic targets.[57]

The final outcome of all of the proposed pathology is that horses experience airway obstruction because of the decreased size of the airways, mucus plugging, and bronchospasm, and this results in the classic clinical signs of RAO/heaves. It is of interest to note that, similar to COPD in humans, horses with RAO have been shown to have systemic signs of disease as well, including increases in resting pulmonary arterial pressure and at least temporary signs of cor pumonale.[61] Systemic stress certainly occurs with blood cortisol increases being seen in the acute stages of RAO exacerbation.[62] Recent studies have shown more increases in inflammatory markers, such as soluble CD14, serum haptoglobin, and serum amyloid A, in horses with RAO than in control groups, again indicating a systemic response.[63,64] In horses with severe, chronic heaves, a paradoxic breathing pattern may be noticed, and diaphragmatic function may be temporarily exhausted[65]; this dysfunction is underlain by skeletal muscle changes in the diaphragm.[66]

RECURRENT AIRWAY OBSTRUCTION: HISTOPATHOLOGY

In addition to the neutrophilic airway inflammation that is detected with BAL cytologic examination, increases in airway wall collagen and elastic fiber content as well as airway smooth muscle have also been documented, and these increases positively correlate with pulmonary resistance in horses with RAO.[67]

CLINICAL SIGNS: RECURRENT AIRWAY OBSTRUCTION

The horse in acute exacerbation of RAO is easy to diagnose when it is accompanied by a clear history of prior episodes of a similar nature. Indeed, it is the repeatability of these episodes of heaves that gives the disease its currently accepted name: recurrent airway obstruction. The classic signs of heaves in a horse with acute exacerbation, from front to back, include flared nostrils, variable mucopurulent nasal discharge, a cough that is often spasmodic, increased expiratory effort, and possibly swaying back and forth with the effort of breathing. Horses with severe heaves often have increased inspiratory effort as well (see later discussion, Lung function). Horses that have suffered from RAO for many years are often thin, from both loss of appetite and the increase in resting energy expenditure due to the very high work of breathing. Indeed, it is possible to calculate that the work of breathing is high enough to approximate the energy expenditure of a horse trotting more than 12 hours per day.[68] Auscultation often reveals both mild crackles and wheezes, and the lung field may be larger than normal on auscultation because of air-trapping and subsequent hyperinflation. When horses are removed from the offending environment, these clinical signs may completely abate and the horse may appear clinically normal unless the disease is sufficiently chronic. In this case, there may be sufficient airway remodeling, fibrosis, or even bronchiectasis or bullae that the horse will appear clinically abnormal despite treatment.

Horses with RAO, even when in remission, exhibit varying degrees of exercise intolerance. During submaximal exercise, which is all that these horses can tolerate, horses with RAO experience hypoxemia, hypercapnea, and hyperlactatemia, as well as a measurable and significant increase in the work of breathing.[69]

CLINICAL SIGNS: INFLAMMATORY AIRWAY DISEASE

Horses with IAD by definition do not have episodes of air hunger or respiratory embarrassment and tend to be younger horses expected to do athletic work. Although horses with IAD are clearly distinguished from the dyspneic horse with RAO, they can be difficult to distinguish from unaffected horses, especially at rest. Subclinical airway disease may result simply in mild abnormalities on auscultation and endoscopy and occasionally in coughing.[70] The prevalence of cough in horses with IAD is hard to estimate, because many studies use the presence of cough as an inclusion criterion.[71,72] Other studies have shown that cough may be seen less than 16% to 50% of the time.[73] On endoscopic examination, excessive airway mucus is often seen, ranging from multiple specks to streams of mucus.[74] Other clinical signs that are frequently noticed include prolonged respiratory recovery, respiratory embarrassment at exercise, worsening of signs during hot, humid weather, and inability to perform work during collection. Racehorses with IAD are typically described as fading during the last quarter of the race (personal observation, Mazan MR, 2015). Interestingly, horses with dorsal displacement of the soft palate (DDSP) have a higher prevalence of IAD than do control horses, bringing into play a chicken-or-egg argument, because it cannot be determined whether IAD is a risk factor for DDSP or if DDSP is a risk factor for IAD.[75]

The extent to which IAD affects performance depends on the use of the horse and the expectations of the owner or trainer. Practitioners who work primarily with pleasure or show horses might report a low incidence of IAD in young horses, but will see more cases as horses age and the disease progresses; this is because these horses do not work sufficiently close to their Vo_{2max} to unmask subclinical IAD. Practitioners working with young horses working near or at Vo_{2max}, such as racehorses, will notice exercise intolerance far more frequently. Indeed, in a National Hunt racing population, excessive mucus was detected endoscopically in 68% of horses and IAD was one of the top 2 reasons cited for horses not running.[76,77] Cough, rather than overt exercise intolerance, is more commonly reported in sport horses other than racehorses.[78]

BREATHING PATTERN: HEAVES/RECURRENT AIRWAY OBSTRUCTION

To understand the deranged breathing of a horse with RAO, it is important to have a clear picture of the way that a normal horse breathes. It is a natural tendency to assume that various species will share a similar basic breathing strategy, but as Koterba and colleagues[79] showed many years ago, horses use their own technique. It is learned in physiology classes that breathing at rest is *from* the relaxed volume of the respiratory system—this is not true in the horse. Instead, after the horse reaches the relaxation volume of the lung, there is a second, *active* phase of expiration, with a return to relaxation volume during a passive phase of inspiration, and then a second *active* phase of inspiration above relaxation volume, and on and on. It is common to think of an abdominal phase of breathing as characterizing the horse with heaves, but in actuality, the abdominal muscles work with the diaphragm even in the normal resting horse. It is likely that this unique strategy is due to the very low chest wall compliance of the horse.

In the horse with heaves, this useful biphasic breathing strategy is either attenuated or lost,[65] and the loss of this species-specific breathing pattern underlies the severe flow limitation that is seen in heaves. Although an evident breathing effort is made with the abdomen in acute heaves, it is not an effective movement, and the actual volume that it delivers is markedly decreased. In some horses, the movement of the abdominal compartment with respect to the thoracic compartment becomes paradoxic, that is, in opposition to the thoracic compartment.[65] In the normal horse, in contrast, increased abdominal effort, for instance, when the horse is galloping, results in large increases in lung volume.[80] Normal horses also have variations to their breathing pattern throughout the day; this natural variability disappears in RAO in exacerbation.[81] Horses with acute exacerbation of heaves often appear to have inspiratory difficulty as well as the expected expiratory difficulty; this can be explained by the occurrence of hyperinflation. With expiratory flow limitation, air becomes trapped and thus useless, and tidal volume and inspiratory capacity decrease; this is analogous to the situation in humans with hyperinflation, wherein an increased inspiratory elastic load is an important contributor to exercise intolerance.[81]

LUNG FUNCTION: INFLAMMATORY AIRWAY DISEASE

Physical airway obstruction due to mucus plugging or epithelial hyperplasia, for instance, and reversible bronchospasm will result in increases in respiratory resistance that cannot be measured at rest in horses with IAD. The reason that increased resistance is usually occult at rest is that the resistances of the multiple small airways, which add in parallel (and thus as reciprocals), are relatively small in comparison with the resistance of the upper airways. Two types of maneuvers are commonly used to parse out the abnormalities, one being an agent that causes bronchospasm, such as histamine or methacholine, and thus creates an increase in airway resistance that is measurable[82,83]; the other being a mechanical provocation, such as inducing increased respiratory frequency and effort with lobeline[65] or endogenous increases in CO_2. With bronchial hyperresponsiveness testing, an increase in airway resistance is measured partially because of a brisk response from hypertrophic airway smooth muscle.[84] An increase in resistance is also measured with provocation when airways are remodeled and narrower than normal airways even at rest: this is because resistance varies inversely with the fourth or fifth power of the radius, and small decreases in radius that are not detectable at rest result in large increases in resistance that physiologic testing can now detect. This low-grade nonseptic airway inflammation does have a negative impact on ventilatory capacity, but that this is more pronounced in racehorses.[23] It has been shown, using bronchiolar biopsy, that oxygen uptake and pulmonary ventilation correlated inversely with the morphologic grade of small airway disease and the height of the bronchiolar epithelium—the last finding suggesting that the extent of obstruction may determine the extent of exercise impairment. Racehorses with IAD have impaired gas exchange during exercise.[85,86] However, other studies have found that horses with obvious evidence of airway inflammation do not necessarily have a history of exercise intolerance, which may reflect the difficulty of diagnosing low-grade respiratory impairment and the trainer's failure to recognize poorer performance than nature intended, however, rather than the benign nature of the underlying disease.

LUNG FUNCTION: RECURRENT AIRWAY OBSTRUCTION

Lung function testing in the horse with clinically evident RAO has traditionally rested on the esophageal balloon ± pneumotachograph method. Although this method is insensitive to the type of small changes that are seen in horses with IAD, the deranged breathing mechanics of horses with RAO can easily be detected with the traditional method. Nonetheless, this method is seldom used outside of the research setting, because calibration and measurement with an esophageal balloon can be tricky to say the least. The idea behind the esophageal balloon method is to get an approximation of maximal pleural pressure (delta Pplmax), which is the driving pressure for breathing. If delta Pplmax is measured in conjunction with flow, then pulmonary resistance and dynamic compliance can be measured, although maximal pleural pressure and pulmonary resistance are most commonly used as indicators of airway obstruction. As a reminder, pulmonary resistance is described by the relationship between the driving pressure of the lung and flow as measured by the pneumotachograph, or by Resistance = Pressure/Flow.

In the horse with RAO in exacerbation, delta Pplmax is markedly increased (more negative), but in remission, these horses may not have any discernable abnormalities on traditional lung function testing. In concert with the markedly increased delta Pplmax, horses with RAO in exacerbation also have increased airway resistance and decreased dynamic compliance.

Other methods of lung function testing (see later discussion, Diagnosis) can be used for clinical diagnosis, including various methods of open plethysmography, forced oscillatory mechanics (FOS), forced expiratory flow-volume curves, volumetric capnography, and tidal breathing flow-volume loops. All of these methods aim to uncover in varying ways the increased airway and pulmonary resistance that is characteristic of heaves and to a lesser extent IAD as well as changes in breathing strategy such as decreased thoracoabdominal asynchrony.

DIAGNOSIS
Clinical Score

Cough, flared nostrils, and abdominal lift all contribute to the phenotype that Robinson[87] used to create a clinical score. Multiple different clinical scoring systems have been used for staging of RAO, but these primary characteristics remain the most important, to the extent that even owners can use these clinical signs as well as historical information to help with the diagnosis of heaves (horse owner–assessed respiratory sign index, or HOARSI).[88] This clinical scoring is useful for moderate to severe cases of RAO, but as Robinson demonstrated, it is not sufficiently sensitive to detect residual low-grade obstruction after treatment with a bronchodilator.[88] A deeper understanding of the disease process, and thus a more refined diagnosis, is achieved through a combination of lung function testing, bronchoalveolar lavage with or without endoscopy, and in some cases, thoracic radiology. In a case where comorbidity is suspected or where there is a question of infectious disease, a full chemistry profile and complete blood count may be useful, but neither is necessary in most cases of RAO/heaves.

Lung Function Testing in Recurrent Airway Obstruction

Although the traditional esophageal balloon/pneumotachograph method is impractical for testing horses in the field, other methods can be used. The method that is best suited to field use is open plethysmography performed with a commercial flow-metric plethysmography system (Ambulatory Monitoring, Inc, Ardsley, NY, USA). With Open Pleth, the horse is outfitted with a pneumotachograph for measurement of flow detected at the nose, and inductance bands at the abdomen and thorax. Briefly, inductance bands detect voltage change when the abdomen and thorax expand and contract with breathing; this change in voltage is interpreted as a change in volume, which is then differentiated with respect to time and thus is expressed as a flow. Measurement of airway obstruction is calculated by the software by subtracting the flow signal generated by the inductance bands from the air flow measured by the pneumotachograph at peak expiration, termed the delta flow. Delta flow increases with bronchoconstriction, as the expected air flow through the pneumotachograph is less than the calculated airflow as measured by the abdominal and thoracic bands. In the horse with clinically evident RAO, a high delta flow can be measured. In the horse with IAD, baseline measurements are usually unremarkable, but increased delta flow is noted in response to agents such as histamine (see later discussion). Respiratory ultrasonic plethysmography, using similar principles, has also been recently reported in the horse.[89]

Lung Function Testing in Horses with Inflammatory Airway Disease

Because the pathology of IAD is far less severe than that of RAO, traditional forms of lung function testing are by definition less diagnostic. In the author's clinic, FOM is most commonly used, because it is most sensitive to small changes in respiratory resistance.[83,90] FOM uses a signal—in the author's clinic, compressed air, but impulse oscillometry can be used as well—that is imposed on the horse's natural breathing. Pressure and flow transducers are used to measure the changes imposed by the horse's respiratory system on the oscillations. The calculated output is total impedance, which can then be apportioned into reactance and resistance, with resistance most commonly used in clinical practice. Delta flow can also be used in conjunction with bronchoprovocation in horses with IAD.

Lung Function Challenge in the Horse with Recurrent Airway Obstruction

The author finds it useful in her clinic to measure delta flow in these horses, administer 450 μg of albuterol by inhaler, or administer N-butylscopolammonium bromide,[91] and in 10 minutes, measure delta flow again. In this way, one can begin to tease out how much of the increase in delta flow is due to bronchospasm and thus is relieved in the short term by use of a bronchodilator, and how much underlying airway remodeling may be contributing to the problem. In horses with RAO in remission, the horse is instead challenged with an agent that will increase airway resistance, such as histamine or methacholine. Horses that are particularly sensitive may react to inhaled water vapor even before exposure to histamine. This method is termed bronchoprovocation, and the dose of histamine at which the horse has predetermined change in a measure of resistance is termed the provocative concentration. Bronchoprovocation has been shown to be the best method for discrimination between healthy control horses and horses with RAO in remission.[88] For FOM, the author looks for a 75% increase in respiratory resistance (termed PCRS75) or a 35% increase in delta flow (PCDF35%). An alternative method of provocation is to induce hyperpnea through rebreathing either with elevation of CO_2 or with lobeline using plethysmography to assess the breathing pattern.[65,92] Normal horses have a normal degree of thoracoabdominal asynchrony at rest (see discussion above), which decreases with disease. Despite the apparent visible increase in abdominal effort in horses with RAO, the thoracic compartment has a higher contribution in affected horses, which is even more apparent during hyperpnea, and thus, a *smaller* degree of thoracoabdominal asynchrony.[89] The resultant change in asynchrony between the thoracic and abdominal compartments has proved to be a sensitive marker of subclinical airway narrowing as well.

Lung Function Challenge in the Horse with Inflammatory Airway Disease

IAD is generally not detectable at rest using the traditional (esophageal balloon) method of lung function testing. Using the FOM technique, more subtle changes can be detected, including frequency dependence of resistance when an input of increasing Hertz is used. Horses with IAD as a group have significantly higher values for respiratory system resistance at the lower frequencies (1–3 Hz) and mild frequency dependence of resistance compared with controls; however, baseline values may still be classified as within normal limits, making this an unreliable method of diagnosis.[21] Likewise, lung resistance decreases with increasing minute ventilation in control horses, but not in horses with IAD.[92] Consequently, without dynamic, frequency-dependent tests of lung function, forced maneuvers, or bronchoprovocation, it seems that one simply fails to document a common feature of small airway obstruction in a horse with IAD because the testing devices are not sufficiently sensitive to these changes.

Horses with clinical signs compatible with IAD, like horses with subclinical RAO, also exhibit signs of airway hyperresponsiveness when they are exposed to nonspecific agents such as histamine aerosol. The basis for airway hyperresponsiveness remains incompletely understood, but is likely a combination of airway wall thickening undetectable by conventional lung function testing, airway inflammation, and autonomic nervous system dysfunction. There is a paucity of information concerning the mediators of airway hyperresponsiveness in horses with IAD. In the author's laboratory, horses with a clinical history and signs compatible with IAD have significantly greater airway reactivity than controls, although some control horses, similar to some humans without asthma, display airway hyperresponsiveness as well. Interestingly, this phenomenon in people is associated with a greater risk of eventual development of asthma[93] and may be tied into the recent finding of signs of IAD being strong risk factors for eventual development of RAO.[30]

Cytologic Diagnosis of Airway Inflammation

Airway inflammation, be it in the less severe disease, IAD, or in the more severe RAO, is best diagnosed with bronchoalveolar lavage. Despite the most recent American College of Veterinary Internal Medicine consensus statement to that effect, some practitioners continue to use the tracheal wash to assess inflammation in both diseases, even though BAL is no harder to perform in the field than is a tracheal wash. It is important to remember that inflammation as defined by greater than 5% neutrophils on BAL versus inflammation defined by greater than 20% neutrophils on tracheal wash do not correlate well; thus, the tracheal wash is unlikely to be a good representation of what is happening in the small airways.[94] Moreover, Derksen and colleagues[95] pointed out more than 2 decades ago that not only did the results of the 2 methods fail to correlate, but also tracheal wash differentials were highly variable in contrast to BAL differentials. In all, the evidence points to the BAL as a superior method of assessing airway inflammation.

The specifics of performing the BAL are well-described elsewhere; however, it is worth mentioning that horses with more severe inflammation are also more likely to experience airway collapse during the procedure.[96] This fact is rarely of clinical importance, but if the airways serving the BAL tube or bronchoscope collapse, it will help to decrease the suction pressure to get a good sample. When inspecting BAL fluid before processing, it is interesting and informative to note that horses with severe heaves will often have a diminished "head" of foamy surfactant as well.

How then, does one diagnose airway inflammation using the bronchoalveolar lavage? It is impossible to make a definitive distinction between IAD and RAO based on BAL cytology, but IAD is generally held to be consistent with mild neutrophilia (>5%), eosinophilia (>0.5%), mastocytosis (2%), or combinations of these in the BAL fluid.[97] The question of whether morphologic differences in BAL identify different IAD syndromes is not clear. In a study from the author's laboratory, horses with neutrophilic BAL tended to be older and have a cough, whereas horses with mastocytosis were more likely to have airway hyperresponsiveness when assessed with histamine bronchoprovocation.[73] Interestingly, a recent study showed that thoroughbred racehorses were more likely to have mastocytosis-eosinophilia with increased amounts of mucus evident in the BAL cytology, whereas standardbreds of the same age were more likely to have neutrophilic inflammation. Neither group was different with respect to exercising hypoxemia or any other physiologic variable, such as exercising heart rate or blood lactate levels.[98] Other studies have also shown that horses with neutrophilic disease were more likely to have greater levels of hypoxemia when exercising.[99]

The BAL cytology of horses with RAO is primarily neutrophilic, at times up to 100% of all cells being neutrophils. Mast cells are rarely identified. Large amounts of mucus are commonly seen, with Curschmann spirals being evident at times. It can be very useful to inspect the mucus in these horses (and indeed in horses with IAD) because many cells may be trapped within mucus, artificially lowering the count if this is ignored. Frequently, hay mold or pollen is found engulfed in alveolar macrophages.

When evaluating BAL cytology for mast cells in particular, it is important to remember that fast Romanowsky stains such as Dif-quick are not suitable.[100] In the author's laboratory, they routinely stain one slide with a fast Romanowsky stain and one side with toluidine blue. This latter stain is easily done by using the first phase of Dif-quick fixative and then leaving the slide in toluidine blue solution for a minimum of 15 minutes. The granules of the mast cells will stain a variety of brilliant magenta colors and will thus be easily identifiable. It is also critical to count a sufficient number of cells, because small differences in mast cells and eosinophils can make or break a diagnosis of IAD. Recent evidence suggests that using ×500 and evaluating 5 dense fields yields the most repeatable results.[101]

Endoscopy

Endoscopy is most useful in ruling out comorbidities that may contribute to exercise intolerance, such as upper airway disease, and is also the best method for assessing mucus accumulation in the trachea.[74] A recent study examined endoscopic assessment of tracheal septum thickness and mucus accumulation and determined that both measurements were useful in distinguishing the horse with RAO from the horse with IAD.[74,102] Tracheal mucus has been associated with cough[103,104] and is very common in stabled horses, with all horses in one study having abnormal findings despite having no clinical complaint.[105] It is important to keep in mind, however, that these were nonracing sport horses; the lower necessary Vo_{2max} accompanying their workload likely masked the subclinical disease that would have affected performance in a racehorse.[106] Indeed, in other studies, poor performance in racehorses has been associated with increased tracheal mucus.[107]

Diagnostic Imaging

Radiographs have been shown to have some correlation with staging of heaves/RAO, especially increases in interstitial and bronchial patterns as well as tracheal thickening.[108] They are most useful, however, in detecting comorbidities such as bronchiectasis,[109] bullae, or pneumothorax from ruptured bullae (personal observation, Mazan MR, 2015) and are not routinely used for diagnosis of heaves in the author's clinic. Radiographs do not correlate well with results of lung function testing or BAL in horses with IAD, and thus, again, are useful only in ruling out comorbidities.[110] Ultrasound may show roughening of the pleura, but is unlikely to be of use in the diagnosis of heaves or IAD.

TREATMENT

The therapeutic goals for treating both RAO and IAD are similar: (1) immediate relief of the bronchospasm that causes cough and excessive respiratory effort with RAO or cough and bronchoconstriction that impairs performance in IAD; (2) reduction of lower airway inflammation, mucus production, and airway plugging; and (3) long-term prevention of episodes of heaves or worsening of IAD by control of lower airway inflammation and airway obstruction.

In order for RAO or IAD to be treated successfully, there must be a treatment strategy with recognizable and achievable goals in place that is approved by both the attending veterinarian and the owner. Owners should also recognize that this may be a chronic problem that may require management of some kind for the life of the horse. Clear expectations of what the outcome of successful treatment will be should also be set in place. It is entirely reasonable, for instance, to expect that a young racehorse would be able to return to racing after a short, targeted period of treatment. The owner of the older horse with heaves, however, must recognize that a much more modest return to light pleasure riding is a reasonable goal.

For both RAO and IAD, although it is important to assess the horse's immediate clinical presentation, it will be equally important to take an in-depth history to try to document environmental triggers. A recent study shows that particulates associated with feeding from a hay net versus feeding from the ground is one of the most important risk factors for the development of airway inflammation.[11] A very thorough inspection and assessment of the horse's environment is also critical to develop a plan to achieve environmental remediation. For instance, if the history suggests that the horse is consistently worse in the spring, whereas clinical signs are abated in the barn in the winter, it suggests that the worst culprits for this horse are the molds and pollens associated with moist warm weather, and the clinician may prescribe clean indoor living for the horse during that period. It is very useful for the owner or trainer to keep a diary for the affected horse, noting when exacerbations occur. Simple interventions, such as opening the barn doors or making sure to feed hay on the ground, can significantly decrease the number of particulates that a horse breathes. Endotoxin levels are lower at the breathing zone in horses at pasture than in stables, which may explain why outdoor living benefits many horses with RAO.[9]

There is strong evidence for the efficacy of treatment of both bronchodilators and glucocorticoids in the treatment of heaves, and there is a reasonably good idea of how and why they work in this disease. This knowledge has largely been extrapolated to the treatment of IAD. For both, the mainstay of treatment has become a combination of environmental remediation, corticosteroid therapy, and bronchodilators.

Corticosteroid Therapy

Corticosteroids remain the cornerstone of successful treatment of both IAD and RAO. Inflammation underlies remodeling of the airways with accompanying airway hyperreactivity, and consequent coughing and expiratory dyspnea. Bronchodilator drugs will help to relieve acute, debilitating bronchospasm, but it is only consistent anti-inflammatory therapy, in conjunction with avoidance of environmental triggers, will break the vicious cycle of inflammation, airway hyperreactivity, and bronchoconstriction. The anti-inflammatory effect of corticosteroids in both RAO and IAD is impressive. Corticosteroids activate glucocorticoid receptors, thus putting into motion a profound inhibition of the arachadonic acid cascade and limiting production of leukotrienes and other inflammatory molecules. Response to steroids can vary considerably from horse to horse.

The choice of whether to use systemic drugs in combination with inhaled drugs or alone may depend on several factors, including severity of disease; finances, as aerosolized drugs and their delivery devices are quite expensive; and known and putative side effects. It is important to remember that corticosteroids can, among other things, adversely affect tissue growth and protein use, impair the barrier function of the intestinal mucosa, cause immune suppression, and suppress adrenal function.

Systemic corticosteroids

Multiple studies have demonstrated the positive effects of corticosteroid drugs on horses with heaves, but the evidence for their use in IAD, despite good clinical response anecdotally, is less robust. Prednisolone and dexamethasone are the corticosteroids used most frequently in the treatment of RAO and IAD. Triamcinolone acetonide has also been shown to relieve airway obstruction in heaves.[111] Triamcinolone, however, is anecdotally more closely associated with the development of laminitis in horses than other corticosteroids. A recent study has shown profound and persistent hyperglycemia and hypertriglyceridemia (3–4 days) in horses after a single injection of triamcinolone, which may explain the anecdotal reports.[112] Thus, its use is discouraged in the treatment of IAD and heaves. Prednisone was also frequently used in the past, but studies have shown therapeutic failures in heaves likely due to the horse's inability to absorb prednisone after oral administration.[113] In a study looking at heaves-affected horses treated with either oral prednisolone (1.0 mg/kg bodyweight) or intramuscular dexamethasone (0.1 mg/kg bodyweight) in conjunction with environmental control, both drugs had similar positive effects on the clinical signs of heaves, endoscopic scores, and blood gases. However, dexamethasone had a more beneficial effect on BAL cytology.[114] In a different study, both prednisolone (2.0 mg/kg bodyweight orally, once per day) and dexamethasone (0.05 mg/kg bodyweight orally, once per day) improved pulmonary function, despite continuous antigen exposure. However, in that study, oral dexamethasone was more effective than oral prednisolone in improving lung function in the affected horses.[115] A recent study also showed that horses suffering from heaves that were treated for 14 days with either isoflupredone acetate (0.03 mg/kg bodyweight, intramuscularly, once a day) or dexamethasone (0.04 mg/kg bodyweight intravenously, once a day) showed improvements in lung function, although BAL fluid samples were not assessed. Isoflupredone, however, resulted in hypokalemia, making it a less than optimal treatment.[116]

Inhaled corticosteroids

The use of inhaled corticosteroids has truly revolutionized the treatment of RAO and IAD. Although initial systemic tapered corticosteroid therapy is often necessary with all but very mild IAD, regular inhaled therapy is essential for long-term success in most cases. The most important factor that limits regular use of inhaled corticosteroids is cost, because drugs such as fluticasone and beclomethasone are very expensive. When assessing the effects of corticosteroids on horses with airway disease, it is important to note what delivery device and drug formulation were used because certain devices deliver more drug to the lower airways, and certain drug formulations, such as QVAR, a proprietary formulation of beclomethasone, have been shown to reach the lower airways more reliably, at least in humans. For this reason, it is difficult to make comparisons of drugs across studies that used different delivery devices. Moreover, the US Food and Drug Administration has phased out the use of chlorofluorocarbon (CFC) propellants in metered dose inhalers (MDIs) in accordance with the Montreal Protocol to protect the ozone layer. Thus, studies using CFC inhalers are not directly comparable to those using the currently available hydrofluoroalkane (HFA) inhalers.

Aerosolized corticosteroids are frequently preferred over systemic to decrease potential side effects. This preference is well-documented in humans, but, although this is a rational approach in horses, there is little documentation to support it. However, using the Aeromask (no longer on the market) and fluticasone propionate at a dose of 2000 μg twice daily, heaves-affected horses were shown to have significant improvement in clinical signs and lung function with no measured detriment to the immune responses.[117] It is not clear to what extent the hypothalamic pituitary adrenal axis (HPA) suppression seen with all doses of beclomethasone 500 mg or greater poses to general health; at any rate, neither chronic HPA suppression nor rebound addisonian crisis has been seen.[118] Likewise, inhaled fluticasone propionate (1500 μg every 12 hours) caused significant decreases in serum cortisol after 7 days.[119] Thus, inhaled corticosteroids certainly have systemic effects; however, it is generally assumed that the effects will be less profound than with systemic therapy. Owners and trainers should be cautioned, however, that "less profound" does not equal lack of detectability. Fluticasone propionate or its matabolites can be detected in blood for a minimum of 72 hours after being given by inhalation and urine for approximately 18 hours after inhalation.[120]

There are few studies of the efficacy of inhaled steroids in horses. Fluticasone propionate is thought to be the most potent, has the longest pulmonary residence time, and causes the least adrenal suppression. On the other hand, newer formulations of beclomethasone dipropionate that incorporate HPA as the propellant have more uniform particle size and are more uniformly mixed. Fluticasone propionate resulted in complete resolution of clinical signs in horses with exacerbation of heaves as well as normalization of pulmonary function tests and significant decrease in BAL neutrophilia in one study,[38] whereas, in another study, distinct improvements in lung function were seen without any changes in BAL neutrophilia.[121] In a recent study, although treatment with inhaled fluticasone hastened improvement of clinical signs and lung function, and even decreased remodeling of airway smooth muscle and subepithelial collagen, response to chronic treatment did not differ from long-term avoidance of environmental triggers.[122]

In the author's clinic, they frequently treat with an initial course of parenteral corticosteroids, typically, a 4-week, decreasing course of prednisolone, followed by inhaled corticosteroids. They use both QVAR and Flovent and the deciding factor as to which one is used is often the cost. For reasons that are not well understood, some horses seem to do better on one drug versus the other, and the clinician must maintain a certain flexibility in choosing drugs.

The long-term goal of corticosteroids is not only to decrease inflammation but to achieve reversal of airway smooth muscle remodeling. This goal can apparently be achieved with both antigen avoidance, using environmental control, and corticosteroids. Antigen avoidance seems to be somewhat better at controlling inflammation, and both antigen avoidance and inhaled fluticasone decrease subepithelial collagen deposition, but inhaled fluticasone seems to accelerate the reversal of smooth muscle remodeling.[122] It would follow, therefore, that the ideal management would incorporate both approaches.

Delivery devices

Devices currently on the market for use in horses include the Aerohippus (Trudell, Ontario, Canada) and the EquineHaler (Equine HealthCare, Horsholm, Denmark). The choice as to which to use is largely determined by cost and by which device will best suit the particular horse in question. A recent study compared the Aerohippus and the EquineHaler using a pressurized MDI and HFA-albuterol to elicit bronchodilation in horses with bronchospasm associated with exacerbation of heaves.[123] Although there was a trend for there to be a larger decrease in pulmonary resistance after treatment with albuterol using the Aerohippus, there were no statistical differences between the 2 devices. Regardless of the type of mask/spacer device used, actual delivery of particles to the lower airways is poor in the horse, as indeed it is even in humans, and the least efficacious means of delivering aerosolized drugs is by nebulization.[124] Unfortunately, strategies that are known to improve lung deposition of aerosolized drugs in humans, such as slow deep breathing and breath-holding, are not practical in the horse. However, keeping the horse calm and the respiratory rate low may help.

Bronchodilators

Bronchodilators, as with corticosteroids, can be administered systemically and via aerosol; however, aerosolization is by far the preferred method. Both β-2 agonists (B2-ARs) (sympathomimetics) and parasympatholytics are used in horses. Of the

B2-ARs commonly used in equine medicine, albuterol, which is known as salbutamol everywhere but in the United States, is primarily administered by inhalation, and clenbuterol is administered orally. For the parasympatholytic agents, ipratropium is administered by inhalation, and atropine and N-butylscopolammonium bromide (Buscopan) are administered parenterally.

It is well-appreciated that the bronchodilation ensuing on treatment with B2-ARs is beneficial to horses with bronchospasm; what is less well appreciated is the ability that these drugs may have to increase ciliary beat frequency and suppress mucus production and release of inflammatory mediators from neutrophils. Parasympatholytics, such as the parenteral atropine and N-butylscopolammonium bromide, and the inhaled ipratropium, block muscarinic acetylcholine receptors, thereby preventing bronchoconstriction. Atropine is the least favored of these drugs, because administration may result in colic secondary to gastrointestinal ileus. Both N-butylscopolammonium bromide and atropine will cause tachycardia, but the former does not cause ileus-associated colic.[125]

Although N-butylscopolammonium bromide can be used for rapid relief of bronchospasm, its effect is only short-lasting.[91] The only longer-lasting systemically administered bronchodilator is clenbuterol, a B2-AR that was approved for use in horses in the United States in 1998 under the brand name Ventipulmin (Boehringer Ingelheim Vetmedica, Inc, St Joseph, MO, USA). Severe toxicities have occurred when improperly compounded clenbuterol was administered to horses.[126] The safety and efficacy of chronic administration of clenbuterol are controversial. Chronic administration of clenbuterol at 2.4 µg/kg (5 days on, 2 days off, for 8 weeks) was reported to have a negative impact on aerobic performance in horses.[127] Tachyphylaxis also appears to be a problem with chronic administration of clenbuterol. For example, a recent study demonstrated that, after 3 weeks of clenbuterol administration at 0.8 µg/kg bodyweight orally, every 12 hours, increased airway reactivity was evident, and the horses were refractory to the bronchodilatory effects of clenbuterol.[128] Reports of the efficacy of clenbuterol are also conflicting. A large study by Erichsen and colleagues[129] showed that 25% of horses had a decrease in clinical signs of heaves when treated with clenbuterol at a dose of 0.8 µg/kg bodyweight, but a second study failed to show any benefit on clinical signs when a much larger dose of 4.0 µg/kg bodyweight was administered.[130] Most horses appear to tolerate the lower doses of clenbuterol well, but with higher doses, horses may have tremors, tachycardia, sweating, and an appearance of anxiousness, among other signs. Together, these findings suggest that the practice of administering clenbuterol to horses to enhance performance is probably misguided at best, and harmful at worst. It is also important to recognize that the recommended duration of treatment is 30 days. Clenbuterol is not appropriate and should not be used as a chronic therapy.

Inhaled Bronchodilators

Short-acting B2-ARs, such as albuterol and fenoterol, are extremely important in treating acute exacerbations of RAO. Albuterol is recognized universally as a rescue drug for both human asthmatics and horses with IAD/RAO. Horses with current exacerbations of RAO labor to breathe and experience paroxysmal coughing; within 15–30 minutes after aerosolized delivery of albuterol, they will experience significant relief. However, the effect wears off within 3 to 6 hours. It is important to remember that the inflammatory condition will persist despite apparent improvement because of transient bronchodilation, and the disease will worsen if the other 2 legs of treatment—corticosteroid (anti-inflammatory) therapy and avoidance of environmental triggers—are not pursued. Regular use of B2 agonists in the absence of anti-inflammatory medication may mask symptoms that would otherwise indicate progressive worsening of the disease, in particular, further airway obstruction with mucus. Albuterol is the most affordable of the short-acting B2 agonists; however, levalbuterol, the R-enantiomer of albuterol, has recently become more affordable (trade name Xopenex). There is a possibility that albuterol may cause unexpected bronchoconstriction due to action of the L-enantiomer. Levalbuterol may prevent this, but paradoxic bronchoconstriction has occurred even with the use of lavalbuterol.[131] Although regular use of inhaled albuterol for 10 days does not result in tachyphylaxis,[132] it may be that longer use would result in treatment failure.

The preponderance of evidence shows that short-acting B2 agonists are not performance enhancing in humans, and there is little evidence to indicate that they are performance-enhancing in horses, with one study showing a small increase in aerobic performance in thoroughbred horses in a treadmill study,[133] while the other failed to show any effect of albuterol administration on aerobic performance in standardbreds on a treadmill.[134] Nonetheless, all equine sporting events ban albuterol, and due care should be taken to stop drug administration before competition, noting that albuterol can be detected in urine for at least 48 hours after administration via MDI. Short-acting B2 agonists can be useful in horses with RAO and underlying airway obstruction to improve the return to training. Short-acting bronchodilators are also useful during lung function testing to assess the reversibility of airway obstruction in horses with RAO. No more than 450 mg of albuterol by inhalation is necessary to bronchodilate most horses, irrespective of the delivery device chosen.

Although aerosolized B2 agonists have a relatively low incidence of side effects, excessive use or sensitive individuals may experience systemic effects, such as trembling, anxiety, and cardiac arrhythmias. The author has noted all these in individuals treated with 900 μg of albuterol, whereas other individuals show no signs of intolerance. Repeated use of the drug tends to decrease side effects as the body downregulates receptors.

Long-acting inhaled B2-ARs therapy
The author treats selected cases of RAO and moderate IAD with long-acting B2-ARs therapy in addition to inhaled corticosteroids, with the initial impression of enhanced performance and quality of life. It cannot be emphasized enough, however, that regular use of long-acting B2-ARs must be accompanied with regular use of inhaled corticosteroids. The most commonly used long-acting B2-ARs are salmeterol and formoterol, whose basic mechanism of action is the familiar cAMP pathway. Their duration of action in horses is 6 to 8 hours.

Inhaled parasympatholytic therapy
The most commonly used inhaled parasympatholytic drug is ipratropium, a quaternary ammonium derivative of atropine that produces bronchodilation lasting approximately 6 hours, which is at least 2 hours longer than albuterol. Although adverse side effects such as thickened mucus, tachycardia, and decreased ciliary beat frequency are possible with parasympatholytics, no such side effects have been reported in horses up to a dose of 1200 μg. Ipratropium cannot be considered a rescue drug, unlike atropine, because it has much longer onset of action; however, the effect may last somewhat longer than atropine. In severely affected horses with RAO, the combination of albuterol and ipratropium may be beneficial.[65]

Mast cell stabilizers
These agents are cromones that block calcium channels, preventing the release of histamine and tryptase, and the subsequent downstream cascade of prostaglandin and leukotriene formulation that eventually cause bronchoconstriction. Sodium

cromoglycate can be efficacious in treating known mast cell–mediated IAD, but will not be of use for treating most horses with neutrophil-mediated disease, and therefore, they are less useful for RAO. Their use, however, requires considerable owner compliance, because the maximum response to this drug occurs at 1 to 2 weeks after beginning treatment.

Environmental remediation

It is important to note that a recent study demonstrated that environmental control was by far the most important means of treating airway inflammation and dysfunction in horses with heaves, and that, indeed, antigen avoidance decreases smooth muscle mass. The barn environment is replete with organic particulate matter, respirable endotoxin, molds, and volatile gases such as ammonia. The worst offenders seem to be hay and straw. Multiple studies have shown that significant improvements can be made by replacing dusty substrates and feed with less dusty substitutes.[135] For instance, pelleted hay and wood shavings are often better than regular hay and straw bedding, but outdoor living, in most cases, is the best. What is not clear to many owners is that even small or transient contacts with hay can initiate severe signs and should be avoided.[136] Indoor arenas present another high dust challenge to the horse, with respirable particulate levels 20 times that which has been recognized to cause respiratory dysfunction in humans. In addition to changing to low dust feeds and beddings, the following recommendations to owners should be made:

- Feed hay from the ground, not from a hay net
- Soak hay well before feeding or use ensiled or baked hay products
- Wet any dusty grain (eg, pellets) before feeding
- Sprinkle aisles with water before sweeping
- Avoid storing hay overhead. If unavoidable, lay a tarp under the hay to avoid dust raining down on the horses
- Use a humectant or hygroscopic agent to reduce dust in the indoor and outdoor arenas
- Remove horses from the barn while cleaning stalls or moving hay
- Do not use blowers to clean aisles
- Remove cobwebs and other dust collectors routinely when horses are out of the barn

An overarching principle that can be derived from the OSHA Dust Control Handbook is that prevention is better than cure. In addition to the well-known presentation of summer pasture-associated RAO in hot, humid southern states, it is important to remember that horses in New England can also have disease that presents primarily in the spring and summer, and that seems to improve when horses are kept temporarily in clean, nondusty indoor environments.

Evaluation of therapeutic outcome

It is important to have a baseline assessment of the horse before initiating therapy. Ideally, this would include auscultation with and without a rebreathing bag, careful physical examination, observation during exercise, and baseline pulmonary function testing (IAD and RAO) and measure of airway reactivity (IAD), or in the case of horses with RAO, postbronchodilator pulmonary function tests and bronchoalveolar lavage. Although historically, pulmonary function testing was available only at a few specialized veterinary pulmonology clinics, user-friendly systems for field-testing are now available, making objective baseline assessments available to practitioners. The goal of a thorough baseline assessment is to facilitate a treatment regimen tailored to the individual horse and to monitor response to therapy. Horses should then be evaluated 1 to 2 months after initiation of therapy to assess response and guide therapy for the upcoming months. If there is poor response to therapy, it is important to do some detective work to determine why treatment has been unsuccessful. For example, it is essential to check the client's technique for using the drug delivery device. Failure to modify the environment may, in some horses, negate any attempts at drug treatment. Some horses with chronic, severe pathologic abnormality may be resistant to corticosteroids or may have irreversible changes in the lungs that prevent response to bronchodilators. Finally, lack of response to therapy may be due to underlying infectious disease and may indicate the need for further diagnostics and perhaps an entirely different approach or concomitant antibiotic use.

REFERENCES

1. Bosshard S, Gerber V. Evaluation of coughing and nasal discharge as early indicators for an increased risk to develop equine recurrent airway obstruction (RAO). J Vet Intern Med 2014;28:618–23.
2. Viel L. Small airway disease as a vanguard for chronic obstructive pulmonary disease. Vet Clin North Am Equine Pract 1997;13(3):549–60.
3. Wagner B. IgE in horses: occurrence in health and disease. Vet Immunol Immunopathol 2009;132(1):21–30.
4. Sweeney CR, Humber KA, Roby KA. Cytologic findings of tracheobronchial aspirates from 66 thoroughbred racehorses. Am J Vet Res 1992;53(7):1172–5.
5. Tremblay GM, Ferland C, Lapointe JM, et al. Effect of stabling on bronchoalveolar cells obtained from normal and COPD horses. Equine Vet J 1993;25(3): 194–7.
6. Millerick-May ML, Karmaus W, Derksen FJ, et al. Local airborne particulate concentration is associated with visible tracheal mucus in thoroughbred racehorses. Equine Vet J 2013;45(1):85–90.
7. Pirie RS. Recurrent airway obstruction: a review. Equine Vet J 2014;46(3): 276–88.
8. Pirie RS, Dixon PM, McGorum BC. Endotoxin contamination contributes to the pulmonary inflammatory and functional response to aspergillus fumigatus extract inhalation in heaves horses. Clin Exp Allergy 2003;33(9):1289–96.
9. Berndt A, Derksen FJ, Robinson NE. Endotoxin concentrations within the breathing zone of horses are higher in stables than on pasture. Vet J 2010;183:54–7.
10. Robinson NE, Karmaus W, Holcombe SJ, et al. Airway inflammation in Michigan pleasure horses: prevalence and risk factors. Equine Vet J 2006;38(4):293–9.
11. Ivester KM, Couetil LL, Moore GE, et al. Environmental exposures and airway inflammation in young thoroughbred horses. J Vet Intern Med 2014;28(3): 918–24.
12. Fortier G, van Erck E, Fortier C, et al. Herpesviruses in respiratory liquids of horses: putative implication in airway inflammation and association with cytological features. Vet Microbiol 2009;139:34–41.
13. Fortier G, Richard E, Hue E, et al. Long-lasting airway inflammation associated with equid herpesvirus-2 in experimentally challenged horses. Vet J 2013;197: 492–5.
14. Cardwell JM, Smith KC, Wood JL, et al. Infectious risk factors and clinical indicators for tracheal mucus in British National Hunt racehorses. Equine Vet J 2014;46(2):150–5.

15. Deaton CM, Marlin DJ, Smith NC, et al. Antioxidant and inflammatory responses of healthy horses and horses affected by recurrent airway obstruction to inhaled ozone. Equine Vet J 2005;37:243–9.
16. Davis MS, Williams CC, Meinkoth JH, et al. Influx of neutrophils and persistence of cytokine expression in airways of horses after performing exercise while breathing cold air. Am J Vet Res 2007;68(2):185–9.
17. Hansen S, Sun L, Baptiste KE, et al. Age-related changes in intracellular expression of IFN-gamma and TNF-alpha in equine lymphocytes measured in bronchoalveolar lavage and peripheral blood. Dev Comp Immunol 2013;39(3):228–33.
18. Lavoie JP, Lefebvre-Lavoie J, Leclere M, et al. Profiling of differentially expressed genes using suppression subtractive hybridization in an equine model of chronic asthma. PLoS One 2012;7(1):e29440.
19. Hughes KJ, Nicolson L, Da Costa N, et al. Evaluation of cytokine mRNA expression in bronchoalveolar lavage cells from horses with inflammatory airway disease. Vet Immunol Immunopathol 2011;140:82–9.
20. Couetil LL, Art T, de Moffarts B, et al. DNA binding activity of transcription factors in bronchial cells of horses with recurrent airway obstruction. Vet Immunol Immunopathol 2006;113:11–20.
21. Hoffman AM, Mazan MR, Ellenberg S. Association between bronchoalveolar lavage cytologic features and airway reactivity in horses with a history of exercise intolerance. Am J Vet Res 1998;59:176–81.
22. Beekman L, Tohver T, Leguillette R. Comparison of cytokine mRNA expression in the bronchoalveolar lavage fluid of horses with inflammatory airway disease and bronchoalveolar lavage mastocytosis or neutrophilia using REST software analysis. J Vet Intern Med 2012;26:153–61.
23. Nyman G, Lindberg R, Weckner D, et al. Pulmonary gas exchange correlated to clinical signs and lung pathology in horses with chronic bronchiolitis. Equine Vet J 1991;23:253–60.
24. O'Callaghan MW, Pascoe JR, Tyler WS, et al. Exercise-induced pulmonary hemorrhage in the horse: results of a detailed clinical, post mortem and imaging study. Equine Vet J 1987;19:411–8.
25. Lakritz J, Wisner ER, Finucane T, et al. Morphologic and morphometric characterization of lung collagen content in clinically normal adult thoroughbreds in race training. Am J Vet Res 1995;56:11–8.
26. Kaup FJ, Drommer W, Damsch S, et al. Ultrastructural findings in horses with chronic obstructive pulmonary disease (COPD). II: Pathomorphological changes of the terminal airways and the alveolar region. Equine Vet J 1990; 22(5):349–55.
27. Pirie RS, Collie DD, Dixon PM, et al. Inhaled endotoxin and organic dust particulates have synergistic proinflammatory effects in equine heaves (organic dust-induced asthma). Clin Exp Allergy 2003;33(5):676–83.
28. Beeler-Marfisi J, Clark ME, Wen X, et al. Experimental induction of recurrent airway obstruction with inhaled fungal spores, lipopolysaccharide, and silica microspheres in horses. Am J Vet Res 2010;71(6):682–9.
29. Marti E, Gerber H, Essich G, et al. The genetic basis of equine allergic diseases. 1. Chronic hypersensitivity bronchitis. Equine Vet J 1991;23(6):457–60.
30. Gerber V, Tessier C, Marti E. Genetics of upper and lower airway diseases in the horse. Equine Vet J 2014. http://dx.doi.org/10.1111/evj.12289.
31. Shakhsi-Niaei M, Klukowska-Rotzler J, Drogemuller C, et al. Replication and fine-mapping of a QTL for recurrent airway obstruction in European Warmblood horses. Anim Genet 2012;43:627–31.

32. Klukowska-Rotzler J, Swinburne JE, Drogemuller C, et al. The interleukin 4 receptor gene and its role in recurrent airway obstruction in Swiss Warmblood horses. Anim Genet 2012;43(4):450–3.
33. Costa LR, Johnson JR, Baur ME, et al. Temporal clinical exacerbation of summer pasture-associated recurrent airway obstruction and relationship with climate and aeroallergens in horses. Am J Vet Res 2006;67(9):1635–42.
34. Derksen FJ, Scott JS, Miller DC, et al. Bronchoalveolar lavage in ponies with recurrent airway obstruction (heaves). Am Rev Respir Dis 1985;132(5): 1066–70.
35. Schmallenbach KH, Rahman I, Sasse HH, et al. Studies on pulmonary and systemic aspergillus fumigatus-specific IgE and IgG antibodies in horses affected with chronic obstructive pulmonary disease (COPD). Vet Immunol Immunopathol 1998;66:245–56.
36. Tahon L, Baselgia S, Gerber V, et al. In vitro allergy tests compared to intradermal testing in horses with recurrent airway obstruction. Vet Immunol Immunopathol 2009;127:85–93.
37. Moran G, Burgos R, Araya O, et al. In vitro bioassay to detect reaginic antibodies from the serum of horses affected with recurrent airway obstruction. Vet Res Commun 2010;34:91–9.
38. Giguere S, Viel L, Lee E, et al. Cytokine induction in pulmonary airways of horses with heaves and effect of therapy with inhaled fluticasone propionate. Vet Immunol Immunopathol 2002;85:147–58.
39. McGorum BC, Dixon PM. Evaluation of local endobronchial antigen challenges in the investigation of equine chronic obstructive pulmonary disease. Equine Vet J 1993;25(4):269–72.
40. Kleiber C, Grunig G, Jungi T, et al. Phenotypic analysis of bronchoalveolar lavage fluid lymphocytes in horses with chronic pulmonary disease. Zentralbl Veterinarmed A 1999;46(3):177–84.
41. Franchini M, Gill U, von Fellenberg R, et al. Interleukin-8 concentration and neutrophil chemotactic activity in bronchoalveolar lavage fluid of horses with chronic obstructive pulmonary disease following exposure to hay. Am J Vet Res 2000;61:1369–74.
42. Ainsworth DM, Matychak M, Reyner CL, et al. Effects of in vitro exposure to hay dust on the gene expression of chemokines and cell-surface receptors in primary bronchial epithelial cell cultures established from horses with chronic recurrent airway obstruction. Am J Vet Res 2009;70(3):365–72.
43. Riihimaki M, Raine A, Art T, et al. Partial divergence of cytokine mRNA expression in bronchial tissues compared to bronchoalveolar lavage cells in horses with recurrent airway obstruction. Vet Immunol Immunopathol 2008;122:256–64.
44. Bullone M, Moran K, Lavoie-Lamoureux A, et al. PI3K and MAPKs regulate neutrophil migration toward the airways in heaves. J Vet Intern Med 2013;27: 164–70.
45. Niedzwiedz A, Jaworski Z, Tykalowski B, et al. Neutrophil and macrophage apoptosis in bronchoalveolar lavage fluid from healthy horses and horses with recurrent airway obstruction (RAO). BMC Vet Res 2014;10:29.
46. Bureau F, Delhalle S, Bonizzi G, et al. Mechanisms of persistent NF-kappa B activity in the bronchi of an animal model of asthma. J Immunol 2000;165(10): 5822–30.
47. Turlej RK, Fievez L, Sandersen CF, et al. Enhanced survival of lung granulocytes in an animal model of asthma: evidence for a role of GM-CSF activated STAT5 signalling pathway. Thorax 2001;56:696–702.

48. Padoan E, Ferraresso S, Pegolo S, et al. Real time RT-PCR analysis of inflammatory mediator expression in recurrent airway obstruction-affected horses. Vet Immunol Immunopathol 2013;156(3–4):190–9.

49. Simonen-Jokinen T, Pirie RS, McGorum BC, et al. Effect of composition and different fractions of hay dust suspension on inflammation in lungs of heaves-affected horses: MMP-9 and MMP-2 as indicators of tissue destruction. Equine Vet J 2005;37(5):412–7.

50. Dacre KJ, McGorum BC, Marlin DJ, et al. Organic dust exposure increases mast cell tryptase in bronchoalveolar lavage fluid and airway epithelium of heaves horses. Clin Exp Allergy 2007;37(12):1809–18.

51. Zhang L, Franchini M, Wehrli Eser M, et al. Increased adenosine concentration in bronchoalveolar lavage fluid of horses with lower airway inflammation. Vet J 2012;193(1):268–70.

52. Winkler GC. Pulmonary intravascular macrophages in domestic animal species: review of structural and functional properties. Am J Anat 1988;181(3):217–34.

53. Schneberger D, Aharonson-Raz K, Singh B. Pulmonary intravascular macrophages and lung health: what are we missing? Am J Physiol Lung Cell Mol Physiol 2012;302(6):498–503.

54. Katavolos P, Ackerley CA, Viel L, et al. Clara cell secretory protein is reduced in equine recurrent airway obstruction. Vet Pathol 2009;46(4):604–13.

55. Yu M, Wang Z, Robinson NE, et al. Inhibitory nerve distribution and mediation of NANC relaxation by nitric oxide in horse airways. J Appl Physiol 1994;76(1):339–44.

56. Abraham G, Kottke C, Dhein S, et al. Agonist-independent alteration in beta-adrenoceptor-G-protein-adenylate cyclase system in an equine model of recurrent airway obstruction. Pulm Pharmacol Ther 2006;19(3):218–29.

57. Venugopal CS, Holmes EP, Polikepahad S, et al. Neurokinin receptors in recurrent airway obstruction: a comparative study of affected and unaffected horses. Can J Vet Res 2009;73(1):25–33.

58. Deaton CM, Marlin DJ, Deaton L, et al. Comparison of the antioxidant status in tracheal and bronchoalveolar epithelial lining fluids in recurrent airway obstruction. Equine Vet J 2006;38(5):417–22.

59. Kirschvink N, Fievez L, Bougnet V, et al. Effect of nutritional antioxidant supplementation on systemic and pulmonary antioxidant status, airway inflammation and lung function in heaves-affected horses. Equine Vet J 2002;34:705–12.

60. Michelotto PV, Muehlmann LA, Zanatta AL, et al. Platelet-activating factor and evidence of oxidative stress in the bronchoalveolar fluid of thoroughbred colts during race training. J Vet Intern Med 2010;24:414–9.

61. Johansson AM, Gardner SY, Atkins CE, et al. Cardiovascular effects of acute pulmonary obstruction in horses with recurrent airway obstruction. J Vet Intern Med 2007;21(2):302–7.

62. Shaba JJ, Behan Braman A, Robinson NE. Plasma cortisol concentration increases within 6 hours of stabling in RAO-affected horses. Equine Vet J 2014;46:642–4.

63. Wagner B, Ainsworth DM, Freer H. Analysis of soluble CD14 and its use as a biomarker in neonatal foals with septicemia and horses with recurrent airway obstruction. Vet Immunol Immunopathol 2013;155:124–8.

64. Lavoie-Lamoureux A, Leclere M, Lemos K, et al. Markers of systemic inflammation in horses with heaves. J Vet Intern Med 2012;26(6):1419–26.

65. Hoffman AM, Oura TJ, Riedelberger KJ, et al. Plethysmographic comparison of breathing pattern in heaves (recurrent airway obstruction) versus experimental bronchoconstriction or hyperpnea in horses. J Vet Intern Med 2007;21(1): 184–92.

66. Gehlen H, Oey L, Rohn K, et al. Pulmonary dysfunction and skeletal muscle changes in horses with RAO. J Vet Intern Med 2008;22(4):1014–21.

67. Setlakwe EL, Lemos KR, Lavoie-Lamoureux A, et al. Airway collagen and elastic fiber content correlates with lung function in equine heaves. Am J Physiol Lung Cell Mol Physiol 2014;307:252–60.

68. Mazan MR, Deveney EF, DeWitt S, et al. Energetic cost of breathing, body composition, and pulmonary function in horses with recurrent airway obstruction. J Appl Physiol 2004;97(1):91–7.

69. Art T, Duvivier DH, Votion D, et al. Does an acute COPD crisis modify the cardiorespiratory and ventilatory adjustments to exercise in horses? J Appl Physiol 1998;84(3):845–52.

70. Bracher V, von Fellenberg R, Winder CN, et al. An investigation of the incidence of chronic obstructive pulmonary disease (COPD) in random populations of swiss horses. Equine Vet J 1991;23(2):136–41.

71. Christley RM, Hodgson DR, Rose RJ, et al. A case-control study of respiratory disease in thoroughbred racehorses in Sydney, Australia. Equine Vet J 2001; 33(3):256–64.

72. Vrins A, Doucet M, Nunez-Ochoa L. A retrospective study of bronchoalveolar lavage cytology in horses with clinical findings of small airway disease. Zentralbl Veterinarmed A 1991;38(6):472–9.

73. Bedenice D, Mazan MR, Hoffman AM. Association between cough and cytology of bronchoalveolar lavage fluid and pulmonary function in horses diagnosed with inflammatory airway disease. J Vet Intern Med 2008;22(4): 1022–8.

74. Koch C, Straub R, Ramseyer A, et al. Endoscopic scoring of the tracheal septum in horses and its clinical relevance for the evaluation of lower airway health in horses. Equine Vet J 2007;39(2):107–12.

75. Courouce-Malblanc A, Deniau V, Rossignol F, et al. Physiological measurements and prevalence of lower airway diseases in trotters with dorsal displacement of the soft palate. Equine Vet J Suppl 2010;38:246–55.

76. Allen KJ, Tremaine WH, Franklin SH. Prevalence of inflammatory airway disease in national hunt horses referred for investigation of poor athletic performance. Equine Vet J Suppl 2006;36:529–34.

77. Wilsher S, Allen WR, Wood JL. Factors associated with failure of thoroughbred horses to train and race. Equine Vet J 2006;38(2):113–8.

78. Mazan M, Hoffman A, Macordes B. Inflammatory airway disease: The clinical picture and effect of discipline. In: Proceedings of a Workshop on Inflammatory Airway Disease: Defining the Syndrome. Newmarket (United Kingdom); R&W Publications: 2002.

79. Koterba AM, Wozniak JA, Kosch PC. Changes in breathing pattern in the normal horse at rest up to age one year. Equine Vet J 1995;27:265–74.

80. Marlin DJ, Schrotert RC, Cashman PM, et al. Movements of thoracic and abdominal compartments during ventilation at rest and during exercise. Equine Vet J Supp 2002;34:384–90.

81. Behan AL, Hauptman JG, Robinson NE. Telemetric analysis of breathing pattern variability in recurrent airway obstruction (heaves)-affected horses. Am J Vet Res 2013;74(6):925–33.

82. Klein HJ, Deegen E. Histamine inhalation provocation test: method to identify nonspecific airway reactivity in equids. Am J Vet Res 1986;47(8): 1796–800.

83. Hoffman AM, Mazan MR. Programme of lung function testing horses with suspected small airway disease. Equine Vet Educ 1999;11:322.

84. Tsurikisawa N, Oshikata C, Tsuburai T, et al. Bronchial reactivity to histamine is correlated with airway remodeling in adults with moderate to severe asthma. J Asthma 2010;47(8):841–8.

85. Couetil LL, Denicola DB. Blood gas, plasma lactate and bronchoalveolar lavage cytology analyses in racehorses with respiratory disease. Equine Vet J Suppl 1999;30:77–82.

86. Courouce-Malblanc A, Pronost S, Fortier G, et al. Physiological measurements and upper and lower respiratory tract evaluation in french standardbred trotters during a standardised exercise test on the treadmill. Equine Vet J Suppl 2002; 34:402–7.

87. Robinson NE. International workshop on equine chronic airway disease. Michigan State University 16-18 June 2000. Equine Vet J 2001;33(1):5–19.

88. Rettmer H, Hoffman AM, Lanz S, et al. Owner-reported coughing and nasal discharge are associated with clinical findings, arterial oxygen tension, mucus score and bronchoprovocation in horses with recurrent airway obstruction in a field setting. Equine Vet J 2014. http://dx.doi.org/10.1111/evj.12286.

89. Haltmayer E, Reiser S, Schramel JP, et al. Breathing pattern and thoracoabdominal asynchrony in horses with chronic obstructive and inflammatory lung disease. Res Vet Sci 2013;95(2):654–9.

90. Richard EA, Fortier GD, Denoix JM, et al. Influence of subclinical inflammatory airway disease on equine respiratory function evaluated by impulse oscillometry. Equine Vet J 2009;41(4):384–9.

91. Couetil L, Hammer J, Miskovic Feutz M, et al. Effects of N-butylscopolammonium bromide on lung function in horses with recurrent airway obstruction. J Vet Intern Med 2012;26(6):1433–8.

92. Pirrone F, Albertini M, Clement MG, et al. Respiratory mechanics in standardbred horses with sub-clinical inflammatory airway disease and poor athletic performance. Vet J 2007;173(1):144–50.

93. Boulet LP, Prince P, Turcotte H, et al. Clinical features and airway inflammation in mild asthma versus asymptomatic airway hyperresponsiveness. Respir Med 2006;100(2):292–9.

94. Malikides N, Hughes KJ, Hodgson DR, et al. Comparison of tracheal aspirates and bronchoalveolar lavage in racehorses. 2. Evaluation of the diagnostic significance of neutrophil percentage. Aust Vet J 2003;81(11):685–7.

95. Derksen FJ, Brown CM, Sonea I, et al. Comparison of transtracheal aspirate and bronchoalveolar lavage cytology in 50 horses with chronic lung disease. Equine Vet J 1989;21(1):23–6.

96. Koblinger K, Hecker K, Nicol J, et al. Bronchial collapse during bronchoalveolar lavage in horses is an indicator of lung inflammation. Equine Vet J 2014;46(1): 50–5.

97. Couetil LL, Hoffman AM, Hodgson J, et al. Inflammatory airway disease of horses. J Vet Intern Med 2007;21(2):356–61.

98. Nolen-Walston RD, Harris M, Agnew ME, et al. Clinical and diagnostic features of inflammatory airway disease subtypes in horses examined because of poor performance: 98 cases (2004-2010). J Am Vet Med Assoc 2013;242(8): 1138–45.

99. McKane SA, Rose RJ, Evans DL. Comparison of bronchoalveolar lavage findings and measurements of gas exchange during exercise in horses with poor racing performance. N Z Vet J 1995;43(5):179–82.

100. Hughes KJ, Malikides N, Hodgson DR, et al. Comparison of tracheal aspirates and bronchoalveolar lavage in racehorses. 1. Evaluation of cytological stains and the percentage of mast cells and eosinophils. Aust Vet J 2003;81(11):681–4.

101. Fernandez NJ, Hecker KG, Gilroy CV, et al. Reliability of 400-cell and 5-field leukocyte differential counts for equine bronchoalveolar lavage fluid. Vet Clin Pathol 2013;42(1):92–8.

102. Wysocka B, Klucinski W. Usefulness of the assessment of discharge accumulation in the lower airways and tracheal septum thickening in the differential diagnosis of recurrent airway obstruction (RAO) and inflammatory airway disease (IAD) in the horse. Pol J Vet Sci 2014;17(2):247–53.

103. Holcombe SJ, Robinson NE, Derksen FJ, et al. Effect of tracheal mucus and tracheal cytology on racing performance in thoroughbred racehorses. Equine Vet J 2006;38(4):300–4.

104. Christley RM, Hodgson DR, Rose RJ, et al. Coughing in thoroughbred racehorses: risk factors and tracheal endoscopic and cytological findings. Vet Rec 2001;148(4):99–104.

105. Gerber V, Robinson NE, Luethi S, et al. Airway inflammation and mucus in two age groups of asymptomatic well-performing sport horses. Equine Vet J 2003; 35(5):491–5.

106. Cardwell JM, Christley RM, Gerber V, et al. What's in a name? Inflammatory airway disease in racehorses in training. Equine Vet J 2011;43(6):756–8.

107. Durando MM, Martin BB, Davidson EJ, et al. Correlations between exercising arterial blood gas values, tracheal wash findings and upper respiratory tract abnormalities in horses presented for poor performance. Equine Vet J Suppl 2006;36:523–8.

108. Tilley P, Sales Luis JP, Branco Ferreira M. Correlation and discriminant analysis between clinical, endoscopic, thoracic X-ray and bronchoalveolar lavage fluid cytology scores, for staging horses with recurrent airway obstruction (RAO). Res Vet Sci 2012;93(2):1006–14.

109. Lavoie JP, Dalle S, Breton L, et al. Bronchiectasis in three adult horses with heaves. J Vet Intern Med 2004;18(5):757–60.

110. Mazan MR, Vin R, Hoffman AM. Radiographic scoring lacks predictive value in inflammatory airway disease. Equine Vet J 2005;37(6):541–5.

111. Lapointe JM, Lavoie JP, Vrins AA. Effects of triamcinolone acetonide on pulmonary function and bronchoalveolar lavage cytologic features in horses with chronic obstructive pulmonary disease. Am J Vet Res 1993;54(8):1310–6.

112. French K, Pollitt CC, Pass MA. Pharmacokinetics and metabolic effects of triamcinolone acetonide and their possible relationships to glucocorticoid-induced laminitis in horses. J Vet Pharmacol Ther 2000;23(5):287–92.

113. Jackson CA, Berney C, Jefcoat AM, et al. Environment and prednisone interactions in the treatment of recurrent airway obstruction (heaves). Equine Vet J 2000;32(5):432–8.

114. Courouce-Malblanc A, Fortier G, Pronost S, et al. Comparison of prednisolone and dexamethasone effects in the presence of environmental control in heaves-affected horses. Vet J 2008;175(2):227–33.

115. Leclere M, Lefebvre-Lavoie J, Beauchamp G, et al. Efficacy of oral prednisolone and dexamethasone in horses with recurrent airway obstruction in the presence of continuous antigen exposure. Equine Vet J 2010;42(4):316–21.

116. Picandet V, Leguillette R, Lavoie JP. Comparison of efficacy and tolerability of isoflupredone and dexamethasone in the treatment of horses affected with recurrent airway obstruction ('heaves'). Equine Vet J 2003;35(4):419–24.
117. Dauvillier J, Felippe MJ, Lunn DP, et al. Effect of long-term fluticasone treatment on immune function in horses with heaves. J Vet Intern Med 2011;25(3):549–57.
118. Rush BR, Worster AA, Flaminio MJ, et al. Alteration in adrenocortical function in horses with recurrent airway obstruction after aerosol and parenteral administration of beclomethasone dipropionate and dexamethasone, respectively. Am J Vet Res 1998;59(8):1044–7.
119. Laan TT, Bull S, van Nieuwstadt RA, et al. The effect of aerosolized and intravenously administered clenbuterol and aerosolized fluticasone propionate on horses challenged with aspergillus fumigatus antigen. Vet Res Commun 2006; 30(6):623–35.
120. Gray BP, Biddle S, Pearce CM, et al. Detection of fluticasone propionate in horse plasma and urine following inhaled administration. Drug Test Anal 2013;5:306–14.
121. Robinson NE, Berney C, Behan A, et al. Fluticasone propionate aerosol is more effective for prevention than treatment of recurrent airway obstruction. J Vet Intern Med 2009;23:1247–53.
122. Leclere M, Lavoie-Lamoureux A, Joubert P, et al. Corticosteroids and antigen avoidance decrease airway smooth muscle mass in an equine asthma model. Am J Respir Cell Mol Biol 2012;47(5):589–96.
123. Bertin FR, Ivester KM, Couetil LL. Comparative efficacy of inhaled albuterol between two hand-held delivery devices in horses with recurrent airway obstruction. Equine Vet J 2011;43(4):393–8.
124. Leach CL, Davidson PJ, Hasselquist BE, et al. Influence of particle size and patient dosing technique on lung deposition of HFA-beclomethasone from a metered dose inhaler. J Aerosol Med 2005;18:379–85.
125. de Lagarde M, Rodrigues N, Chevigny M, et al. N-butylscopolammonium bromide causes fewer side effects than atropine when assessing bronchoconstriction reversibility in horses with heaves. Equine Vet J 2014;46:474–8.
126. Thompson JA, Mirza MH, Barker SA, et al. Clenbuterol toxicosis in three quarter horse racehorses after administration of a compounded product. J Am Vet Med Assoc 2011;239(6):842–9.
127. Kearns CF, McKeever KH. Clenbuterol diminishes aerobic performance in horses. Med Sci Sports Exerc 2002;34:1976–85.
128. Read JR, Boston RC, Abraham G, et al. Effect of prolonged administration of clenbuterol on airway sensitivity and sweating in horses with inflammatory airway disease. Am J Vet Res 2012;73:140–5.
129. Erichsen DF, Aviad AD, Schultz RH, et al. Clinical efficacy and safety of clenbuterol HCl when administered to effect in horses with chronic obstructive pulmonary disease (COPD). Equine Vet J 1994;26(4):331–6.
130. Traub-Dargatz JL, McKinnon AO, Thrall MA, et al. Evaluation of clinical signs of disease, bronchoalveolar and tracheal wash analysis, and arterial blood gas tensions in 13 horses with chronic obstructive pulmonary disease treated with prednisone, methyl sulfonmethane, and clenbuterol hydrochloride. Am J Vet Res 1992;53(10):1908–16.
131. Broski SE, Amundson DE. Paradoxical response to levalbuterol. J Am Osteopath Assoc 2008;108:211–3.
132. Mazan MR, Lascola K, Bruns SJ, et al. Use of a novel one-nostril mask-spacer device to evaluate airway hyperresponsiveness (AHR) in horses after chronic administration of albuterol. Can J Vet Res 2014;78(3):214–20.

133. Bailey J, Colahan P, Kubilis P, et al. Effect of inhaled beta 2 adrenoceptor agonist, albuterol sulphate, on performance of horses. Equine Vet J Suppl 1999;30:575–80.
134. Mazan MR, Hoffman AM. Effects of aerosolized albuterol on physiologic responses to exercise in standardbreds. Am J Vet Res 2001;62:1812–7.
135. Kirschvink N, Di Silvestro F, Sbai I, et al. The use of cardboard bedding material as part of an environmental control regime for heaves-affected horses: in vitro assessment of airborne dust and aeroallergen concentration and in vivo effects on lung function. Vet J 2002;163:319–25.
136. Fairbairn SM, Lees P, Page CP, et al. Duration of antigen-induced hyperresponsiveness in horses with allergic respiratory disease and possible links with early airway obstruction. J Vet Pharmacol Ther 1993;16:469–76.

Update on Exercise-Induced Pulmonary Hemorrhage

Stacey Sullivan, BVSc, MVS, MANZCVS*,
Kenneth Hinchcliff, BVSc, MS, PhD

KEYWORDS

- Equine • Bleeding • Performance • Epistaxis • Welfare

KEY POINTS

- EIPH is caused by pulmonary capillary stress failure. High-intensity exercise causes large magnitude increases in pulmonary vascular pressure and markedly negative pleural pressure that result in mechanical disruption of the pulmonary capillary wall. The role of pulmonary veno-occlusive remodeling in the pathogenesis of EIPH is an area of current active research.
- Horses with moderate to severe EIPH have an unequivocal diminution of race performance. Horses with moderate to severe EIPH detected on tracheobronscopic examination are less likely to win races, finish further behind the winner, and are less likely to be in the top 90th percentile of money earners than horses with mild EIPH or no EIPH. A single episode of EIPH grades 1, 2, or 3 does not affect the lifetime athletic performance of thoroughbred race horses. Severe (grade 4) EIPH and epistaxis might affect career longevity.
- Furosemide is the only medication proved to be efficacious to reduce or prevent EIPH during strenuous exercise. Currently, there is insufficient evidence to determine if any other medications used for EIPH are effective for reducing the frequency of detection or severity of EIPH.
- There is some evidence that EIPH might be progressive. However, most horses with EIPH do not experience a reduction in lifetime performance and horses with EIPH successfully transition to other athletic pursuits after retirement from racing. EIPH is only rarely identified as the primary cause of exercise-associated sudden death.

INTRODUCTION

Exercise-induced pulmonary hemorrhage (EIPH) is an important disease of horses that perform high-intensity athletic activity. EIPH is most frequently identified in Thoroughbred and Standardbred racehorses performing high-speed exercise. EIPH is

Funding Sources: None.
Conflict of Interest: None.
Equine Centre, Faculty of Veterinary and Agricultural Sciences, The University of Melbourne, 250 Princess Highway, Werribee, Victoria 3030, Australia
* Corresponding author.
E-mail address: staceyls@unimelb.edu.au

considered a major issue for the racing industry because of the high prevalence of the condition, the association with reduced short-term athletic performance, the widespread use of furosemide as prophylaxis of EIPH in some racing jurisdictions, and concerns of the impact of EIPH on the overall health and welfare of equine athletes. During the last 10 years, important advances have been made in understanding the pathogenesis and risk factors for EIPH and the impact of the disease on performance and career. This article summarizes the most recent advances in EIPH.

HOW COMMON IS EXERCISE-INDUCED PULMONARY HEMORRHAGE?

EIPH has been identified in virtually all breeds of horses used for flat racing, harness racing, hurdle and steeplechase racing, polo, western performance disciplines, eventing, show jumping, and dressage. The prevalence of EIPH varies according to the type of exercise performed, the population of horses examined, the criteria used to define EIPH (epistaxis vs tracheobronchoscopic severity grade vs cytologic evidence of EIPH), and the frequency of examinations. Using tracheobronchoscopy performed within 2 hours of racing, approximately 43% to 75% of Thoroughbred racehorses exhibit blood within the trachea after a single examination.[1–4] With repeated examinations, the prevalence of EIPH increases to greater than 85%.[4,5] The prevalence of endoscopically evident EIPH in horses performing other pursuits, such as dressage or jumping, has not been comprehensively evaluated with the exception of polo ponies, where 11% to 46% of horses used for polo were found to have EIPH after competition.[6,7]

Cytologic methods of detecting EIPH commonly reveal a higher prevalence of disease than when tracheobronchoscopy or epistaxis is used to diagnose EIPH. This is primarily because of the length of time red blood cell (RBC) breakdown products persist in respiratory fluids and presumably, but not demonstrably, the greater sensitivity of examination of bronchoalveolar lavage (BAL) fluid to detect evidence of hemorrhage. Although the presence of RBCs, effete RBCs, or hemosiderophages is prima facie evidence of hemorrhage into the airways, the concentration of these cells in BAL fluid that is clinically important has not been determined.

Almost 100% of Thoroughbred horses in race training have evidence of blood in the lower airways, which is interpreted as evidence of EIPH.[8] In contrast, endurance horses in competitive training have none or less than 1% of hemosiderophages on evaluation of BAL wash samples, indicating the prevalence of clinically important EIPH in endurance horses is probably low.[9] Epistaxis, arguably the most severe manifestation of EIPH, occurs relatively infrequently in 1.1% to 3.5% of Thoroughbred and Standardbred horses after racing. The incidence of epistaxis in horses performing athletic endeavors other than racing is not documented.

HOW DOES EXERCISE-INDUCED PULMONARY HEMORRHAGE OCCUR?

Currently, the accepted pathophysiologic mechanism of EIPH is stress failure of the pulmonary capillaries caused by excessive transmural pressure created by very high intracapillary pressure (predominantly caused by high blood pressure) and low intra-alveolar pressure (generated by negative intrapleural pressures associated with inspiration) produced during exercise.[10]

Strenuous exercise in horses is associated with marked increases in pulmonary vascular pressures. Mean pulmonary arterial pressure increases from resting levels of 25 mm Hg to greater than 95 mm Hg during maximal exercise on a treadmill at speeds of greater than or equal to 14 m/s on a 5% incline.[11,12] Pulmonary artery wedge pressure (which approximates pulmonary venous pressure) and estimated pulmonary capillary pressures similarly increase in magnitude during strenuous exertion. This three- to four-fold increase in pulmonary vascular pressures occurs primarily because of an increase in cardiac output.[13] Under experimental laboratory conditions, the critical mean pulmonary arterial pressure above which mechanical disruption of the pulmonary capillaries occurs is 75 to 100 mm Hg, lower than that observed in most galloping horses.[14] Injury to the blood-gas barrier seems to be rapidly reversed once the pulmonary vascular pressure decreases to levels observed in nonexercising horses.[10] Consistently more breaks per millimeter occur in dorsocaudal lung regions than in cranioventral lung lobes.[14] Unlike dogs and humans, the dorsocaudal lung regions of horses receive relatively greater pulmonary blood flow during exercise than cranioventral lung lobes.[15] This likely contributes to the vulnerability of pulmonary capillaries to rupture and accounts for the typical dorsal distribution of lesions in horses with EIPH.

In addition to marked increases in intravascular pressures, pleural (alveolar) pressures become more negative during exercise. Pleural pressures are an important component of transmural pressure that creates shear forces across pulmonary capillaries. Pleural pressures in normal horses during inspiration decrease from approximately −0.7 kPa (−5.3 mm Hg) at rest, to −8.5 kPa (64 mm Hg) during strenuous exercise.[16] Experimentally induced partial inspiratory and expiratory upper airway obstruction results in markedly more negative pleural pressures and increase in estimated transmural capillary pressures above that of the critical breaking point of pulmonary capillaries.[17] This suggests dynamic conditions of the upper respiratory tract contribute to pulmonary capillary stress failure and EIPH in some horses. EIPH, usually of lesser severity, also occurs in horses during prolonged submaximal exercise (trotting at 40%–60% maximum oxygen consumption) where mean pulmonary arterial (ie, intravascular) pressure does not typically exceed the critical breaking point of greater than 75 mm Hg. In these situations, excessive transmural pressure is thought to primarily arise from the contribution of very negative pleural pressures because of altered inspiratory/expiratory breathing mechanics.[16]

Ultrastructural evidence of pulmonary capillary stress failure has been identified in three horses exercised on a treadmill[10] and in experimental perfusion studies of equine lungs.[14] Typical ultrastructural and histologic findings of pulmonary capillary stress failure include (1) disruption of the capillary endothelium and alveolar epithelium; (2) RBCs within the alveoli and interstitium; and (3) RBCs, platelets, and macrophages closely associated with areas of endothelial and epithelial discontinuity. Recent research has focused on a newly identified histologic lesion, termed veno-occlusive remodeling, which occurs primarily in the caudodorsal lung region of horses with EIPH. Veno-occlusive remodeling refers to remodeling of small diameter (100–200 μm outer diameter) intralobular pulmonary veins. Remodeling is characterized by deposition of collagen around pulmonary veins and marked medial smooth muscle hypertrophy and intimal hyperplasia within the pulmonary vein wall.[18,19] These structural lung changes are thought to confer altered mechanical properties (namely, an increase in stiffness) to the pulmonary veins that potentially have important physiologic consequences. It is theorized that narrowing and occlusion of the pulmonary vein wall, which is essentially considered an adaptive structural change to repeated bouts of strenuous exercise, could further increase intravascular pressures upstream at the pulmonary capillaries and contribute to capillary stress failure. This is supported by the finding that pulmonary veins, and to a lesser extent pulmonary arteries, in the caudodorsal lung regions of raced horses with EIPH are stiffer than those from unexercised horses.[20] The amount of exercise necessary to induce these changes has not been determined. Two weeks of intense exercise did not result in alterations of mRNA and protein expression expected to precede structural changes to the pulmonary veins in an initial study.[21] The role of veno-occlusive remodeling in EIPH requires further investigation.

Lower airway inflammation has long been suspected to play a role in the development or progression of EIPH but without empirical evidence to support this contention. There are two potential ways in which inflammation could contribute to EIPH: lower airway inflammation and bronchoconstriction have the potential to cause intrathoracic airway obstruction and, therefore, more negative intra-alveolar (pleural) pressures contributing to development of EIPH; and presence of blood in the alveolar and interstitial spaces potentially causes inflammation and fibrosis, which could perpetuate EIPH. An association has been detected between the presence of lower airway inflammation and EIPH in racehorses, although whether the inflammation was a cause or effect of EIPH is unclear[22,23] and mild pulmonary inflammation increased the severity of EIPH in an experimental model of airway inflammation achieved by instillation of 0.1% acetic acid into the distal bronchi.[24] These findings provide the basis for suggestion of a role of small airway disease in development of EIPH. Other investigators have also found that single and multiple instillations of blood into the airways causes a mild, transient inflammation response (increase in type 2 pneumocytes), which generally resolves by 14 days.[25] Although results are somewhat conflicting between research groups, intra-alveolar instillation of blood per se does not seem to consistently cause the pulmonary fibrosis typically seen in severe cases of EIPH. Presence of hemosiderin within the interstitial space (rather than alveolar space) has recently been identified as a crucial factor in the development of fibrosis that could be important in perpetuation or progression of EIPH. No association has been detected between EIPH and lower airway bacterial agents, such as Streptococcus spp or Pasturella like spp.[22] Although the weight of evidence suggests lower airway inflammation contributes to EIPH in some horses, it is important to understand many horses with EIPH show no evidence of lower airway inflammation, highlighting that EIPH is a complex disease.

The role of genetics in the development of EIPH is one avenue of research that has until recently been largely underinvestigated. The heritability (h^2) of epistaxis in populations of Thoroughbred racehorses in South Africa, Australia, United Kingdom, and Hong Kong has been evaluated over the last 10 years using pedigree analysis.[26–28] Epistaxis, presumably caused by EIPH, has been found to have a small to moderate heritability (estimate of 0.3–0.5), which is similar to the heritability of other diseases, such as superficial digital flexor injury and distal limb fracture. The genetic contribution to the risk of developing EIPH has not been evaluated in horses with bleeding of varying severity. Based on current evidence, it is likely that the expression of EIPH in individual horses is multifactorial, with an underlying genetic predisposition modulated by other genes and environmental factors.

WHAT ARE THE RISK FACTORS FOR EXERCISE-INDUCED PULMONARY HEMORRHAGE?

Risk factors for EIPH or epistaxis have been investigated in multiple studies of Thoroughbred and Standardbred racehorses in the United Kingdom, Australia, South Africa, Brazil, Japan, Hong Kong, and the United States. Although some risk factors seem common to EIPH and epistaxis, the risk factors for either condition are not identical. As a general rule, the more intense the exercise or higher the speed attained, the greater the proportion of horses detected with EIPH or epistaxis. The prevalence of EIPH is higher after racing, as compared with breezing or training.[2,29] Epistaxis is most common after racing.[29,30] Horses competing in steeplechase or hurdles racing are at greater risk of epistaxis than horses competing in flat races or other disciplines.[30–32] There is no consistent association between sex and EIPH,[1,2,33] but epistaxis has occurs more often in male horses. This is postulated to reflect that mares and fillies are more often retired to breeding earlier in their career than geldings.

Cumulative measures of racing volume, often reported as number of racing starts, duration of racing career, number of years spent racing, and age, have long been identified as important risk factors for EIPH and epistaxis. For example, horses with greater than or equal to 50 starts were 1.78 times more likely to have endoscopically evident grade 1 and higher EIPH.[33] Horses racing for greater than 2 years are more likely to show epistaxis.[34] These factors likely represent increased exposure time for disease development. Although age is often identified as a risk factor for bleeding,[1,2,22,27,30–32] studies examining this association invariably fail to control for number of racing starts or used too few horses. The age of a horse per se is probably not an important risk factor when compared with other indices of racing volume, such as racing starts or time spent racing, which more accurately represent the pathogenesis of EIPH.

Cool ambient environmental temperature, reported as temperatures less than 20°C, or winter/spring season have also been repeatedly identified as risk factors for EIPH and epistaxis in Standardbred and Thoroughbred racehorses.[27,33–35] Horses that race at temperatures less than 20°C are 1.9 times more likely to be diagnosed with endoscopically evident EIPH after a race.[33] Most racehorses train at cooler environmental temperatures than that at which they race. Cold-induced airway hyperresponsiveness (bronchoconstriction) or impaired conditioning of cold air during exercise are two possible mechanisms that could plausibly cause musosal inflammation or altered breathing mechanics that might contribute to altered extravascular pressures during exercise. However, the pathophysiologic basis and clinical relevance of cool air to EIPH are unclear.

WHAT IS THE IMPACT OF EXERCISE-INDUCED PULMONARY HEMORRHAGE ON PERFORMANCE?

Historically, there were conflicting results of the impact of EIPH on performance. Associations were detected with inferior or superior racing performance, or no association was detected at all.[1,2,36,37] These conflicting results were generated from studies that used different statistical methods, populations of horses, study methodologies, and diagnostic criterion and the lack of methodologically robust, large-scale studies evaluating the association between EIPH and performance. Over the last 10 years, the impact of EIPH on short- and long-term performance has been investigated in better-quality studies, making the impact of EIPH on athletic performance clearer.

EIPH is an important cause of reduced athletic performance during a race. The impact of EIPH during a single race was evaluated in a prospective, cross-sectional study of 744 Australian Thoroughbred racehorses competing in Melbourne, Victoria. The study evaluated 52% of the racing population at the time and was representative of the broader population of horses racing at that time in terms of performance and earnings. Horses were not medicated with furosemide. This study found that Thoroughbred racehorses with endoscopically visible EIPH of severity grade 2 and higher are four times less likely to win and two times less likely to win or finish in the first three race positions.[3] Horses with EIPH severity 1 and lower are three times more likely to be in the top 90th percentile or higher for earnings.[3] Horses with EIPH of grade 2 and higher finished significantly further behind the winner than did horses with EIPH grade 1 and lower.[3] These findings were corroborated in a second similarly conducted study in 1000 South African Thoroughbred racehorses.[38] South African racehorses without

EIPH were two times more likely win races, finished an average of one length ahead of horses with EIPH, and were two times more likely to be in the highest decile in race earnings.[38]

Investigating the effects of EIPH on long-term performance is challenging because of the need to define the disease classification of all horses under standardized conditions and to follow horses for a prolonged period of time, preferably their entire career. The effect of EIPH on long-term performance can be evaluated from two perspectives. The first is "what is the relationship between EIPH diagnosed on a single occasion and subsequent future athletic performance?" The second is "how does EIPH progress over a horse's career and what is the impact of this on long-term performance?" The relationship between EIPH diagnosed on single occasion and lifetime performance was assessed in the 744 Australian Thoroughbred racehorses when all horses had retired from competitive racing. There was no association between a single episode of EIPH severity grade 1, 2, and 3 and career duration, earnings, or total number of starts, wins, or placings achieved during a horse's career.[38] Horses with severe (grade 4) EIPH were found to have shorter career durations, fewer earnings, and fewer starts than horses without EIPH.[38] This could have been caused by a biologic effect of EIPH grade 4 on performance or management decisions based on the knowledge of the endoscopic examination. Other studies have also found associations between epistaxis and fewer career earnings[39] and reduced duration of racing career.[40]

To the authors' knowledge, studies that serially evaluate EIPH over their entire career under standardized racing conditions have not yet been performed. One retrospective, descriptive study of 822 New Zealand Thoroughbred racehorses competing in Hong Kong evaluated EIPH on multiple occasions until retirement.[29] EIPH-positive and -negative horses competed in a similar number of racing starts during their career, and horses with epistaxis retired because of the condition.[29] Days to retirement and career longevity were found to be longer for EIPH-positive horses,[29] which is speculated to be caused by greater exposure time for disease development rather than a lack of effect of the condition on performance. The conclusions of this study have been questioned and are limited by its retrospective nature, nonstandardized conditions in which examinations were performed and conducted, and nonrandom selection of horses for inclusion in the study. Much remains to be investigated on the effect of EIPH on a horse's long-term athletic performance.

WHAT TREATMENTS ARE EFFECTIVE FOR EXERCISE-INDUCED PULMONARY HEMORRHAGE?

A wide variety of medications have been used to treat EIPH. Most medications address a putative pathophysiologic mechanism and/or an etiologic factor that has been implicated in the development of the disease during the last 40 years. The aims of treatment include a reduction in the severity of bleeding and prevention of any potential adverse pulmonary sequelae (eg, pulmonary inflammation, infection, or fibrosis). Despite substantive efforts to identify alternative, effective treatments for EIPH, currently the only medication demonstrated to be efficacious for prophylaxis of EIPH in high-quality randomized controlled trials and meta-analyses is furosemide. The following summarizes the quality and quantity of evidence available for furosemide and various other medications used to treat EIPH in racehorses.

Furosemide has been used for more than 40 years to reduce the occurrence or severity of EIPH. The mechanism of action to reduce or prevent EIPH is not known. Furosemide is a loop diuretic that has been demonstrated to attenuate the increased right atrial, pulmonary arterial, venous, and capillary pressures considered important in the development of pulmonary capillary stress failure during exercise.[41] Furosemide also has direct effects on the pulmonary veins to relax venous smooth muscle. Although race-day use of furosemide is banned in many racing jurisdictions outside the United States and Canada, the medication is commonly administered to horses with EIPH during training to reduce EIPH severity. Some studies have reported conflicting results of the effectiveness of furosemide for EIPH. This is because of differences in study design or methodology and/or low statistical power of individual trials to detect an effect or difference. There is now high-quality evidence from randomized, blinded, placebo-controlled trials conducted under racing conditions in large numbers of horses that furosemide is effective in reducing the incidence and severity of EIPH.[4,42] Recently, a systematic review and meta-analysis of 11 studies evaluating efficacy of furosemide for EIPH in 5653 horses unequivocally demonstrated a positive effect of furosemide to reduce EIPH in Thoroughbred and Standardbred racehorses.[43] There is currently insufficient information to determine the optimal dosage and timing of administration of furosemide before exercise.[43] Additionally, combinations of furosemide with other medications, such as clenbuterol, carbazachrome, or nasal strips, have not been found to be any more effective than furosemide administered alone.[44–46]

Medications used to treat pulmonary arterial hypertension in humans have also been evaluated to treat EIPH in experimental studies in small numbers of horses exercising on a treadmill. These studies characteristically have low statistical power and, being conducted on a treadmill, have unknown relevance to actual racing conditions. Low statistical power is a critical deficiency because it means that failure to detect an effect is not the same as demonstration of no effect. Studies with low power provide little information of drug efficacy unless included in a large meta-analysis.[47]

Vasodilators investigated to date include phosphodiesterase inhibitors (sildenafil, E4021), angiotensin-converting enzyme inhibitors (enalapril), α_2-adrenergic agonists (clonidine, guanabenz), and nitric oxide analogues (nitroglycerin, L-NAME, inhaled nitric oxide).[48–51] EIPH in horses does not mimic pulmonary hypertension in humans in that horses do not suffer from pathologically elevated pulmonary vascular pressures at rest. None of these medications have convincingly demonstrated a significant reduction in pulmonary artery pressure or a reduction in EIPH when evaluated in horses exercising on a treadmill. Although it is possible that these medications could be effective for EIPH, studies examining their effectiveness have suffered from low statistical power to detect an effect. Currently, there is no evidence of efficacy of these medications for EIPH and the level of evidence for their use is low.

Pentoxifylline, another nonselective phosphodiesterase inhibitor, has also been used for its hemorrheologic properties to increase RBC deformability and decrease blood viscosity. This medication was not found to affect the pulmonary capillary pressure of exercising horses and did not affect the prevalence of EIPH in one small experimental study.[52] Aminocaproic acid (ACA) is a potent inhibitor of fibrin degradation, and has been used to hypothetically reduce EIPH severity by preventing clot degradation. Although exercise induces changes in blood coagulation and fibrinolysis, multiple studies have found that horses with EIPH do not have defects in coagulation or increased fibrinolysis.[53] Moreover, breaks in capillary endothelium rapidly seal following reduction of pulmonary vascular pressures.[10] Several studies, using small numbers of horses (N = 6–8), have found no effect of ACA 2, 5, or 7 g administered intravenously 4 hours before exercise to alter EIPH in horses exercising on a treadmill.[54–56] Likewise, conjugated estrogens (Premarin, 25 mg intravenously 2 hours before exercise) have not been found to alter EIPH severity.[56] There is no evidence that ACA or conjugated estrogens, by inhibiting fibrinolysis or via any other purported anti-inflammatory effects, alter the frequency of detection or severity of EIPH in racehorses. Given that horses with EIPH do not have prolonged coagulation times, use of vitamin K for bleeding is not expected to be effective. Likewise, there is no evidence of efficacy of aspirin, hesperidin or citrus bioflavinoids (28 g orally for 90 days), vitamin C, or carbazochrome salicylate (100 mg intravenously before exercise) to prevent or reduce EIPH.[46,57]

External nasal dilator strips were developed to reduce collapse of the nasal passage, decrease upper airway resistance, and reduce changes in pleural pressures that contribute to high pulmonary transmural pressure. Although several studies using small numbers of horses (N = 6–23 horses) have demonstrated a statistically significant reduction in BAL RBC number, other studies have not identified any change in pulmonary gas exchange or endoscopically visible EIPH detected after exercise.[45,58–61] The clinical benefit of nasal dilators for EIPH has yet to be demonstrated in high-quality randomized controlled field trials.

Airway obstruction, either intrathoracic or extrathoracic, increases airway resistance and results in more negative intrathoracic (pleural) pressure during inspiration to maintain tidal volume and alveolar ventilation.[17] It is intuitive that conditions causing partial inspiratory obstruction (eg, left laryngeal hemiplegia) might exacerbate EIPH; however, potential associations between upper airway obstruction and EIPH or epistaxis largely have not been investigated. A single study of limited numbers of racehorses in Hong Kong found the occurrence of epistaxis in horses with left laryngeal hemiplegia was no different to matched cohorts before surgery, but after surgery horses were more likely to experience epistaxis.[40]

There is a widely held belief among clinicians treating EIPH in racehorses that inflammatory conditions of the lower airways contribute to development or perpetuation of bleeding. Consequently, many racehorses are treated with medications intended to decrease airway inflammation and relieve bronchoconstriction. Few studies have thoroughly and systematically evaluated this association, and no studies have evaluated the potential benefit of using inhaled, parenteral, or enteral corticosteroids on occurrence of EIPH. Low-allergenic bedding (shredded paper) used to prevent EIPH has no apparent effect on the prevalence of the condition.[62] Concentrated equine serum reportedly decreased BAL RBC numbers in a single study sponsored by the pharmaceutical company and using a small number of horses running on a treadmill.[63] The clinical importance of a decrease in BAL RBC number is unknown, and further studies in large numbers of horses exercising under racing conditions have not been published supporting the initial positive findings of the preliminary trials. No studies have investigated the impact of rest on EIPH occurrence, but rest is one treatment that likely prevents further bleeding and the subsequent development of interstitial inflammation, hemosiderin accumulation, fibrosis, and bronchial angiogenesis.

IS EXERCISE-INDUCED PULMONARY HEMORRHAGE A PROGRESSIVE DISEASE?

There is evidence that EIPH is a progressive disease. Horses without EIPH that have not raced or exercised strenuously do not show the typical gross postmortem and histologic lesions characteristic of horses with moderate to severe EIPH. Typical histopathologic lesions identified in horses with moderate to severe EIPH include bronchiolitis, bronchial angiogenesis, veno-occlusive remodeling, and fibrosis.[64] EIPH is often identified on postmortem evaluations of horses that die suddenly during racing,[65] and it has been suggested that some cases of race-associated sudden death are fulminant cases of EIPH.[66]

SUMMARY

EIPH is a disease that affects horses performing high-intensity exercise. The proximate cause of EIPH is pulmonary capillary stress failure. The pathophysiologic basis of the disease involves very high exercising pulmonary capillary pressures and very low pleural pressures created during exercise. An early and important pathologic lesion is veno-occlusive remodeling; however, whether this finding is cause or consequence of EIPH is not yet known. Moderate to severe EIPH is associated with inferior performance during a single race and there is evidence that severe EIPH and epistaxis are associated with shorter career duration. There is high-quality evidence that furosemide is effective for reducing the severity of EIPH. Currently, there is moderate-quality evidence that EIPH is a progressive disease.

REFERENCES

1. Pascoe J, Ferraro GL, Cannon JH, et al. Exercise-induced pulmonary haemorrhage in racing Thoroughbreds: a preliminary study. Am J Vet Res 1981;42:703–6.
2. Raphel CF, Soma LR. Exercise induced pulmonary haemorrhage in Thoroughbreds after racing and breezing. Am J Vet Res 1982;43:1123–7.
3. Hinchcliff KW, Jackson MA, Morley PS, et al. Association between exercise-induced pulmonary haemorrahge and performance in Thoroughbred racehorses. J Am Vet Med Assoc 2005;227:768–74.
4. Hinchcliff KW, Morley PS, Guthrie AJ. Efficacy of furosemide for prevention of exercise-induced pulmonary haemorrhage in Thoroughbred racehorses. J Am Vet Med Assoc 2009;235:76–82.
5. Sweeney CR, Soma LR, Maxson AD, et al. Effects of furosemide on the racing times of thoroughbreds. Am J Vet Res 1990;51:772–8.
6. Moran G, Carrillo R, Campos B, et al. Evaluación endoscópica de hemorragia pulmonar inducida por el ejercicio en equinos de polo. Archivos de Medicina Veterinaria 2003;35:109–13.
7. Voynick BT, Sweeney CR. Exercise induced pulmonary hemorrhage in polo and racing horses. J Am Vet Med Assoc 1986;188:301–2.
8. McKane SA, Canfield PJ, Rose RJ. Equine bronchoalveolar lavage cytology: survey of Thoroughbred racehorses in training. Aust Vet J 1993;70:401–4.
9. Fraipont A, Van Erck E, Ramery E, et al. Subclinical diseases underlying poor performance in endurance horses: diagnostic methods and predictive tests. Vet Rec 2011;169:154.
10. West JB, Mathieu-Costello O, Jones JH, et al. Stress failure of pulmonary capillaries in racehorses with exercise-induced pulmonary haemorrhage. Equine Vet J 1993;26:441–7.
11. Manohar M, Hutchens E, Coney E. Pulmonary haemodynamics in the exercising horse and their relationship to exercise-induced pulmonary haemorrhage. Br Vet J 1993;149:419–28.
12. Manohar M, Goetz TE. Pulmonary vascular pressures of exercising Thoroughbred horses with and without endoscopic evidence of EIPH. J Appl Physiol 1996;81:1589–93.
13. Manohar M, Goetz TE. Pulmonary vascular resistance of horses decreases with moderate exercise and remains unchanged as workload is increased to maximal exercise. FASEB J 1999;13:A1112.
14. Birks EK, Mathieu-Costello O, Fu Z, et al. Very high pressures are required to cause stress failure of pulmonary capillaries in Thoroughbred racehorses. J Appl Physiol 1997;82:1584–92.

15. Erickson HH, Bernard SL, Glenny RW, et al. Effect of furosemide on pulmonary blood flow distribution in resting and exercising horses. J Appl Physiol 1999; 86:2034–43.
16. Jones JH, Cox KS, Takahashi T, et al. Heterogeneity of intrapleural pressures during exercise. Equine Vet J 2002;34:391–6.
17. Ducharme NG, Hackett RP, Gleed RD, et al. Pulmonary capillary pressure in horses undergoing alteration of pleural pressure by imposition of various upper airway resistive loads. Equine Vet J 1999;31:27–33.
18. Derksen FJ, Williams KJ, Pannirselvam RR, et al. Regional distribution of collagen and haemosiderin in the lungs of horses with exercise-induced pulmonary haemorrhage. Equine Vet J 2009;41:586–91.
19. Williams KJ, Derksen FJ, de Feijter-Rupp H, et al. Regional pulmonary veno-occlusion: a newly identified lesion of equine exercise-induced pulmonary hemorrhage. Vet Pathol 2008;45:316–26.
20. Stack A, Derksen FJ, Williams KJ, et al. Lung region and racing affect mechanical properties of equine pulmonary microvasculature. J Appl Physiol 2014;117: 370–6.
21. Stack A, Derksen FJ, Sordillo LM, et al. Effects of exercise on markers of venous remodeling in lungs of horses. Am J Vet Res 2013;74:1231–8.
22. Newton JR, Wood JL. Evidence of an association between inflammatory airway disease and EIPH in young Thoroughbreds during training. Equine Vet J Suppl 2002;(34):417–24.
23. Michelotto PV, Muehlmann LA, Zanatta AL, et al. Pulmonary inflammation due to exercise-induced pulmonary haemorrhage in Thoroughbred colts during race training. Vet J 2011;190:e3–6.
24. McKane SA. Experimental mild pulmonary inflammation promotes the development of exercise-induced pulmonary haemorrhage. Equine Vet J 2010;42:235.
25. Derksen FJ, Williams KJ, Uhal BD, et al. Pulmonary response to airway instillation of autologous blood in horses. Equine Vet J 2007;39:334.
26. Velie BD, Raadsma HW, Wade CM, et al. Heritability of epistaxis in the Australian Thoroughbred racehorse population. Vet J 2014;202(2):274–8.
27. Weideman H, Schoeman SJ, Jordaan GF, et al. Epistaxis related to exercise induced pulmonary haemorrhage in South African Thoroughbreds. J S Afr Vet Assoc 2003;74:127–31.
28. Welsh CE. Heritability of musculoskeletal conditions and exercise induced pulmonary haemorrhage in Thoroughbred racehorses. University of Glasgow. 2014.
29. Preston SA, Riggs CM, Singleton MD, et al. Descriptive analysis of longitudinal endoscopy for exercise induced pulmonary haemorrhage in Thoroughbred racehorses training and racing at the Hong Kong Jockey Club. Equine Vet J 2014. http://dx.doi.org/10.1111/evj.12326.
30. Cook WR. Epistaxis in the racehorse. Equine Vet J 1974;6:45–58.
31. Takahashi T, Hiraga A, Ohmura H, et al. Frequency of and risk factors for epistaxis associated with exercise-induced pulmonary haemorrhage in horses: 251,609 race starts (1992-1997). J Am Vet Med Assoc 2001;218:1462–4.
32. Newton JR, Rogers K, Marlin DJ, et al. Risk factors for epistaxis on British racecourses: evidence for locomotory impact-induced trauma contributing to the aetiology of exercise-induced pulmonary haemorrhage. Equine Vet J 2005;37:402–11.
33. Hinchcliff KW, Morley PS, Jackson MA, et al. Risk factors for exercise-induced pulmonary haemorrhage in Thoroughbred racehorses. Equine Vet J 2010;42: 228–34.

34. Lapointe JM, Vrins A, McCarvill E. A survey of exercise-induced pulmonary hae-morrhage in Quebec Standardbred racehorses. Equine Vet J 1994;26:482–5.
35. Costa MF, Thoassian A. Evaluation of race distance, track surface and season of the year on exercise-induced pulmonary haemorrhage in flat racing thorough-breds in Brazil. Equine Vet J Suppl 2006;(36):487–9.
36. Birks EK, Shuler KM, Soma LR, et al. EIPH: postrace endoscopic evaluation of Standardbreds and Thoroughbreds. Equine Vet J 2002;34:375–8.
37. Morley PS, Bromberek JL, Saulez MN, et al. Exercise-induced pulmonary hae-morrhage impairs racing performance in Thoroughbred racehorses. Equine Vet J 2014. http://dx.doi.org/10.1111/evj.12368.
38. Sullivan SL, Anderson GA, Morley PS, et al. Prospective study of the association between exercise induced pulmonary haemorrhage and long term performance in Thoroughbred racehorses. Equine Vet J 2014. http://dx.doi.org/10.1111/evj.12263.
39. Thomas AD, Green MJ, Morris T, et al. Prevalence, recurrence, risk factors and effect on performance of epistaxis in racing Thoroughbreds in the UK. 914, 849. (2001–2010).
40. Mason BJ, Riggs CM, Cogger N. Cohort study examining long-term respiratory health, career duration and racing performance in racehorses that undergo left-sided prosthetic laryngoplasty and ventriculocordectomy surgery for treat-ment of left-sided laryngeal hemiplegia. Equine Vet J 2013;45:229–34.
41. Manohar M, Goetz TE, Sullivan E, et al. Pulmonary vascular pressures of strenu-ously exercising Thoroughbreds after administration of varying doses of fruse-mide. Equine Vet J 1997;29:298–304.
42. Pascoe J, Macabe A, Franti C, et al. Efficacy of furosemide in the treatment of exercise-induced pulmonary haemorrhage in Thoroughbred racehorses. Am J Vet Res 1985;46:2000–3.
43. Sullivan SL, Whittem T, Morley PS, et al. A systematic review and meta-analysis of furosemide for exercise induced pulmonary haemorrhage in Thoroughbred and Standardbred racehorses. Equine Vet J 2014. http://dx.doi.org/10.1111/evj.12373.
44. Manohar M, Goetz TE, Rothenbaum P, et al. Clenbuterol administration does not enhance the efficacy of furosemide in attenuating the exercise-induced pulmo-nary capillary hypertension in Thoroughbred horses. J Vet Pharmacol Ther 2000;23:389–95.
45. Kindig CA, McDonough P, Fenton G, et al. Efficacy of nasal strip and furosemide in mitigating EIPH in Thoroughbred horses. J Appl Physiol 2001;91:1396–400.
46. Perez-Moreno CI, Couetil LL, Pratt SM, et al. Effect of furosemide and furosemide-carbazochrome combination on exercise-induced pulmonary haemorrhage in Standardbred racehorses. Can Vet J 2009;50:821–7.
47. Hinchcliff KW, Couetil LL, Knight PK, et al. Exercise induced pulmonary hemor-rhage in horses: ACVIM Consensus Statement (Draft). 2014. Available at: http://www.acvim.org/Portals/0/PDF/ACVIM%20Consensus%20statement%20EIPH%20draft%20for%20comment.pdf. Accessed November 21, 2014.
48. Colahan PT, Jackson CA, Rice B, et al. The effect of sildenafil citrate administra-tion on selected physiological parameters of exercising Thoroughbred horses. Equine Vet J 2010;42:606–12.
49. Kindig CA, McDonough P, Finley MR, et al. NO inhalation reduces pulmonary arte-rial pressure but not hemorrhage in maximally exercising horses. J Appl Physiol 2001;91:2674–8.
50. Durando M, Perry B, Murray B, et al. Effect of a lung-directed type v phosphodi-esterase inhibitor and nitric oxide on exercise-induced pulmonary hemorrhage in thoroughbred racehorses. J Vet Intern Med 2004;18:375–460.

51. Durando MM, Hyman SS, Birks EK. Effects of e4021 and nitric oxide, alone and in combination with furosemide, on exercise-induced pulmonary hemorrhage in maximally exercising horses. J Vet Intern Med 2003;17:369–460.
52. Manohar M, Goetz TE, Rothenbaum P, et al. Intravenous pentoxifylline does not enhance the pulmonary haemodynamic efficacy of frusemide in strenuously exercising Thoroughbred horses. Equine Vet J 2001;33:354–9.
53. Giordano A, Meazza C, Salvadori M, et al. Thromboelastometric profiles of horses affected by exercise-induced pulmonary hemorrhages. Vet Med Int 2010.
54. Buchholz BM, Murdock A, Bayly WM, et al. Effects of intravenous aminocaproic acid on exercise-induced pulmonary haemorrhage (EIPH). Equine Vet J 2010; 42:256–60.
55. Durando MM, Birks EK. Effect of aminocaproic acid on the severity of exercise-induced pulmonary hemorrhage. J Vet Int Med 2008;22:823–4.
56. Epp TS, Edwards KL, Poole DC, et al. Effects of conjugated oestrogens and aminocaproic acid upon exercise-induced pulmonary haemorrhage (EIPH). Equine Comp Exerc Physiol 2008;5:95–103.
57. Sweeney CR, Soma LR. Exercise-induced pulmonary hemorrhage in Thoroughbred horses: response to furosemide or hesperidin-citrus bioflavinoids. J Am Vet Med Assoc 1984;185:195–7.
58. McDonough P, Kindig CA, Hildreth TS, et al. Effect of furosemide and the equine nasal stripon exercise-induced pulmonary haemorrhage and time-to-fatigue in maximally exercising horses. Equine Comp Exerc Physiol 2004;1:177–84.
59. Lester G, Clark C, Rice B, et al. Effect of timing and route of administration of furosemide on pulmonary hemorrhage and pulmonary arterial pressure in exercising Thoroughbred racehorses. Am J Vet Res 1999;60:22–8.
60. Valdez SC, Nieto JE, Spier SJ, et al. Effect of an external nasal dilator strip on cytologic characteristics of bronchoalveolar lavage fluid in Thoroughbred racehorses. J Am Vet Med Assoc 2004;224:558–61.
61. Geor RJ, Ommundson G, Fenton G, et al. Effects of an external nasal strip and frusemide on pulmonary haemorrhage in Thoroughbreds following high intensity exercise. Equine Vet J 2001;33:577–84.
62. Mason D, Collins E, Watkins K. Effect of bedding on the incidence of exercise induced pulmonary haemorrhage in racehorses in Hong Kong. Vet Rec 1984; 115:268–9.
63. Epp TS, McDonough P, Myers DE, et al. The effectiveness of immunotherapy in treating exercise-induced pulmonary hemorrhage. J Equine Vet Sci 2009;29: 527–32.
64. O'Callaghan MW, Pascoe JR, Tyler WS, et al. Exercise-induced pulmonary haemorrhage in the horse: results of a detailed clinical, post mortem and imaging study. II. Gross lung pathology. Equine Vet J 1987;19:389–93.
65. Lyle CH, Uzal FA, McGorum BC, et al. Sudden death in racing Thoroughbred horses: an international multicentre study of post mortem findings. Equine Vet J 2011;43:324–31.
66. Gunson DE, Sweeney CR, Soma LR. Sudden death attributable to exercise induced pulmonary haemorrhage in racehorses: 9 cases (1981-1983). J Am Vet Med Assoc 1988;193:102–6.

Thoracic Trauma in Horses

Kim A. Sprayberry, DVM[a],*, Elizabeth J. Barrett, DVM, MS[b]

KEYWORDS

- Traumatic injury • Pleural physiology • Thoracic • Lacerations • Sharp trauma
- Blunt trauma • Pneumothorax • Rib fractures • Flail chest

KEY POINTS

- Traumatic injuries involving the thorax can be superficial, necessitating only routine wound care, or they may extend to deeper tissue planes and disrupt structures immediately vital to respiratory and cardiac function.
- Diagnostic imaging should be considered part of a comprehensive examination at admission and is indicated for follow-up monitoring for later-onset complications, such as hemothorax and pneumothorax.
- Entry of gas into the pleural cavity obliterates the subatmospheric pressure state and creates pneumothorax and lung collapse.
- Rib fractures and pulmonary and cardiac contusion are sequelae of blunt trauma.
- Wounds in any area of the thorax that could allow introduction of air into the pleural cavity must be assessed for that potentiality in addition to the routine concerns that are germane to assessment of any wound.
- Horses generally respond well to diligent monitoring, intervention for complications, and appropriate medical or surgical care after sustaining traumatic wounds of the thorax.

REVIEW OF THORACIC FUNCTION IN NORMAL BREATHING

Normal breathing necessitates proper functioning of the brainstem respiratory centers, central and peripheral chemoreceptors, stretch receptors in the lung, the phrenic nerve arising from the C5–C7 spinal cord segments,[1] neuromuscular junctions with the diaphragm and intercostal muscles, and a competent thoracic wall. Inhalation ensues when contraction of the diaphragm and external intercostal muscles expand the dimensions of the thorax, creating subatmospheric pressure in the lower airways and alveoli and inducing passive flow of air from the atmosphere into the lungs. During inspiration at rest, the negative pressure developed in the alveoli is only approximately

[a] Animal Science Department, Cal Poly University San Luis Obispo, 1 Grand Ave, San Luis Obispo, CA 93407, USA; [b] Hagyard Equine Medical Institute, 4250 Ironworks Pike, Lexington, KY 40511, USA
* Corresponding author.
E-mail address: kspraybe@calpoly.edu

Vet Clin Equine 31 (2015) 199–219
http://dx.doi.org/10.1016/j.cveq.2014.12.001
0749-0739/15/$ – see front matter © 2015 Elsevier Inc. All rights reserved.

1 mm Hg lower than atmospheric pressure, but this modest gradient effectively draws air through the nasal passages and conducting airways down into the alveoli.[2] Expiration is passive, resulting from air flowing back out of the lungs as the lung recoils back to original dimensions. When all components function normally, the thorax and lungs cycle rhythmically and efficiently through expansion and recoil phases, air flows into and out of the alveoli, and gas exchange takes place across the interface between pulmonary capillaries and alveoli.

The thorax is a complex body cavity, conformed to maximize breathing efficiency. The lungs lie inside the pleural cavity, a closed, membrane-bound space lying inside the larger thoracic cavity. In the pleural cavity, pressure is always approximately 4 mm Hg lower (ie, more negative) than the alveolar pressure.[2] This "negative-pressure" state is maintained independently from the subatmospheric alveolar pressures created by thoracic expansion during inspiration. The vacuum in the closed pleural space causes the lungs to remain in a state of partial expansion and fill the larger thoracic cavity during all phases of the breathing cycle, including expiration. The negative pressure or vacuum is maintained by the inherent tendencies of the thoracic wall and lungs to recoil away from each other: the elastic recoil properties of lung tissue make it tend to deflate and contract away from the inner aspect of the thoracic wall, while the elastic recoil tendencies of the thoracic wall compel it to spring outward and away from the lungs. The balance of the outward pull of the thoracic wall and the inward pull of the lungs creates a vacuum of approximately -4 mm Hg, which is maintained as a constant because the pleural space is closed and has no communication with the alveoli or atmosphere. This vacuum keeps the transmural pressure across the lungs positive and prevents them from completely collapsing, even during forced expiration. During forced expirations such as coughing, sneezing, or exertional breathing, contraction of the abdominal and internal intercostal muscles actually creates intervals of positive pressure in the pleural cavity, but the pressure is still the same 4 mm Hg lower than alveolar pressure at any given moment.

Counteracting the tendency of the chest wall and lungs to recoil away from each other is the cohesive effect of the small volume of serous fluid in the pleural cavity. The intermolecular attraction of water molecules in this fluid holds the visceral and parietal pleural surfaces together, so that despite their tendency to move away from the chest wall, the lungs are mechanically coupled to and follow the chest wall excursions. Because the lung and chest wall are thus held in contact, the pleural cavity should be understood to be a potential space rather than an actual cavity, in health.

The pleural cavity is separated into right and left cavities by the mediastinum, a septum composed of adipose and other loose connective tissue. Within the mediastinum lie the heart, great vessels, nerves, and segments of the trachea and esophagus. The mediastinum is said to be incomplete or open in horses because of communicating fenestrations in the parietal pleura, especially that covering the caudal and ventral portions of the mediastinum.[3] These small stomata create a functional communication between the 2 pleural cavities and enable a penetrating wound on one side of the chest to cause bilateral pneumothorax. Chronic inflammation in the pleural cavity, as with pleuropneumonia, causes the pores to become sealed with fibrin and fluid, lessening the likelihood that pneumothorax and lung collapse will ensue in the contralateral hemithorax when a transthoracic drain is placed.

Traumatic injuries of the thorax can affect soft tissue or bone (ie, the ribs, sternum, shoulder, or proximal forelimb bones), and often involve both. They have the potential to disrupt respiratory function by directly injuring respiratory structures, introducing infection, or disrupting the physiologic vacuum state found in the pleural cavity. In addition to infection and pain, potential problems with any wounds, loss of integrity in the thorax can lead to immediate pulmonary and cardiac impairment. This article reviews the various types of thoracic injury and their management.

INITIAL EVALUATION OF THE HORSE WITH KNOWN OR POSSIBLE THORACIC INJURY

As with many types of evaluations, physical examination of a horse in which a traumatic event was observed or suspected should begin with a visual assessment of the animal from across the stall if the situation permits. This enables the examiner to obtain a global perspective of the horse's demeanor, posture, and respiratory pattern. If it can be done safely, it is often informative to observe the horse breathing from a dorsal perspective; climbing onto a hay bale or some stable surface and observing the motion of both lateral thoracic walls simultaneously from a dorsal view may reveal asymmetry, local bony deformation, focal concavity, splinting, paradoxic chest wall motion, or a differing range of excursion between the 2 sides during breathing. The examiner also should carefully (digitally) examine the thoracic planes for early development of subcutaneous emphysema and for crepitus. In foals, detection of the edema that forms around rib fractures is facilitated by wetting the foal's hair with warm water or alcohol.

Initial assessment of deep wounds is indicated and may prompt measures to occlude a full-thickness perforation of the chest wall before the remainder of the physical examination is completed. Wounds that perforate the chest wall should be made airtight by covering with a self-adherent occlusive barrier (eg, Ioban [Ioban incise drape; 3M, Minneapolis, MN], V.A.C. drape [KCI Animal Health, San Antonio, TX]) or kitchen plastic wrap, suturing, or packing with sterile bandaging materials.[4] Once entry of air into the pleural cavity has been ceased, a more careful and thorough evaluation of the wound or wounds can be undertaken. A horse that has any combination of tachypnea, dyspnea, nostril flaring, restlessness, or discolored (cyanotic) mucous membranes in this setting should be suspected of having pneumothorax, and intervention for this (described in a later section) should take precedence over methodical completion of the examination.

Not only should the heart rate and respiratory rate be determined, but also, importantly, the character of the sounds should be assessed and recorded. Dullness or absence of lung sounds ventrally should point the examiner to check for hemothorax or pleural effusion, whereas dullness or absence of sounds dorsally (in a standing animal) may indicate pneumothorax. Making a note of the cardiac rhythm and clarity of sounds at initial evaluation and during follow-up examinations enables later-onset changes to be detected promptly. Life-threatening hemopericardium, hemothorax, or pneumothorax can develop gradually in the hours to days after injury.

Initial laboratory work depends on the horse's cardiopulmonary status. For horses with acute thoracic trauma that have signs of distress or shock, a minimum database of complete blood count, total protein concentration, arterial blood gas analysis, and lactate concentration is indicated. Part or all of this testing may need to be run serially to assess response to interventions. A horse being evaluated for chronic draining tract or pleuropneumonia from a previous thoracic injury likely would not need laboratory work to assess hemodynamic stability, but would warrant running a hemogram, fibrinogen, and microbial culture.

One of the most important components of the examination is diagnostic imaging. Both radiographic and sonographic imaging are important, but in the emergent situation, ultrasound has the advantage as a rapid, point-of-care, first-line imaging modality. This is because sonography so sensitively detects fluid accumulations, which usually indicates a site of hemorrhage in a trauma patient. Ultrasound enables determination of the magnitude and laterality of both bony and soft-tissue lesions in real time. With sonographic imaging, the concerns of beam centering, phase of respiration, and overexposure or underexposure are moot, and the sensitivity of imaging is not diminished in the ventral thoracic fields because of overlying musculature and small lung volume. An abbreviated imaging examination technique called focused assessment with sonography for trauma (FAST) is a standardized 4-point imaging protocol for detection of fluid accumulation in body cavities that can be performed quickly, on the order of several minutes. Protocols and views have been modified and standardized by body cavity, and the diagnostic expediency in critically injured patients afforded by FAST techniques has gained a great deal of attention in small animal and human emergency medicine.[5,6] A modification of FAST used for thoracic imaging (TFAST in veterinary medicine; EFAST for extended FAST in human medicine) allows the examiner to quickly detect or rule out pneumothorax and accumulation of pericardial or pleural fluid as manifestations of thoracic injury. A similar protocol, fast local abdominal sonography in horses (FLASH), has gained attention in emergency evaluation of horses with colic.[7] Multiple studies in human emergency medicine show bedside ultrasound to be at least equivalent to and often better than chest radiography at revealing pneumothorax or hemothorax in trauma patients.[8–10] Curvilinear ultrasound transducers operating in the range of 2.5 to 5.0 MHz are most suitable for thoracic imaging in the horse. Linear transducers used for reproductive work also can be used; images yielded by linear probes are higher in resolution and detail, but have low penetrance and more skill with sonography may be needed to interpret the rectangular images. Curvilinear transducers are needed for imaging obese horses.

In general, radiography for evaluation of thoracic disease is more useful in small animals and foals than in adult horses. In smaller animals, it is useful in detecting fractures, lung changes, and cardiac changes. In a recent report, radiography was used to diagnose and monitor osteomyelitis, with and without underlying fracture, at the rib costochondral junctions in 3 septic foals.[11] Pneumomediastinum is an example of a soft-tissue change that can be seen only radiographically[12] and that evades sonographic detection because of its midsagittal location, deep to aerated lung. For similar reasons, radiography must be used to image any horses with subcutaneous emphysema over the thorax. Radiography and contrast fistulography can be necessary for locating radiolucent foreign bodies, such as wood fragments in deep tissue planes in or around the thorax.

Thoracoscopy is an adjunctive imaging technique useful in evaluation of some cases of thoracic trauma (**Fig. 1**). Endoscopic imaging in the chest can be used as a diagnostic tool to locate foreign bodies or as a therapeutic aid to determine the best site for thoracotomy or placement of a chest drain. The procedure can be performed in standing sedated or recumbent anesthetized horses. During thoracoscopy, a state of pneumothorax and lung collapse is induced on the operated side, enabling better viewing of and access to thoracic structures. Whether the horse is standing or under general anesthesia, serial arterial blood gas evaluation is indicated, and equipment and supplies needed for prompt intervention for hypoxemia should be positioned in easy reach (eg, equipment for supplementation of oxygen by nasal insufflation, equipment for positive pressure ventilation, and instruments needed for quick cessation of the procedure). Thoracoscopic techniques have been described elsewhere.[13,14] In brief, for standing procedures, the horse should be restrained in stocks. Detomidine infusion (0.8 μg/kg/min; or, for a 450-kg horse, 12 mg detomidine in 250 mL of 0.9% saline given at 2 drops per second with a 150-drop/mL drip set, or to effect) induces satisfactory sedation and analgesia when combined with local anesthesia for standing procedures.[15] Local anesthesia can be delivered directly at the site

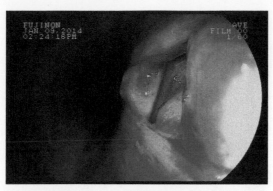

Fig. 1. Thoracoscopic photograph of the site of chest wall perforation in a horse with penetrating thoracic trauma. (*Courtesy of* Dr. Amelia Munsterman.)

of trocar placement or by means of regional anesthesia of the intercostal nerves. For procedures to be performed under general anesthesia, the horse is positioned in dorsal recumbency or in lateral recumbency with the affected lung up. Special consideration is given to adequacy of tissue oxygenation, and if needed, the dependent lung can be mechanically ventilated. For either technique, the initial telescope insertion site is placed dorsally, in intercostal space 10, 11, or 12, just ventral to the insertion of the epaxial muscles. A 1.5-cm–long incision is made through the skin and subcutaneous tissue, and a teat cannula is advanced through the incision and pleura, creating the pneumothorax. Additional trocar sites are determined with the telescope, depending on the purpose of the surgery and what needs to be inspected visually. Care should be taken to place the portals in the middle of the intercostal space to allow maximum mobility of the instruments. Closure of the skin after removal of the trocars is routine. A certain degree of discomfort will be seen when the pneumothorax is induced in a standing horse; if the horse becomes moderately or severely uncomfortable or dyspneic, the procedure should be stopped and the pneumothorax reversed.

A last but important aspect of evaluation concerns the wounded horse's abdomen. Although intra-abdominal tissue injuries are not unusual in horses with thoracic injury, they are usually less conspicuous during the initial evaluation and rush to stabilize the thoracic wounds. However, abdominal organ injury is a substantial cause of death in horses hospitalized for thoracic injuries,[16] and the abdomen also should be evaluated sonographically for areas of free fluid or other manifestations of hemorrhage or internal organ injury, as soon in the examination as possible. Fractures or trauma to the sixth rib, or any ribs caudal to it, should especially incite careful clinical and sonographic evaluation of abdominal organs.[17]

LACERATIONS AND SHARP OR PENETRATING TRAUMA

The most common cause of laceration or penetration of the thorax is collision with other objects.[16] Commonly reported causes include impalement on objects, such as fencing or stakes (wooden or metal), tree branches, or metal (such as parts of horse trailers in vehicle accidents); goring by horned animals; or injury by debris flying at high velocity in tornadoes or hurricanes (**Fig. 2**). Gunshot wounds also cause thoracic wall perforation, and will be considered separately. The most important sequelae of lacerations and penetrating trauma in the thoracic area are wound infection, subcutaneous

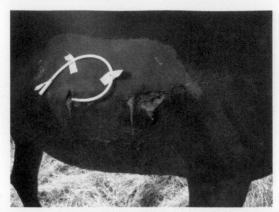

Fig. 2. Mare with entry and exit wounds from a tree branch impalement that tracked along the external aspect of the ribs but did not penetrate the pleural cavity. The wounds were assessed for depth, ultrasound was used to confirm that the pleural cavity was not penetrated, and a catheter was left indwelling to facilitate wound lavage and drainage.

emphysema, pneumothorax, foreign body embedment, chronic fistula from imbedded foreign body or osteomyelitis, and pleuritis or pleuropneumonia.

After careful cleansing and aseptic preparation, wounds should be explored carefully with a sterile probe to ascertain depth and extent. Any irrigation should be done under low pressure to avoid compacting fluids or infective material into the depths of a wound that does or may communicate with the pleural cavity. Debridement and surgical closure should be undertaken where appropriate, but areas in which extensive avulsion of skin or muscle has occurred or where there is heavy contamination must be left to heal by second intention or delayed primary closure. Negative-pressure wound therapy is well-reported in human medicine, although it is relatively new in equine medicine[18]; this approach to wound management may find particular application in management of thoracic wounds in horses. Tension sutures and drains should be placed where needed to support closure and primary healing. The horse should be given a broad-spectrum combination of antimicrobials that includes antianaerobe activity, a nonsteroidal anti-inflammatory medication and other analgesics for multimodal analgesia if needed, and tetanus prophylaxis should be boosted.

SUBCUTANEOUS EMPHYSEMA

Deep lacerations or puncture wounds in the axillary and pectoral regions can give rise to subcutaneous emphysema (**Fig. 3**). During movement, forelimb motion draws air into these wounds while they are agape, and muscle contractions push air from the wound cavity into the surrounding tissue planes. The volume of air entering the subcutaneous tissues in this manner can become substantial, and the resulting subcutaneous emphysema may become marked as air dissects along neurovascular bundles and muscle fascia, extending up into the shoulders, neck, throat, and head. In extreme cases, the volume of air accumulating around the larynx can endanger breathing to the extent of necessitating a tracheostomy. Performing the tracheostomy can be greatly complicated by severe emphysema, and placing a jugular intravenous catheter can likewise be rendered difficult to impossible. The stretched skin and crepitant underlying tissues can be very painful, and horses may become irritable or defensive to handling or touching of the affected areas.

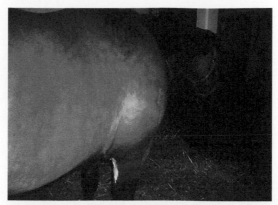

Fig. 3. Mare with severe subcutaneous emphysema over the neck, shoulders, and thorax from an innocuous appearing puncture wound in the right axilla (where white dressing has been applied).

After cleansing and exploration, the portions of the axillary or pectoral wound that cannot be sutured should be occluded with packing secured with tape wrapped around the horse's neck and shoulders or with a stent bandage. The horse's movement should be limited. The treatment goal is to prevent additional air from entering the wound while allowing time for the present emphysema to resolve. Most horses do not require further intervention for subcutaneous emphysema. Attention to digital pulse intensity and provision of supplemental sole support, if indicated, should be part of serial monitoring and care. Extensive subcutaneous emphysema can take several weeks to completely resolve once the entry wound has sealed.

PNEUMOTHORAX

Pneumothorax refers to air that has entered the pleural cavity, and is a serious complication of thoracic injury. With traumatic pneumothorax, air can enter the pleural space by means of penetrating wounds that perforate the thoracic wall, wounds that puncture or tear the lung, wounds that lead to subcutaneous emphysema and pneumomediastinum, esophageal rupture, and puncture or tearing of the trachea.[17] In other veterinary species and humans, iatrogenic pneumothorax has been reported secondary to thoracocentesis,[19] tube thoracostomy,[20] bronchoscopy,[21] diagnostic transtracheal aspiration, surgery of the respiratory tract,[17] mechanical ventilation,[22–24] orthopedic surgery of the vertebral column,[25] nasogastric intubation,[26,27] acupuncture,[28] needle myelography,[29] thoracoscopy,[30] and many other diagnostic and therapeutic scenarios.[23]

In horses, penetrating wounds can involve any part of the thoracic cage, including the axillary or pectoral regions. Although traumatic pneumothorax from pectoral injury is possible and does occur, injuries in the pectoral region less commonly extend to intrathoracic structures because of the abundant musculature covering this area, the parabolic shape of the anterior part of the thorax, and the narrow thoracic opening between the first ribs.[31] It is important to remember that when a long branch or stake enters one part of the chest and exits another, air can enter through either or both of the sites. The size and external appearance alone of a wound should not be used to determine depth of penetration or predict consequences (**Fig. 4**).[12]

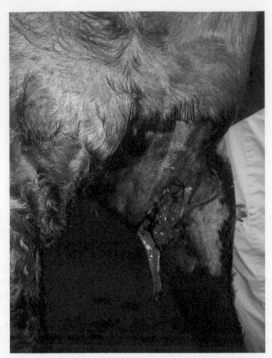

Fig. 4. Horse with a deep, penetrating laceration of the medial aspect of the cubital joint. Despite this wound's appearance as affecting chiefly the medial aspect of the forelimb, it should be assessed for extension into the anterior aspect of the left pleural cavity at the time of admission. This type of wound can be anticipated to lead to subcutaneous emphysema, and even after wound packing or closure, the horse should be monitored for later-onset pneumomediastinum and possibly pneumothorax. (*Courtesy of* Dr. Amelia Munsterman.)

Pneumothorax is classified as open or closed, and as traumatic, spontaneous, or iatrogenic. In large-animal medicine, it is most useful to designate a pneumothorax as open, meaning air has entered the cavity through a wound in the thoracic wall and there is a defect in the parietal pleura, or closed, meaning the chest wall is intact and air has entered from some part of the respiratory tract through a defect in the visceral or mediastinal pleura. With the latter, the air may be escaping from lung punctured by a broken rib, a tearing injury of the lower trachea, or extension of pneumomediastinum into the pleural cavity, to name a few examples.[32] A third type of pneumothorax, which can arise from either an open or closed pneumothorax, is referred to as tension pneumothorax. The term tension pneumothorax refers to progressive increase in gas tension (pressure) when a tear in either the parietal pleura or the visceral pleura acts as a ball-and-valve apparatus, drawing air into the pleural cavity with each inspiration but preventing outflow during expiration. Whereas pleural pressure in an open pneumothorax will reach and equilibrate with atmospheric pressure, the pressure in tension pneumothorax will eventually become supra-atmospheric. This type of pneumothorax has a more malignant clinical course, because the patient must contend with not only the loss of normal lung expansion and gas exchange that result from simple pneumothorax, but also with rapidly progressive cardiovascular compromise caused by increasingly positive pressure in the pleural cavity. As pleural pressure becomes progressively less negative and eventually positive, venous return decreases, along with cardiac output and mean systemic pressure, leading to tachycardia, hypoxemia, acidosis, and hypotension. Tension pneumothorax can be recognized by progressively increasing respiratory excursions, increasing respiratory effort, distress, hypoxemia, and hypotension.[4,24,33,34]

In humans, upright radiographic views of the thorax are used to determine the extent of pneumothorax.[35] A pneumothorax is considered to be small when the apex-to-cupola distance is less than 3 cm and large when the apex-to-cupola distance is greater than 3 cm (the cupola is the dome-shaped area at the superior extent of the chest wall).[36] Earlier reports determined that approximately 1.5% of the volume of a pneumothorax can be reabsorbed per 24-hour period,[37,38] suggesting that a pneumothorax in which free air occupied 20% of a pleural cavity would take approximately 16 days for complete resolution. Free pleural air is gradually reabsorbed into pulmonary lymphatics and capillaries.

In quadripedal animals, such as horses, quantifying a pneumothorax, radiographically or otherwise, has not been reported to the authors' knowledge, but standing lateral radiographs could be used to similar effect. Alternatively, sonographic detection of the "lung point" has long been used (if not reported) by equine veterinarians in critical care, and also is used by human emergency room physicians to grade a pneumothorax when ultrasound is used instead of radiography.[8,39] The lung point is the point along the chest wall at which the "glide sign" meets free gas in an animal with pneumothorax. Glide sign refers to the sliding of the visceral pleura along the parietal pleura as the lung expands and deflates during breathing. In a standing horse, with the ultrasound transducer being moved from dorsal to ventral in an intercostal space, the lung point is the point at which the static reverberation echo from the dorsal cap of free gas first meets sliding lung movement in the same frame. Marking this point along successive rib spaces enables the collapsed lung's dorsal extent to be determined and some estimation of severity to be made. The decision of whether to place a cannula or tube in the affected pleural cavity and remove the free air, however, is chiefly made on the basis of the animal's demeanor, mucous membrane color, heart and respiratory rates, arterial blood gas values, and pulse oximetry.

Horses admitted with tachypnea, dyspnea, tachycardia, altered mucous membrane color, or other vital sign abnormalities should be stabilized with a resuscitative fluid protocol and supplemental oxygen (initial flow rate, 15 L/min) while full examination is ongoing and while laboratory results are pending.

Management of open pneumothorax first demands occlusion of the wound and prevention of further entry of air into the pleural cavity. Wounds can be sutured, or occluded with packing or an airtight membrane. A muscle pedicle flap also has been used successfully to close a thoracic wound.[40] A horse with a simple open or closed pneumothorax that is mild or early may have no clinical signs and require only wound care, wound occlusion, and monitoring. A more moderate degree of pneumothorax leading to tachypnea and hypoxemia may necessitate reinflating the lung by reestablishing vacuum in the affected hemithorax. A 3 × 3-inch patch of hair is clipped in a dorsal aspect of the 11th through 15th intercostal space, the skin is aseptically prepared, and the thoracic wall is blocked down to parietal pleura with lidocaine or carbocaine.[4,41] With sterile technique, a stab incision is made through the skin, and a small-bore tube (a blunt-tipped teat cannula, 10-gauge to 14-gauge intravenous [IV] catheter, or 16-French or 24-French trocar catheter) is introduced into the skin incision and advanced into the pleural cavity. The catheter stylet or trocar is removed once the pleural cavity is accessed. Often a small popping sensation is appreciated as the instrument passes through the parietal pleura, and the horse may flinch. If a teat cannula (blunt-tipped) or IV catheter is used, air is removed by repeated aspiration with a stopcock and large syringe or by attaching a suction unit. If a trocar catheter is used, a catheter-tipped 35-mL or 60-mL syringe can be pushed into the flared end of the catheter and used to aspirate air, or a "Christmas tree" adapter can be used to attach the catheter to suction tubing. Reestablishment of vacuum in the pleural space and consequent reexpansion of the lung can be confirmed by placing an ultrasound transducer next to the catheter or cannula and observing the moving lung surface (the glide sign) reentering and filling the dorsal portion of the pleural cavity. The gliding lung also can be felt moving across the embedded portion of the cannula or catheter just before it is withdrawn. One or 2 simple interrupted skin sutures should be preplaced next to the cannula or catheter, and the device removed. In horses with uncomplicated open or closed pneumothorax, effective occlusion of the wound and 1-time removal of the free pleural gas may be sufficient to resolve the problem. In others, such as those with a tension pneumothorax, leaving an indwelling tube with attached Heimlich valve or other sterile 1-way device for continuous removal of pleural air is necessary until the internal site of air leakage has become sealed (**Fig. 5**).

Administration of 100% oxygen gas increases the rate of reabsorption of pleural air by inducing "nitrogen washout," or movement of N_2 in the pleural free air down its concentration gradient into the alveoli, where it is exhaled. The evidence for efficacy of this treatment is mixed, with positive results reported in some studies and no difference reported in others.[42–44] Without a horse being on a ventilator, it is impossible to attain an inspired oxygen fraction (Fio$_2$) of 100%, so this is not a feasible intervention for resolving pneumothorax in horses. However, the goal of administering oxygen via nasal insufflation to a horse with pneumothorax is simply to raise Fio$_2$ and saturate hemoglobin, which is accomplished with an arterial oxygen pressure (Pao$_2$) of 100 mm Hg and can be achieved in most adult horses with nasopharyngeal oxygen flows of 5 to 15 L per minute.[45] The Fio$_2$ achieved in horses with pulmonary injury from smoke inhalation in a structure fire could be expected to be less favorable.[46]

Horses with a chronic draining tract following previous thoracic injury have either a persisting foreign body fragment or a bone sequestrum. Debridement, exploration with a sterile probe, and imaging with a contrast fistulogram or thoracoscopy, may be needed to track the suppuration to its origin in these horses. Antimicrobial

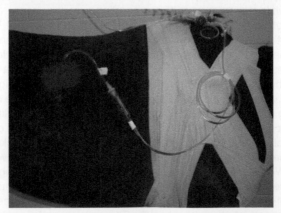

Fig. 5. Thoracostomy tube and Heimlich valve secured in place in the dorsal aspect of the right pleural cavity in a horse with tension pneumothorax. (*Courtesy of* Dr. Dwayne Rodgerson.)

administration can help reduce the volume of drainage from these wounds, but removal of the foreign body is necessary to permanently resolve the fistular drainage.

PLEUROPNEUMONIA

Extension of a laceration or sharp trauma across the thoracic wall tracks microbes and blood in the pleural cavity and can lead to pleuritis or pleuropneumonia. Careful debridement of the wound and ensuring that wound fluids and inflammatory debris have a route for egress to the outside of the chest wall is therefore an important aspect of wound care.[33] Placement of Penrose drains in the subcutaneous planes of the chest wall around the wound tract or use of negative-pressure wound management[18] may be helpful in facilitating this, along with effective infection control. An empirically selected broad-spectrum antimicrobial regimen that includes antianaerobe activity is often successful at limiting infection, but in instances in which persisting or recurrent pyrexia and inflammatory hemogram changes are found on serial monitoring, the chest should be sonographically imaged again. If pleuropneumonia is diagnosed, pleural fluid should be drained by placing a trocar catheter in the thoracic wall, and the fluid should undergo microbial culture and sensitivity testing. Pleuropneumonia was the leading nontraumatic cause of pneumothorax in one study,[17] and animals with pleuropneumonia-related pneumothorax may have a poorer prognosis for survival.[17,35]

GUNSHOT WOUNDS

Gunshot wounds in the thorax constitute a special classification of penetrating wound. Bullet contact with the heart is likely to be fatal, but otherwise, the initial evaluation and stabilization of a gunshot horse should proceed as described for other types of penetrating thoracic trauma. The horse should be examined for an exit wound, and both entry and exit wounds should be cleansed and occluded. The animal's respiratory and cardiac function should be assessed while bloodwork is pending, and findings of tachycardia or dyspnea would warrant including arterial blood gases and possibly lactate concentration and oximetry. Common complications are hemothorax and pneumothorax. Removal of bullets from other areas of the body is not always associated with improved outcomes in human medicine, and once complications, if any, have been addressed and the horse is stabilized, monitoring, provision of a broad-spectrum antimicrobial regimen, and pain control often yield a favorable outcome without surgical intervention to remove the bullet. Gunshot wounds in horses have been well described in this volume recently,[47] and the reader is referred to this and other sources[48–50] for further information.

BLUNT TRAUMA

Blunt trauma is characterized by tissue injury arising from transfer of energy across a body surface without disruption of the skin. The more dense the tissue, the more kinetic energy will be absorbed, making solid organs more susceptible to blunt trauma injury than hollow organs and filled hollow organs (such as intestines) more susceptible to injury than empty hollow organs. Horses sustain blunt trauma in falls; vehicular accidents; collision with buildings, trees, fencing, jumps, or other animals; and kicks, among other scenarios.

Considering the sequence of events of energy transfer in a trailer accident can help elucidate how forcible contact damages tissues. Vehicle accidents can be considered to cause 3 impacts.[51] First, the vehicle or trailer impacts another object as it comes to an abrupt halt in the crash; the kinetic energy is absorbed by the vehicle, and the metal is deformed. Second, the forward motion of the unrestrained animal's body, traveling at the same speed as the vehicle, is arrested as it impacts the framework of the trailer or pavement if it is ejected from the trailer; the kinetic energy is absorbed by the trailer and by the animal's body, deforming metal and body parts. The third impact is the animal's internal organs' collision against the body framework; the organs continue their forward motion until stopped by the surrounding anatomic structures, and tissue structure is deformed or altered. In the body, such rapid deceleration forces cause the brain to move forward against the skull, abdominal organs to collide with the abdominal walls and pelvis, and thoracic contents to collide against the chest wall. Thoracic organs also are compressed by the advancing diaphragm and weight of the viscera behind it. During the third impact, differential movement among adjacent structures leads to generation of shear forces, causing stretching and linear shearing between adjacent relatively fixed and free structures. An example of this type of injury is seen in aortic rupture associated with blunt thoracic trauma. The distal portion of the aorta is fixed to the thoracic portion of the spine and decelerates much more quickly than the mobile aortic arch; this may result in aortic disruption or rupture in the proximal portion of the descending aorta, a common blunt trauma injury in humans, along with tearing of the lower trachea by this same mechanism.[52] For this reason, in a horse that has sustained blunt thoracic trauma, detection of crepitus in the neck or chest area in the absence of external wounds should prompt endoscopic evaluation of the trachea to investigate for tearing or rupture from this mechanism.

Common sequelae of blunt thoracic trauma in humans include thoracic cage fractures, hemothorax, pneumothorax, lung contusions, myocardial contusion, diaphragm rupture, and aortic rupture.[53] Rib fractures are usually from birth injury in foals, but are a sequela of blunt trauma in the adult horse.[16,33] In foals, blunt thoracic injury can result from kicks, being stepped on by an adult horse, and collisions with structures or other animals. Treatment for blunt thoracic trauma varies with associated injuries and presence and degree of respiratory compromise. Pain control and serial imaging of the body cavity interiors over the ensuing 3 to 4 days after the injury are indicated to detect late-onset hemorrhage or other changes in the thoracic cavity.

Rib Fractures

Rib fractures can represent a particular challenge to manage because, aside from the ribs' role in ventilation being affected, the fractured bone ends can cause multiple associated soft-tissue complications that can be life-threatening. Most horses have 18 pairs of ribs, and fracture of one or even several on one side of the thorax does not appear to significantly impair ventilation, although they likely cause considerable discomfort. The fractured rib ends, on the other hand, can lacerate blood vessels in the thoracic wall and cause hemothorax, contuse lung, puncture lung and cause pneumothorax, lacerate the diaphragm, puncture the pericardium, contuse myocardium, and puncture myocardium. The more cranial ribs are more robust in constitution and protected by more overlying soft tissue, and considerable force is needed to cause fractures. Fractures in this area are a harbinger of substantial blunt force trauma to other organs, and can be expected to lacerate vasculature, tear intercostal muscles, and disrupt or lacerate diaphragmatic insertions.

The most common equine presentation for rib fractures is that of a neonatal foal, in which rib fractures are nearly always birth injuries.[54,55] Rib fractures can often be detected during physical examination in newborn foals, with a focus of swelling, tenderness to digital pressure, or crepitus appreciable overlying the injured structures. Foals sometimes grunt or groan when the injured ribs are palpated, and a clicking sensation may be felt in the fractured ribs as they lift and fall with the underlying lung excursions. Signs in adult horses with broken ribs are similar, with the fractures detected by focal swelling, tenderness, and crepitus, along with lethargy and lameness or altered gait in one or both forelimbs.[56] The fractures can best be investigated sonographically. Ultrasound imaging is considered an extension of the physical examination at the authors' practice. In either an adult horse or a foal being scanned for thoracic injury, the hair should be wetted with warm rubbing alcohol and the transducer (the authors prefer a 5-MHz microconvex probe or 7-MHz to 10-MHz linear probe) moved from dorsal to ventral in the relevant intercostal spaces. Sites of fracture can usually be found by finding sites of pulmonary contusion; once this echogenic lesion in the lung has been discovered, the transducer is moved from the intercostal space at that site onto the top of the rib, and the fracture, often with a surrounding hematoma, can usually be appreciated (**Fig. 6**). In addition to revealing the fracture, this imaging may additionally reveal hemothorax, pneumothorax, and, importantly, will enable assessment of the proximity between the fractured bone ends and the beating myocardium. The latter finding allows for surgical fixation to be scheduled promptly, after physiologic stabilization of the animal.

The goal of fluid administration in a horse or foal with hemothorax is to support systemic perfusion while tolerating some degree of hypotension. Intracavitary hemorrhage does not always necessitate blood transfusion: if hemorrhage is acute but ceases, the effects of hypovolemia (tachycardia, sweating, restlessness or agitation, hypotension) can be managed with crystalloids alone in most instances. Transfusion is indicated when augmentation of the hematocrit is needed to support global tissue oxygenation. Clinical indicators of insufficiency in the circulation's oxygen-carrying capacity are tachycardia, tachypnea, lethargy, altered mucous membrane color (pale to greyish or white), and hyperlactatemia that are sustained in the face of fluid support. Other values that point to decreased oxygen delivery in the context of hemorrhage are indicators of low mixed venous oxygen saturation or high extraction ratios. A difference of more than 30% between arterial and venous saturations or an oxygen extraction ratio higher than 40-50 are useful measures of estimates of tissue oxygen status. Sonographic detection of swirling movements in the extravasated blood in the body cavity confirms that active hemorrhage is ongoing, and this should also be factored into a decision to administer blood.[57] Blood lactate over 4 mmol/L, venous partial pressure of oxygen less than 30 mm Hg, venous hemoglobin saturation less than 50%, and oxygen extraction ratio over 40% are all useful indicators of insufficient tissue oxygenation in the context of acute loss of oxygen carrying capacity.

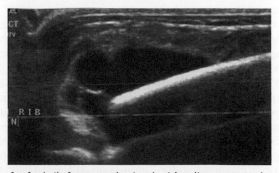

Fig. 6. Sonogram of a foal rib fracture obtained with a linear-array ultrasound transducer. Notice the hematoma that has developed and is organizing around the distracted rib end. The hematoma helps protect adjacent lung or myocardium from puncture. (*Courtesy of* Dr. Jami Whiting and Dubai Equine Hospital.)

Rib fractures in adult horses may occur as the result of open or closed chest trauma, such as falls, kicks, or automobile accidents. All rib fractures may have accompanying complications, such as pneumothorax or hemothorax. Diagnosis is made by physical examination, radiograph, and ultrasonography. Treatment includes pain control and management of the secondary complications, as detailed previously in this article. Fracture fixation in an adult horse is not always feasible, and is usually unnecessary with isolated or minimally displaced fractures.[33] Displaced fractures can be debrided or minimally resected to prevent further local trauma from rib edges. In horses in which the fractured ends are severely displaced or in which fractures have created flail chest, surgical repair techniques and anesthetic considerations similar to those described for foals may be warranted. The horse should be stabilized before surgical intervention, and careful attention should be paid to monitoring of oxygenation and ventilator adequacy while the horse is under anesthesia.[58] Reports of the anesthetic management of adult horses with rib fractures and traumatic pneumothorax or hemothorax detail these considerations.[56,59]

On the basis of retrospective studies, as many as 20% of foals can have some form of thoracic trauma during birth, including fractured ribs or costochondral dislocation.[55] The most common site of fracture is at the costochondral junction or immediately proximal to it. The percentage of foals admitted to referral centers that have fractured ribs (65%) is even higher.[54,55] Most foals have minimally displaced fractures that heal uneventfully and without intervention. However, as in adult horses, fractured ribs have the potential to lead to a number of potentially fatal complications. Hemothorax from ruptured thoracic vessels or cardiac puncture, pneumothorax, diaphragmatic rupture and herniation of viscera, and perforation of lung or the gastrointestinal tract can occur. Surgical repair is usually withheld unless there is potential for life-threatening complications. These risks are heightened where 2 or more ribs are fractured, the affected ribs are more cranial and overlie the heart (ribs 3–5), or a substantial degree of displacement and movement is seen with respiration.

Multiple techniques can successfully be used in surgical repair of fractured ribs in foals.[60–62] Thoracocentesis may be performed before surgery to reduce pneumothorax or address hemothorax. Foals with hemothorax may need to be hemodynamically stabilized before anesthesia with partial-volume resuscitative fluids and possibly fresh whole blood to replace circulatory volume and augment oxygen-carrying capacity. The severity of pain associated with rib fractures in humans, who can articulate their symptoms, is not trivial. Multimodal analgesic techniques are useful in adult horses and foals with rib fractures, and can begin before surgery with some combination of regional anesthesia of intercostal nerves, systemic nonsteroidal anti-inflammatory drugs, and opioids. A broad-spectrum regimen of antimicrobials should also be started, as the extravasated blood may serve as a medium for microbial colonization.

If sedation is necessary before anesthetic induction, a benzodiazepine derivative (diazepam, 0.1 mg/kg, IV; or midazolam, 0.1-0.2 mg/kg, IV) combined with butorphanol (0.05-0.1 mg/kg, intramuscularly or IV) can be used. Ketamine (1–2 mg/kg, IV) is a suitable induction drug, and isoflurane or sevoflurane are suitable for anesthetic maintenance. Positive pressure ventilation, with or without positive end expiratory pressure (PEEP), can be used for foals with persistent hypercapnia and hypoxemia. As a strategy for improving oxygenation while minimizing adverse hemodynamic effects, the lowest PEEP necessary and a relatively small tidal volume (4–6 mL/kg) should be used. Opioid drugs should be used with restraint and monitoring in horses with traumatic thoracic, as they cause respiratory depression and, when used serially, reduced intestinal tract motility.

Multiple surgical techniques have been described and include external coaptation with splints and cerclage wire,[58] internal fixation with 2.7-mm reconstruction plates and cerclage wire,[60] nylon suture,[62] or nylon cable ties.[61] The foal is placed in lateral recumbency with the affected ribs uppermost. In cases in which ribs are fractured on each side of the thorax, the more critically affected side is repaired first, after which the foal is repositioned for repair of the other side. In instances in which there is additional thoracic or abdominal trauma, the foal is then moved to dorsal recumbency and the abdomen entered routinely to repair diaphragmatic hernia or intestinal damage as needed. An external fixation technique, coaptation with splints, is accomplished by placing stainless steel suture material percutaneously around the affected ribs, proximal and distal to the fracture site, and fixing the wires to cast or splint material molded to the external surface of the rib cage. Care must be taken to pass the stainless steel suture directly adjacent to the visceral side of the rib and avoid piercing or contacting intrathoracic structures, or pleural infection will result. In the authors' hands, internal fixation has been the best option for providing stable fixation in complicated rib fracture cases.

The choice of which ribs to repair is dictated by fracture location, the risk for myocardial puncture as revealed by imaging, and surgeon experience. Often, fixation of 2 or 3 critically located ribs has a stabilizing effect on adjacent ribs, and the foal is afforded sufficient protection and pain relief to heal well postoperatively. For internal fixation with any technique, the ribs can be approached through incisions made directly over each fracture (**Fig. 7**) or a single incision placed strategically to be slid over and expose multiple affected ribs. Once the fracture site is adequately exposed, the fractures can be reduced by use of towel clamps applied to the bone fragments. The ends do not need to meet precisely, but the sharp edges should be directed away from the thoracic cavity. Manipulation of the rib fragment distal to the costochondral junction must be done with great care, as the cartilage in this area is easily macerated, and this can make it difficult to find purchase for a screw. Typically, the fractures remain stable once they have been reduced, but if not, an assistant can provide traction until the coaptation has been placed.

When 2.7-mm reconstruction plates are used, 4 to 6 cortices of fixation on each fragment end are recommended. The plate is contoured to the rib and slightly overbent at the fracture site. Extreme care is taken to avoid drilling past the inner cortex of the rib, which could lead to further thoracic trauma. After the screws are placed, 2 to 4 stainless steel cerclage wires (18-gauge to 22-gauge) are placed encircling the rib and plate. This wire prevents the screws from pulling out of the cortex. Although this is the most common method used in most hospitals, 2 alternate techniques have been described. One

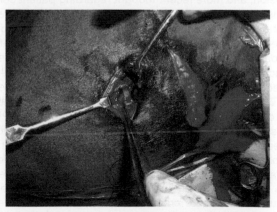

Fig. 7. Intraoperative photograph of a foal undergoing internal fixation surgery for a fractured rib. (*Courtesy of* Dr. Dwayne Rodgerson.)

group[62] described successful use of the Securos Cranial Cruciate Ligament Repair System and 80-pound nylon strand. The nylon strand is passed through holes drilled in the cranial aspect of the proximal and distal fracture fragments in a figure-8 pattern through the medullary cavity of the rib. The strand is secured with a specialized crimp clamp. Other investigators[61] have reported use of gas-sterilized nylon cable ties. Initially, the holes were drilled as they would be for plates, from lateral to medial through the full thickness of the rib in both the proximal and distal aspects of the rib. The cable tie is passed through the drill holes, and is tightened and trimmed as closely to the cable tie lock as possible. More recently, one of the investigators of that report (D.R.) drilled to place the cable ties from cranial to caudal through the rib, which allows for easier placement of the tie. The subcutaneous tissues and skin are closed routinely, and air is evacuated from the pleural cavity with a teat cannula. A Foley catheter is placed in the pleural cavity as described earlier, with a Heimlich valve or other 1-way device attached to allow for continuous evacuation of the thoracic cavity over the ensuing few days. Broad-spectrum antimicrobials are continued and stall rest is enforced for 4 to 6 weeks or until the fractures are healed as assessed with ultrasound. Typically, implants are left to remain in place for the life of the horse unless some complication develops (eg, drainage or sequestrum formation). In those instances, implant removal is routine.

Flail Chest

When a rib is fractured at 2 sites along its length, the segment of rib between the fractures becomes mechanically isolated from the segments proximal and distal to it. When 2 or more contiguous ribs are each fractured in 2 (or more) places, an island of chest wall is thus created that becomes functionally uncoupled from the rest of the chest wall. This area moves in the opposite direction from the rest of the wall during respiratory excursions, such that when the thoracic wall is expanding outward during inhalation, the island of chest wall is pulled inward by the developing negative pressure and when the thoracic wall is recoiling inward during exhalation, the flail segment moves outward because of the positive pressure. This is referred to as paradoxic motion of the thoracic wall, or flail chest.

Flail chest disrupts the ribs' and lateral chest walls' contribution to thoracic expansion and breathing, and this has traditionally been deemed the most important mechanism of patient compromise with this injury. However, most of the pleural cavity expansion during breathing at rest is created by diaphragmatic contraction, not lateral chest wall expansion, and more recent thought regarding patient compromise is that pulmonary contusion plays the chief role in determining the degree of respiratory compromise that develops with flail chest. The degree of force required to fracture equine ribs, especially the more cranial ribs, is considerable, and the blunt transfer of this force across the chest wall causes substantial soft-tissue injury to adjacent pulmonary parenchyma. Extravasation of blood from pulmonary vessels into the interstitium causes decreased lung alveolar volume, decreased compliance, and gas diffusion impairment with consequent ventilation:perfusion mismatch and hypoxemia.[4]

In recognition of this, management of flail chest in humans and small animals is increasingly conservative. An initial period of mechanical ventilation is a frequent component of treatment in humans. This is not a feasible intervention in adult horses, but oxygen supplementation by nasal insufflation is supportive and helpful in both foals and larger animals. In nearly all instances, restricting movement and administering analgesics and gastroprotectants yields a favorable outcome. A flail segment created by fractures in the more cranial ribs (through approximately #7, on either side) especially warrants careful and repeated evaluation for underlying pulmonary, cardiac, or diaphragmatic injury and may be an indication for surgical stabilization of the chest wall. In selected cases, surgical fixation of rib fractures in the absence of flail chest is indicated.[56] As with the other types of thoracic injury discussed, serial arterial blood gas monitoring is helpful in assessing whether supplemental oxygen is needed. Values of Pao_2 less than 60 mm Hg or a pulse oximeter reading less than 90% are indicative of hypoxemia and the need for oxygen supplementation.

Diaphragmatic Rupture

Tearing and rupture of the diaphragm can be a consequence of blunt trauma or a direct injury from fractured ribs. Diaphragmatic tears typically occur along the ventral midline, just dorsal to the xiphoid process. Acquired hernias can arise secondary to trauma to the thorax or a sudden increase in intra-abdominal pressure, such as develops during parturition, abdominal distension, strenuous exercise, or a fall. The borders of the tear often have thin, roughened edges, may or may not be accompanied by hemorrhage, and may be inflamed, especially in acute cases.[63,64] Chronic acquired diaphragmatic tears have smooth, fibrous, and thickened edges and may be accompanied by visceral adhesions.

Definitive diagnosis of a diaphragmatic hernia can be difficult, and is often made during surgery.[65] The horse's history may include some event causing increased intra-abdominal pressure, such as dystocia. Abnormal physical examination findings are often nonspecific or associated with abdominal pain, exercise intolerance, or respiratory distress.[62–64] Thoracic ultrasound and radiography may be useful in preoperative identification of diaphragmatic hernia.[64–66] Gas-filled and fluid-filled tubular or sacculated structures may be visualized in the thorax on ultrasound, indicating the presence of small or large intestine. Intestinal motility and excessive pleural fluid also may be observed.

Diaphragmatic hernias should be repaired surgically, as conservative management appears to end in euthanasia.[67,68] Forms of surgical approach that have been described for diaphragmatic hernia repair include a cranioventral midline incision, lateral thoracotomy through rib resection, flank approach, and thoracoscopy.[67,69]

The cranioventral midline approach can provide adequate exposure of the diaphragm in foals, but in adult horses access to defects in the dorsal part of the muscle is limited.[67,69] Tilting the surgery table to position the horse in reverse Trendelenburg position or to move viscera laterally, away from the lesion, may aid in improving access.[63] In addition, extending the cranioventral midline incision 15 to 20 cm lateral and parallel to the last rib at the level of the xiphoid process, as well as exteriorizing the ascending and descending colon, can improve access to the lesion.[69] Defects can be closed directly by suturing with heavy synthetic absorbable or nonabsorbable suture material, or by using omentum, peritoneum, transversus abdominus muscle, or synthetic mesh.[70] Combinations of these techniques can strengthen the repair. The investigators (D.R., E.B.) use long-handled instruments and staplers, and use a loop suture to avoid the first knot to simplify suturing of dorsal tears.[71,72]

When it is clinically sound, delaying repair of acute hernias allows fibrous tissue to form at the margins of the defect, ensuring that sutures will hold the tissue in position.[73] A 2-stage repair can be performed in which initially entrapped viscera is removed from the hernia via ventral midline exposure and the second procedure is performed as a standing laparoscopy to repair the defect in the diaphragm.[74] However, delaying surgery carries the risk of enabling further entrapment of viscera. Diaphragmatic tears with fresh, friable edges can be repaired with synthetic mesh.

Anesthesia of horses with diaphragmatic rupture is complicated by hypoventilation and decreased oxygenation.[70] The surgeon may be alerted to search for a diaphragmatic defect by the anesthetist noting rapid systemic deterioration after induction or when the horse is being placed in dorsal recumbency. These problems are related to the volume of viscera displaced into the thorax and compressing the lung, which leads to hypoventilation and alveolar collapse. To compensate for these effects, mechanical ventilation should be used intraoperatively, and 100% oxygen should be provided perioperatively. Serial blood gas evaluations should be used to determine whether interventions are effective in supporting global tissue oxygenation. Finally, removing abdominal contents from the thoracic cavity as quickly as possible will allow the lung to reinflate. Chronically affected lungs should be reinflated slowly to prevent reflex pulmonary edema. The postoperative care of these patients is similar to that of patients with colic, but may necessitate resolution of pneumothorax before recovery.

SUMMARY

Traumatic injuries involving the thorax can be superficial, necessitating only routine wound care, or they may extend to deeper tissue planes and disrupt structures immediately vital to respiratory and cardiac function. Diagnostic imaging, especially ultrasound, should be considered part of a comprehensive examination, both at admission and during follow-up. In addition to pulmonary injury, thoracic wounds also can carry injury to cardiac tissue, vascular structures, and abdominal organs, and any of these complications will contribute to or determine the clinical course and outcome. Penetrating or sharp wounds of the thoracic wall may permit direct entry of gas into the pleural cavity through a tear in the parietal pleura. Blunt injury can cause extreme shear forces that create tears in the trachea or lower airways, permitting gas to dissect along tissue planes and enter the mediastinum or pleural cavity. Entry of gas into the pleural cavity obliterates the physiologic state of vacuum and creates pneumothorax and lung collapse. Wounds in any area of the respiratory system that could allow introduction of air in the pleural cavity must be assessed for that potentiality in addition to the routine concerns that are germane to assessment of any wound. Horses generally respond well to diligent monitoring, intervention for complications, and appropriate medical or surgical care after sustaining traumatic wounds of the thorax.

REFERENCES

1. Sisson S. Nervous system of the horse. In: Sisson S, editor. A textbook of veterinary anatomy. Philadelphia: WB Saunders Co; 1910. p. 695–6.
2. Sherwood L, Klandorf H, Yancey P. Respiratory systems. In: Sherwood L, Klandorf H, Yancey P, editors. Animal physiology: from genes to organisms. 2nd edition. Belmont (CA): Brooks/Cole; 2013. p. 518–20.
3. Budras K, Sack WO, Röck S, et al. Thoracic cavity. In: Budras K, Sack WO, Röck S, et al, editors. Anatomy of the horse. 5th edition. Hannover (Germany): Schlutersche Verlagsgesellschaft mbH & Co KG; 2009. p. 60.
4. Radcliffe RM, Ducharme NG, Divers TJ, et al. Treating thoracic injuries. Comp Cont Ed Equine Ed 2009;4:208–23.
5. Lisciandro GR, Lagutchik MS, Mann KA, et al. Evaluation of a thoracic focused assessment with sonography for trauma (TFAST) protocol to detect pneumothorax and concurrent thoracic injury in 145 traumatized dogs. J Vet Emerg Crit Care 2008;18:258–69.
6. Tayal VS, Beatty MA, Marx JA, et al. FAST (focused assessment with sonography in trauma) accurate for cardiac and intraperitoneal injury in penetrating anterior chest trauma. J Ultrasound Med 2004;23:467–72.
7. Busoni V, De Busscher V, Lopez D, et al. Evaluation of a protocol for fast localised abdominal sonography of horses (FLASH) admitted for colic. Vet J 2011;188: 77–82.

8. Zhang M, Liu Z, Yang J, et al. Rapid detection of pneumothorax by ultrasonography in patients with multiple trauma. Crit Care 2006;10:R112.
9. Ball CG, Kirkpatrick AW, Laupland KB, et al. Factors related to the failure of radiographic recognition of occult posttraumatic pneumothoraces. Am J Surg 2005; 189:541–6.
10. Madill JJ. In-flight thoracic ultrasound detection of pneumothorax in combat. J Emerg Med 2010;39:194–7.
11. Cesarini C, Macieira S, Girard C, et al. Costochondral junction osteomyelitis in 3 septic foals. Can Vet J 2011;52:772–7.
12. Hance SR, Robertson JT. Subcutaneous emphysema from an axillary wound that resulted in pneumomediastinum and bilateral pneumothorax in a horse. J Am Vet Med Assoc 1992;200:1107–10.
13. Vachon AM, Fischer AT. Thoracoscopy in the horse: diagnostic and therapeutic indications in 28 cases. Equine Vet J 1998;30:467–75.
14. Fischer AT, Vachon AM. Thoracoscopy. In: Fischer AT, editor. Equine laparoscopy. Philadelphia: WB Saunders Co; 2002. p. 255–64.
15. Peroni JF, Rondenay Y. Analgesia and anesthesia for equine laparoscopy and thoracoscopy. In: Fischer AT, editor. Equine laparoscopy. Philadelphia: WB Saunders Co; 2002. p. 119–30.
16. Laverty S, Lavoie JP, Pascoe JR, et al. Penetrating wounds of the thorax in 15 horses. Equine Vet J 1996;28:220–4.
17. Boy MG, Sweeney CR. Pneumothorax in horses: 40 cases (1980-1997). J Am Vet Med Assoc 2000;216:1955–9.
18. Gemeinhardt KD, Molnar JA. Vacuum-assisted closure for management of a traumatic neck wound in a horse. Equine Vet Educ 2005;17:27–33.
19. Heidecker J, Huggins JT, Sahn SA, et al. Pathophysiology of pneumothorax following ultrasound-guided thoracentesis. Chest 2006;130:1173–84.
20. Josephson T, Nordenskjold CA, Larsson J, et al. Amount drained at ultrasound-guided thoracentesis and risk of pneumothorax. Acta Radiol 2009;50:42–7.
21. Relave F, David F, Leclère M, et al. Thoracoscopic lung biopsies in heaves-affected horses using a bipolar tissue sealing system. Vet Surg 2010;39: 839–46.
22. Hsu CW, Sun SF. Iatrogenic pneumothorax related to mechanical ventilation. World J Crit Care Med 2014;3:8–14.
23. Celik B, Sahin E, Nadir A, et al. Iatrogenic pneumothorax: etiology, incidence and risk factors. Thorac Cardiovasc Surg 2009;57:286–90.
24. Reuter JD, Fowles KJ, Terwilliger GA, et al. Iatrogenic tension pneumothorax in a rabbit (Oryctolagus cuniculus). Contemp Top Lab Anim Sci 2005;44:22–5.
25. Grand JG, Bureau SC. Video-assisted thoracoscopic surgery for pneumothorax induced by migration of a K-wire to the chest. J Am Anim Hosp Assoc 2011; 47:268–75.
26. Gladden J. Iatrogenic pneumothorax associated with inadvertent intrapleural NGT misplacement in two dogs. J Am Anim Hosp Assoc 2013;49:e1–6. http://dx.doi.org/10.5326/JAAHA-MS-6091.
27. de Aguilar-Nascimento JE, Kudsk KA. Use of small-bore feeding tubes: successes and failures. Curr Opin Clin Nutr Metab Care 2007;10:291–6.
28. Conway N, Sreenivasan S. The acupunctured lung. Am J Emerg Med 2014;32: 111.e1. http://dx.doi.org/10.1016/j.ajem.2013.08.026.
29. Unlüer EE, Akyol PY, Karagöz A, et al. A deadly complication of superficial muscular needle electromyography: bilateral pneumothoraces. Case Rep Med 2013;2013:861787.

30. Peroni JF, Horner NT, Robinson NE, et al. Equine thoracoscopy: normal anatomy and surgical technique. Equine Vet J 2001;33:231–7.
31. Peroni J. Thoracic trauma: gasping for air. Proceedings. ACVS Symposium. Chicago. Nov 3–5, 2011;52–4.
32. Sharma A, Jindal P. Principles of diagnosis and management of traumatic pneumothorax. J Emerg Trauma Shock 2008;1:34–41.
33. Holcombe SJ, Laverty S. Thoracic trauma. In: Auer JA, Stick JA, editors. Equine surgery. Philadelphia: WB Saunders; 1999. p. 382–5.
34. Nelson D, Porta C, Satterly S, et al. Physiology and cardiovascular effect of severe tension pneumothorax in a porcine model. J Surg Res 2013;184:450–7.
35. Collins CD. Quantification of pneumothorax size on chest radiographs using interpleural distances: regression analysis based on volume measurements from helical CT. Am J Roentgenol 1995;165:1127–30.
36. Baumann MH, Strange C, Heffner JE, et al. Management of spontaneous pneumothorax. An American College of Chest Physicians Delphi consensus statement. Chest 2001;119:590.
37. Flint K, Al-Hillawi AH, Johnson NM. Conservative management of spontaneous pneumothorax. Lancet 1984;2:687–8.
38. Kircher LT, Swartzel RL. Spontaneous pneumothorax and its treatment. J Am Med Assoc 1954;155:24–9.
39. Lichtenstein D, Mezière G, Biderman P, et al. The "lung point": an ultrasound sign specific to pneumothorax. Intensive Care Med 2000;26:1434–40.
40. Stone WC, Trostle SS, Gerros TC. Use of a primary muscle pedicle flap to repair a caudal thoracic wound in a horse. J Am Vet Med Assoc 1994;205:828–30.
41. Radcliffe RM. Thoracic injury in horses. In: Orsini JA, Divers TJ, editors. Equine emergencies: treatment and procedures. 4th edition. St Louis (MO): WB Saunders; 2012.
42. Northfield TC. Oxygen therapy for spontaneous pneumothorax. Brit Med J 1971; 4:86.
43. Zierold D, Lee SL, Subramanian S, et al. Supplemental oxygen improves resolution of injury-induced pneumothorax. J Pediatr Surg 2000;35:998–1001.
44. Shaireen H, Rabi Y, Metcalfe A, et al. Impact of oxygen concentration on time to resolution of spontaneous pneumothorax in term infants: a population based cohort study. BMC Pediatr 2014;14:208. http://dx.doi.org/10.1186/1471-2431-14-208.
45. Wilson DV, Schott HC II, Robinson NE, et al. Response to nasopharyngeal oxygen administration in horses with lung disease. Equine Vet J 2006;38:219–23.
46. Kemper T, Spier S, Barratt-Boyes SM, et al. Treatment of smoke inhalation in five horses. J Am Vet Med Assoc 1993;202:91–4.
47. Munsterman A, Hanson RR. Trauma and wound management: gunshot wounds in horses. Vet Clin North Am Equine Pract 2014;30:453–66 Cook VL, Hassel DM, editors.
48. Mellick MA, Adreani CM. Management of a gunshot wound in a mare. Can Vet J 2008;49:180–2.
49. Hanson RR. Complications of equine wound management and dermatologic surgery. Vet Clin North Am Equine Pract 2008;24:663–96.
50. Vatistas NJ, Meagher DM, Gillis CL, et al. Gunshot injuries in horses: 22 cases (1971-1993). J Am Vet Med Assoc 1995;207:1198–200.
51. National Safety Council defensive driving video series. Available at: www.nsc.org/products_training/Training/driverimprovementtrng/Pages/DDC4.aspx. Accessed August 31, 2014.

52. Wanek S, Mayberry J. Blunt thoracic trauma: flail chest, pulmonary contusion, and blast injury. Crit Care Clin 2004;20:21–81.
53. Shorr RM, Crittenden M, Indeck M, et al. Blunt thoracic trauma. Analysis of 515 patients. Ann Surg 1987;206:200–5.
54. Sprayberry KA, Bain FT, Seahorn TL, et al. Fifty-six cases of rib fractures in neonatal foals hospitalized in a referral center intensive care unit from 1997–2001. Presented at the 47th Annual Convention of the American Association of Equine Practitioners. San Diego (CA), November 25–28, 2001. 395–99.
55. Schambourg MA, Laverty S, Mullim S, et al. Thoracic trauma in foals: post mortem findings. Equine Vet J 2003;35:78–81.
56. Peters ST, Hopkins A, Stewart S, et al. Myocardial contusion and rib fracture repair in an adult horse. J Vet Emerg Crit Care 2013;23:663–9.
57. Divers TJ. Monitoring tissue oxygenation in the ICU patient. Clinical techniques in equine practice. Orsini JA, ed. Saunders Elsevier 2003;2:138–44.
58. Lugo J, Carr EA. Thoracic disorders. In: Auer JA, Stick JA, editors. Equine surgery. 4th edition. St Louis (MO): Elsevier Saunders; 2012. p. 655–7.
59. Chesnel MA, Aprea F, Clutton RE. Anesthetic management of a horse with traumatic pneumothorax. Can Vet J 2012;53:648–52.
60. Bellezzo F, Hunt RJ, Provost R, et al. Surgical repair of rib fractures in 14 neonatal foals: case selection, surgical technique and results. Equine Vet J 2004;36:557–62.
61. Downs C, Rodgerson D. The use of nylon cable ties to repair rib fractures in neonatal foals. Can Vet J 2011;52:307–9.
62. Kraus BM, Richardson DW, Sheridan G, et al. Multiple rib fracture in a neonatal foal using a nylon strand suture repair technique. Vet Surg 2005;34:399–404.
63. Pauwels FF, Hawkins JF, MacHarg MA, et al. Congenital retrosternal (Morgagni) diaphragmatic hernias in three horses. J Am Vet Med Assoc 2007;231:427–32.
64. Santschi EM, Juzwiak JS, Moll DH, et al. Diaphragmatic hernia repair in three young horses. Vet Surg 1997;26:242–5.
65. Hart SK, Brown JA. Diaphragmatic hernia in horses: 44 cases (1986-2006). J Vet Emerg Crit Care 2009;19:357–62.
66. Kelmer G, Kramer J, Wilson DA. Diaphragmatic hernia: etiology, clinical presentation and diagnosis. Comp Cont Ed Equine Ed 2008;328–36.
67. Roelvink ME, Sloet van Oldruitenborgh-Oosterbaan MM, Calsbeek HC. Chronic diaphragmatic hernia in the horse. Equine Vet Educ 1993;5:255–8.
68. Malone ED, Farnsworth K, Lennox T, et al. Thoracoscopic-assisted diaphragmatic hernia repair using a thoracic rib resection. Vet Surg 2001;30:175–8.
69. Freeman DE. Small intestine. In: Auer JA, Stick JA, editors. Equine surgery. 4th edition. St Louis (MO): Elsevier Saunders; 2012. p. 438–9.
70. Kelmer G, Kramer J, Wilson DA. An in-depth look: diaphragmatic hernia: treatment, complications and prognosis. Comp Cont Ed Equine Ed 2008;3:37–45.
71. McMaster MA, Spirito M, Munsterman AS, et al. Surgical repair of a diaphragmatic tear in a Thoroughbred broodmare. J Equine Vet Sci 2014. http://dx.doi.org/10.1016/j.jevs.2014.07.009.
72. Romero A, Rodgerson DH, Kay TA, et al. Diaphragmatic hernias in 25 cases (2001-2006). Presented at the 52nd Annual Convention of the American Association of Equine Practitioners. San Antonio (TX), December 2–6, 2006;565–6.
73. Dabareiner RM, White NA. Surgical repair of a diaphragmatic hernia in a racehorse. J Am Vet Med Assoc 1999;214:1517–8.
74. Röcken MI, Mosel G, Barske K, et al. Thoracoscopic diaphragmatic hernia repair in a warmblood mare. Vet Surg 2013;42:591–4.

Index

Note: Page numbers of article titles are in **boldface** type.

http://dx.doi.org/10.1016/S0749-0739(15)00013-9
0749-0739/15/$ – see front matter © 2015 Elsevier Inc. All rights reserved.
vetequine.theclinics.com

Printed and bound by CPI Group (UK) Ltd, Croydon, CR0 4YY

03/10/2024

01040490-0005